Muscular Dystrophy

METHODS IN MOLECULAR MEDICINE™

John M. Walker, Series Editor

68. **Molecular Analysis of Cancer,** edited by *Jacqueline Boultwood and Carrie Fidler,* 2002
67. **Meningococcal Disease:** *Methods and Protocols,* edited by *Andrew J. Pollard and Martin C. J. Maiden,* 2001
66. **Meningococcal Vaccines:** *Methods and Protocols,* edited by *Andrew J. Pollard and Martin C. J. Maiden,* 2001
65. **Nonviral Vectors for Gene Therapy:** *Methods and Protocols,* edited by *Mark A, Findeis,* 2001
64. **Dendritic Cell Protocols,** edited by *Stephen P. Robinson and Andrew J. Stagg,* 2001
63. **Hematopoietic Stem Cell Protocols,** edited by *Christopher A. Klug and Craig T. Jordan,* 2001
62. **Parkinson's Disease:** ***Methods and Protocols,*** edited by *M. Maral Mouradian,* 2001
61. **Melanoma Techniques and Protocols:** ***Molecular Diagnosis, treatment, and Monitoring,*** edited by *Brian J. Nickoloff,* 2001
60. **Interleukin Protocols,** edited by *Luke A. J. O'Neill and Andrew Bowie,* 2001
59. **Molecular Pathology of the Prions,** edited by *Harry F. Baker,* 2001
58. **Metastasis Research Protocols:** ***Volume 2, Cell Behavior In Vitro and In Vivo,*** edited by *Susan A. Brooks and Udo Schumacher,* 2001
57. **Metastasis Research Protocols:** ***Volume 1, Analysis of Cells and Tissues,*** edited by *Susan A. Brooks and Udo Schumacher,* 2001
56. **Human Airway Inflammation:** *Sampling Techniques and Analytical Protocols,* edited by *Duncan F. Rogers and Louise E. Donnelly,* 2001
55. **Hematologic Malignancies:** *Methods and Protocols,* edited by *Guy B. Faguet,* 2001
54. ***Mycobacterium tuberculosis*** **Protocols,** edited by *Tanya Parish and Neil G. Stoker,* 2001
53. **Renal Cancer:** *Methods and Protocols,* edited by *Jack H. Mydlo,* 2001
52. **Atherosclerosis:** ***Experimental Methods and Protocols,*** edited by *Angela F. Drew,* 2001
51. **Angiotensin Protocols,** edited by *Donna H. Wang,* 2001
50. **Colorectal Cancer:** ***Methods and Protocols,*** edited by *Steven M. Powell,* 2001
49. **Molecular Pathology Protocols,** edited by *Anthony A. Killeen,* 2001
48. **Antibiotic Resistance Methods and Protocols,** edited by *Stephen H. Gillespie,* 2001
47. **Vision Research Protocols,** edited by *P. Elizabeth Rakoczy,* 2001
46. **Angiogenesis Protocols,** edited by *J. Clifford Murray,* 2001
45. **Hepatocellular Carcinoma:** ***Methods and Protocols,*** **edited by** *Nagy A. Habib,* 2000
44. **Asthma:** ***Mechanisms and Protocols,*** **edited by** *K. Fan Chung and Ian Adcock,* 2001
43. **Muscular Dystrophy:** ***Methods and Protocols,*** **edited by** *Katherine B. Bushby and Louise Anderson,* 2001
42. **Vaccine Adjuvants:** ***Preparation Methods and Research Protocols,*** edited by *Derek T. O'Hagan,* 2000
41. **Celiac Disease:** ***Methods and Protocols,*** edited by *Michael N. Marsh,* 2000
40. **Diagnostic and Therapeutic Antibodies,** edited by *Andrew J. T. George and Catherine E. Urch,* 2000
39. **Ovarian Cancer:** ***Methods and Protocols,*** edited by *John M. S. Bartlett,* 2000
38. **Aging Methods and Protocols,** edited by *Yvonne A. Barnett and Christopher R. Barnett,* 2000
37. **Electrochemotherapy, Electrogenetherapy, and Transdermal Drug Delivery:** *Electrically Mediated Delivery of Molecules to Cells,* edited by *Mark J. Jaroszeski, Richard Heller, and Richard Gilbert,* 2000
36. **Septic Shock Methods and Protocols,** edited by *Thomas J. Evans,* 2000
35. **Gene Therapy of Cancer:** ***Methods and Protocols,*** edited by *Wolfgang Walther and Ulrike Stein,* 2000

METHODS IN MOLECULAR MEDICINE™

Muscular Dystrophy

Methods and Protocols

Edited by

Katharine M. D. Bushby

Department of Human Genetics, School of Biochemistry and Genetics, University of Newcastle upon Tyne, Newcastle upon Tyne, UK

and

Louise V. B. Anderson

Department of Neurobiology, Medical School, University of Newcastle upon Tyne, Newcastle upon Tyne, UK

Humana Press **Totowa, New Jersey**

Softcover reprint of the hardcover 1st edition 2001
999 Riverview Drive, Suite 208
Totowa, New Jersey 07512

Production Editor: Jason S. Runnion
Cover design by Patricia F. Cleary

This publication is printed on acid-free paper. ∞
ANSI Z39.48-1984 (American Standards Institute) Permanence of Paper for Printed Library Materials.

For additional copies, pricing for bulk purchases, and/or information about other Humana titles, contact Humana at the above address or at any of the following numbers: Tel.: 973-256-1699; Fax: 973-256-8341; E-mail: humana@humanapr.com or visit our Website: http://humanapress.com

10 9 8 7 6 5 4 3 2 1

Library of Congress Cataloging in Publication Data

Muscular dystrophy: methods and protocols / edited by Katharine Bushby
and Louise V. B. Anderson.
p. ; cm. -- (Methods in molecular medicine ; 43)
Includes bibliographical references and index.
ISBN 978-1-61737-140-0 e-ISBN 978-1-59259-138-1
1. Muscular dystrophy--Molecular aspects--Laboratory manuals. I. Bushby, Katharine.
II. Anderson, Louise V. B. III. Series.
[DNLM: 1. Muscular Dystrophies--genetics. 2. Genetic Screening. 3. Genetics,
Biochemical. 4. Muscular Dystrophies--diagnosis. WE 559 M9853 2000]
RC935.M7.M874 2000
616.7'48042--dc21

00-053902
CIP

Preface

The term "muscular dystrophy" (MD) describes a group of primary genetic disorders of muscle that often have a distinctive and recognizable clinical phenotype, accompanied by characteristic, but frequently not pathognomonic, pathological features. Research into the molecular basis of the MDs by a combination of positional cloning and candidate gene analysis has provided the basis for a reclassification of these disorders, with genetic and protein data augmenting traditional clinically based nomenclature. These findings have brought insights into the molecular pathogenesis of MD, with an increasing number of potential pathways involved in arriving at a dystrophic phenotype. Some common themes can be recognized, however, including the involvement of five members of the dystrophin-associated complex (dystrophin and four sarcoglycans) in different types of MD, and the involvement of two nuclear envelope proteins in producing an Emery-Dreifuss MD phenotype. Other disease-associated genes appear to cause MD in a completely unrelated way, such as the involvement of calpain 3 in a form of limb-girdle muscular dystrophy.

Section 1 of *Muscular Dystrophy: Methods and Protocols* reviews traditional strategies used to identify MDs. Meantime, techniques developed as a result of the research strategies described previously have become an integral part of the management of many patients with MD and their families, and these techniques are addressed in Sections 2 (DNA-based tests) and 3 (protein-based analyses). The continued effort to translate this enhanced understanding into a molecular cure or treatment for MD is reviewed in Section 4. *Muscular Dystrophy: Methods and Protocols* concentrates on those methods most likely to be relevant to clinical practice and most commonly applied to try to answer the questions that MD raises.

Katharine M. D. Bushby
Louise V. B. Anderson

Contents

Contributors

LOUISE V. B. ANDERSON • *Department of Neurobiology, Medical School, University of Newcastle upon Tyne, Newcastle upon Tyne, UK*

EGBERT BAKKER • *Department of Human Genetics, Leiden University Medical Centre, Leiden, The Netherlands*

RITA J. BALICE -GORDON • *Department of Biochemistry and Molecular Biology, University of Southern California, Los Angeles, CA*

RUMAISA BASHIR • *Department of Molecular Genetics, Biology of Disease, University of Durham, Thornaby, Stockton-on Tees, UK*

JACQUES BECKMANN • *Genethon, Evry, France*

CARSTEN G. BÖNNEMANN • *Department of Pediatrical Cardiology, Center for Child Medicine, Georg-August-Universität Göttingen, Göttingen, Germany*

ROBERT H. BROWN, JR. • *MDA Clinic, Massachusetts General Hospital, Boston, MA*

KATHARINE M. D. BUSHBY • *Department of Human Genetics, School of Biochemistry and Genetics, University of Newcastle Upon Tyne, Newcastle upon Tyne, UK*

ANN CURTIS • *Department of Molecular Genetics, School of Biochemistry and Genetics, University of Newcastle Upon Tyne, Newcastle upon Tyne, UK*

JOHAN T. DEN DUNNEN • *MGC-Department of Human Genetics, Leiden University Medical Center, Leiden, The Netherlands*

C. DE TOMA • *Laboratiore de Biochimie et Genetique Moleculaire, Paris , France*

GEORGE DICKSON • *Division of Biochemistry, School of Biological Sciences, University of London, Egham, Surrey, UK*

JONATHAN K. DORE • *Regional Genetic Service, St. Mary's Hospital, Manchester, UK*

MATTHEW G. DUNCKLEY • *Division of Biochemistry, School of Biological Sciences, University of London, Egham, Surrey, UK*

MARK EVANS • *Hutzel Hospital, Detroit, MI*

RUNE R. FRANTS • *Department of Human Genetics, Leiden University Medical Centre, Leiden, The Netherlands*

DAVID GARDNER-MEDWIN • *Flocktons, Heddon on the Wall, Northumberland, UK*

James Giron • *Children's Research Institute, Department of Molecular Genetics, Washington, DC*

Pascale Guicheney • *CRVA-Department Gencell, France*

Daisy Haggerty • *Department of Molecular Genetics, School of Biochemistry and Genetics, University of Newcastle Upon Tyne, Newcastle Upon Tyne, UK*

Ruth Harrison • *Department of Human Genetics, School of Biochemistry and Genetics, University of Newcastle Upon Tyne, Newcastle upon Tyne, UK*

Anne Helbling-Leclerc • *CRVA-Department Gencell, France*

Eric P. Hoffman • *Children's Research Institute, Department of Molecular Genetics, Washington, DC*

Marc Jeanpierre • *Laboratoire de Biochimie Genetique, Paris, France*

Margaret A. Johnson • *Department of Neurology, Medcial School, University of Newcastle upon Tyne, Newcastle upon Tyne, UK*

Helen M. Kingston • *Regional Genetic Service, St. Mary's Hospital, Manchester, UK*

Louis M. Kunkel • *Division of Genetics, Departments of Neurology, The Childrens' Hospital, Boston, MA*

Qui Lu • *Neuromuscular Unit, Royal Postgraduate School, Hammersmith Hospital, London, UK*

Vincenzo Nigro • *Istituto di Patologia Generale e Oncologia, Seconda Universita Degli, Studi di Napoli, Napoli, Italy*

Maria Rita Passos-Bueno • *Instituto de Biologia, Universidade de Sao Paulo, Sao Paulo, Brazil*

Frederica Piccolo • *Laboratiore de Biochimie et Genetique Moleculaire, Paris, France*

Sita Reddy • *Department of Biochemistry and Molecular Biology, University of Southern California, Los Angeles, CA*

Mark M. Rich • *Department of Biochemistry and Molecular Biology, University of Southern California, Los Angeles, CA*

Isabelle Richard • *Genethon, Evry, France*

Caroline A. Sewry • *Neuromuscular Unit, Royal Postgraduate School, Hammersmith Hospital, London, UK*

Daniela Toniolo • *Istituto di Genetica Biochimica ed Evoluzionistica, Pavia, Italy*

Silvère M. van der Maarel • *Department of Human Genetics, Leiden University Medical Centre, Leiden, The Netherlands*

Mariz Vainzof • *Instituto de Biologia, Universidade de Sao Paulo, Sao Paulo, Brazil*

Mayana Zatz • *Instituto de Biologia, Universidade de Sao Paulo, Sao Paulo, Brazil*

I

Background

1

Application of Molecular Methodologies in Muscular Dystrophies

Katharine M. D. Bushby and Louise V. B. Anderson

The term "muscular dystrophy" (MD) describes a group of primary genetic disorders of muscle that often have a distinctive and recognizable clinical phenotype, accompanied by characteristic, but frequently not pathognemonic, pathological features. Research into the molecular basis of the MDs by a combination of positional cloning and candidate gene analysis has provided the basis for a reclassification of these disorders, with genetic and protein data augmenting traditional clinically based nomenclature (**Table 1**). These findings have brought insights into the molecular pathogenesis of MD, with an increasing number of potential pathways involved in arriving at a dystrophic phenotype. Some common themes can be recognized, however, including the involvement of five members of the dystrophin-associated complex (dystrophin and four sarcoglycans) in different types of MD (**Fig. 1**: *1*), and the involvement of two nuclear envelope proteins in producing an Emery-Dreifuss MD phenotype *(2)*. Other disease-associated genes appear to cause MD in a completely unrelated way, such as the involvement of calpain 3 in a form of limb-girdle muscular dystrophy *(3)*.

Section 1 of this book reviews traditional strategies used to identify MDs. Meantime, techniques developed as a result of the research strategies described above have become an integral part of the management of many patients with MD and their families, and these techniques are addressed in Sections 2 (DNA-based tests) and 3 (protein-based analyses). The continued effort to translate this enhanced understanding into a molecular cure or treatment for MD is reviewed in **Subheading 4**.

This book concentrates on those methods most likely to be relevant to clinical practice: thus, although linkage analysis has often been a crucial step in

From: *Methods in Molecular Medicine, vol. 43: Muscular Dystrophy: Methods and Protocols*
Edited by: K. M. D. Bushby and L. V. B. Anderson © Humana Press Inc., Totowa, NJ

Table 1
Muscular Dystrophy Genes and Proteins

Muscular dystrophy (MD)	Abbreviation	Alternative names	Gene location
Duchenne MD	DMD	Dystrophinopathy	Xp21
Becker MD	BMD	Dystrophinopathy	Xp21
Emery-Dreifuss MD	EDMD		Xq28
Dominant Emery-Dreifuss MD	AD-EDMD		1q11
Limb-girdle MD type 1A	LGMD1A		5q
Limb-girdle MD type 1B	LGMD1B		1q11
Limb-girdle MD type 1C	LGMD1C		3p25
Limb-hirdle MD type 1D	LGMD1D		6q22
Limb-girdle MD type 1E	LGMD1E		7q
Limb-girdle MD type 2A	LGMD2A	Calpainopathy	15q15
Limb-girdle MD type 2B	LGMD2B	Dysferlinopathy	2p13
Miyoshi myopathy	MM	Dysferlinopathy	2p13
Miyoshi-type MD	MMD		10
α-Sarcoglycanopathy	SGCA	LGMD2D, SCARMD2	17q21
β-Sarcoglycanopathy	SGCB	LGMD2E	4q12
γ-Sarcoglycanopathy	SGCC	LGMD2C, SCARMD1	13q12
δ-Sarcoglycanopathy	SGCD	LGMD2F	5q33
Limb-girdle MD type 2G	LGMD2G		17q11
Limb-girdle MD type 2H	LGMD2H		9q31
Limb-girdle MD type 2I	LGMD2I		19q13-3
Merosin-negative congenital MD			6q22
Congenital MD with rigid spine			1p35
Fukuyama congenital MD	FCMD		9q31
Congenital Myopathy (or ?MD)			12q13
Facioscapulohumeral MD	FSHD		4q35
Myotonic dystrophy	DM		19q13
Myotonic dystrophy type 2	DM2		3q
Oculopharyngeal MD	OPMD		14q11
Epidermolysis bullosa simplex + MD	MD-EBS		8q24

Additional loci for many of these phenotypes (e.g., autosomal recessive and dominant LGMD, merosin-positive CMD, FSHD) probably exist, as inferred from the exclusion of all the known loci in additional large families.

Table 1 *(continued)*
Muscular Dystrophy Genes and Proteins

Recessive/ dominant	Protein	Other names	Location of protein
r	Dystrophin		Plasma membrane
r	Dystrophin		
r	Emerin		Nuclear membrane
d	Lamin A/C		Nuclear membrane
d	Myotilin		Sarcomeric
d	Lamin A/C		Nuclear membrane
d	Caveolin 3		Plasma membrane
d	? Homolog of band 4.1		? Plasma membrane
d	?		
r	Calpain 3		? Cytoplasm/nucleus
r	Dysferlin		Plasma membrane
r	Dysferlin		
r	?		
r	α-Sarcoglycan	adhalin, A2 50DAG,	Plasma membrane
r	β-Sarcoglycan	A3b	Plasma membrane
r	γ-Sarcoglycan	35DAG, A4	Plasma membrane
r	δ-Sarcoglycan		Plasma membrane
r	Telethonin		Sarcomeric
r	?		
r	?		
r	Laminin α2-chain	Merosin	Basal lamina/ extracellular matrix
r	?		
r	Fukutin		Secreted extracellularly ?
r	Integrin α7-chain		Plasma membrane
d	?		
d	Myotonin protein kinase	DMPK	Various, according to antibody
d	?		
d	Poly(A) binding protein-2	PABP2	Nucleus
r	Plectin 1	PLEC1	Basement membranes

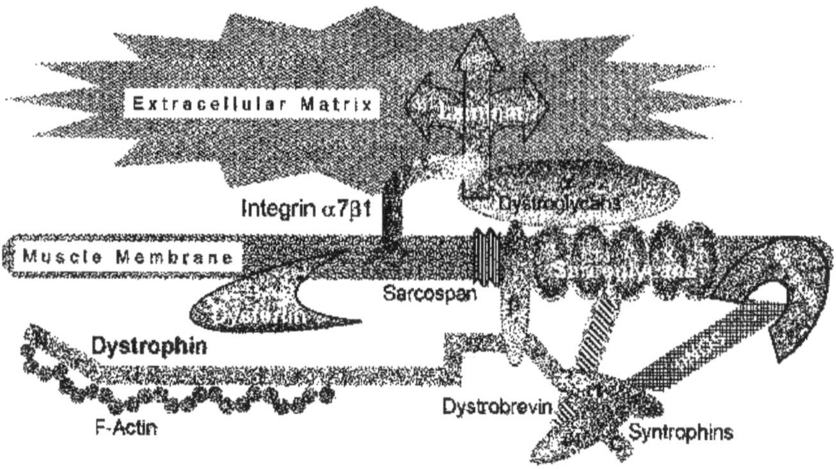

Fig. 1. Schematic diagram of the proteins that are located at or near the muscle plasma membrane, and are implicated in muscle disease (*see* **Table 1**).

moving toward a molecular definition of these disorders, in the clinical context it is generally of limited value in only a small number of defined situations. Even when a disease gene has been identified, the types of mutation(s) encountered in a specific disease influence the practical availability of genetic testing (**Table 2**). For example, in myotonic dystrophy a single type of mutation (triplet-repeat expansion) is present in most affected individuals. Most patients with facioscapulohumeral MD can be shown to carry a DNA deletion, variable in size, but detectable using a single DNA probe (*see* Chap. 18). In both of these disorders, therefore, a relatively straightforward analysis can be employed to identify the majority of affected individuals, although in neither case is the molecular pathology of the disease understood. In the dystrophinopathies, the predominance of a particular type of mutation (intragenic deletion) simplifies the analysis in the majority of families (*see* Chap. 6). The continued need to apply a range of different tests, to provide as complete an answer as possible to the questions of carrier testing and prenatal diagnosis in these conditions means that, although such testing is widely available, it may remain complex (Chaps. 19 to 23). In other disorders, e.g., the limb-girdle muscular dystrophies *(4)*, a range of point mutations have been described. This emphasizes the need to integrate DNA and protein-based diagnosis in these disorders whenever possible; techniques for finding unknown point mutations in multiexon genes will undoubtedly continue to improve, but the current situation is that protein analysis, in the first instance, usually on muscle biopsy samples, is much more practical for most individuals in the clinical setting (*5*; **Section 2**). Mutation

Table 2
Types of Mutation Found in the Muscular Dystrophies:

Whole gene/adjacent genes deleted	Rare cause of DMD
Single/multiple exons deleted	Common in DMD: rare in other MDs
Single/multiple exons duplicated	Seen in DMD
Single/few base pairs removed	Common in LGMDs, EDMD, CMD, rare in DMD
Single/few base pairs inserted	Common in LGMDs, EDMD, CMD, rare in DMD
Base substitution (variable in type and position)	Common in LGMDs, EDMD, CMD, rare in DMD
Expanded triplet motif	DM (all cases)
Contracted repetitive elements	FSHD (but gene responsible not known)

detection directed by the results of such protein analysis is a much more viable option, in order to define the mutation in an individual case, to confirm the diagnosis and offer genetic counseling or prenatal diagnosis. If treatments based on the modification of specific gene defects ever come into clinical practice, then the requirement to define the mutation in every case will become absolute.

However, there should be a degree of caution applied to the use of the ever-increasing number of molecular tests available. The advisedness of proceeding with testing is a concern faced regularly by those involved in counseling patients and families affected with genetic diseases. Specific discussions in this area relate to the issue of carrier testing in childhood or to the application of presymptomatic testing for late-onset disorders, especially given the continued imprecision of such techniques in predicting the timing of onset or severity of the disorder in question. Just because a test may be technically possible, it is not necessarily appropriate to everyone's situation, needs, or wishes, and certainly should not be applied without informed counseling and consent. Genetic issues may be uniquely sensitive, and concerns about confidentiality and autonomy of decision-making need to be taken seriously. The rush to employ these new methodologies, with their emphasis so often on prevention, should not be used to appear to devalue the people affected with these conditions or to distract the clinician, or indeed the broader society, from the need to address other aspects of their rights.

Accepting these caveats, and the need for these tests to be approached with counseling and sensitivity, the authors have drawn together in this book methods that may be of use in each specific disease. Faced with a diagnosis of a genetic disease, a number of questions are commonly encountered, relating to the exact nature of the disorder, its cause and likely progression, the risk of it happening again either to the individual or to the wider family, and the prospects for prevention and cure. The methods described here are those most commonly applied to try to answer these questions in families with MD.

References

1. Ozawa E., Noguchi, S., Mizuno, Y., Hagiwara, Y., and Yoshida, M. (1998) From dystrophinopathy to sarcoglycanopathy: evolution of a concept of muscular dystrophy. *Muscle Nerve* **21,** 421–438.
2. Bonne, G., di Barletta, M. R., Varnous, S., Becane, H., Hammouda, E., Merlini, L., et al. (1999) Mutations in the gene encoding lamin A/C cause autosomal dominant Emery-Dreifuss muscular dystrophy. *Nature Genet.* **21,** 285–288.
3. Richard, I., Broux, O., Allamand, V., Fougerousse, F., Chiannilkulchai, N., Bourg, N., et al. (1995) Mutations in the proteolytic enzyme calpain 3 cause limb-girdle muscular dystrophy type 2A. *Cell* **81,** 27–40.
4. Bushby, K. (1999) Making sense of the limb-girdle muscular dystrophies. *Brain* **122,** 1403–1420.
5. Anderson, L. V. B. and Davison, K. (1999) Multiplex western blotting for the analysis of muscular dystrophy proteins. *Am. J. Pathol.* **154,** 1017–1022.

2

Clinical Examination as a Tool for Diagnosis

Historical Perspective

David Gardner-Medwin

The purpose of diagnosis, since the days of classical Greece, when the concept was introduced, has been to provide a basis for prognosis and for the prescription of a regimen of management. Prognosis, i.e., explaining to the patient and family what the future holds, remains the central purpose of medicine, encapsulated in the private consultation. All other matters, including such important things as investigation as an aid to diagnosis and treatment as a component of management, are peripheral to this.

It is only in the past 50 yr that serious attention has been given to genetic prognosis, and for only half that period have most clinicians devoted the scientific care and compassion to this aspect of prognosis that justify the use of the term "genetic counseling." Indeed, as far as the muscular dystrophies (MDs) are concerned, it is the need for accurate genetic counseling that has been the spur to defining the diagnostic categories with precision.

Only occasional case reports of what is now called MD can be identified in the literature before the 1850s. Then Meryon in England, Aran and Duchenne in France, and Wachsmuth and Griesinger in Germany began to recognize the progressive degenerative diseases of muscle, distinguished neuropathic from myopathic muscle disease and developed systems of clinical, pathological, and electrical examination of muscles, which enabled them to begin to classify and name disorders. The term "progressive muscular dystrophy" was introduced by Erb in 1891 *(1)* for progressive myopathic degenerations. Although these early authors clearly recognized the hereditary nature of many of their cases, the concept of genetically determined disease did not become central to

From: *Methods in Molecular Medicine, vol. 43: Muscular Dystrophy: Methods and Protocols*
Edited by: K. M. D. Bushby and L. V. B. Anderson © Humana Press Inc., Totowa, NJ

the understanding of these disorders until the rediscovery of Mendel's work and the defining of the Mendelian modes of inheritance, in the first decade of this century; the idea that sporadic cases were somehow different in nature lingered on in the minds of some doctors until the 1960s. By about 1910, most of the commoner types of MD had been approximately identified, and then, for more than 30 yr, no further significant progress was made. Bell (1943) *(2)* attempted a genetic classification, revealing an unsatisfactory correlation between modes of inheritance and the then-recognized clinical types. Walton and Nattrass (1954) *(3)* began the modern process of attempting to combine clinical and genetic criteria in their classification. The introduction of the estimation of blood aldolase and creatine kinase (CK) activity, in the 1960s, and, shortly afterwards, the introduction of histochemical examination of muscle biopsies (which brought to light several previously unidentifiable congenital myopathies), provided two valuable new tools for differential diagnosis. Furthermore, the use of CK estimation in carriers of the Duchenne gene introduced a useful (though fallible) technique for the scientific study of the carrier state and its genetic implications.

By the early 1980s, before the molecular genetics revolution, matters stood thus: The MDs formed a discrete group of muscle disorders, readily distinguishable on clinical, histological, enzyme assay, and electromyographic grounds from the neuropathic disorders, the histochemically identifiable congenital myopathies, the endocrine myopathies, polymyositis, and various rarer myopathies. Within the group of true MDs, the clinical diagnosis was based on three criteria: the precise distribution of affected muscles, weak and wasted or, in some cases, hypertrophic; the related criteria of the age at the onset of symptoms and the rate of progression of the symptoms; and the mode of inheritance, when this was evident from the family history. Sporadic cases were naturally relatively difficult to identify. Muscle histology and serum CK activity were valuable adjuncts, electromyography was less so.

All these criteria, by then refined by much study and scientific discourse, resulted in a classification that included the X-linked Duchenne (DMD), Becker and Emery-Dreifuss muscular dystrophy (EDMD) types, the autosomal dominant facioscapulohumeral (FSHD), scapulohumeral, distal and oculopharyngeal types, as well as the multisystem disorder, myotonic dystrophy. It was among the autosomal recessive (AR) types, so often presenting as sporadic cases, that the most difficulty was encountered; the provisional categories of these were the limb-girdle muscular dystrophy (LGMD) types, presenting in childhood or adult life, and the congenital muscular dystrophy (CMD) types, together with some rarer forms, distal and Fukuyama CMDs.

The names of many of these types clearly indicate the primary diagnostic importance of detailed recording of the distribution of affected muscles; the distinction between DMD and BMD, and between the CMD and LGMD types, depended on the timing and progression of symptoms. The problem with the AR types was that there seemed to be no consistent or clearly definable patterns of selective muscle involvement by which these might be positively identified or subdivided, nor was laboratory investigation sufficiently helpful to solve the problem. Indeed, it was recognized that at least one autosomal dominant form of LGMD existed, although its identification in the sporadic case was never secure. Distinction of LGMD from BMD or from the Duchenne carrier state, in which proximal muscular weakness sometimes occurs, was a particular problem, and serious errors in the consequent genetic advice were not uncommon.

In recent years, many new categories of AR MD have been identified by their genetic linkage to particular loci, and, more recently still, by their specific molecular pathology. In many cases, this has made it possible to recognize for the first time characteristic patterns of selective muscle involvement, not previously discernible among the muddled group of LGMDs. Whether every LGMD type will ultimately prove to be clinically recognizable, it is too early to say, but, at present, this looks unlikely. Because most of the MDs have characteristic patterns of selective muscle involvement, it should not be assumed to be axiomatic that all of them must.

This is not the place to describe in detail the precise patterns of muscle involvement that characterize the various classical types of MD. These may be found in clinical texts such as those by Walton, Karpati, and Hilton-Jones (1994) ***(4)***. A resumé would be valueless and potentially dangerous, because the essence of clinical diagnosis of these disorders lies in the details. For inspiration in the techniques involved the works of Duchenne (1870) ***(5)*** and Gowers (1881) ***(6)*** can be recommended.

The advent of molecular genetics has transformed the diagnosis and classification of the MDs as later chapters in this book show. The chief consequences can be listed as follows:

1. Molecular diagnosis has confirmed the validity of many previously identified entities, for example, DMD, BMD, EDMD, FSHD and myotonic dystrophies.
2. It has provided a firm basis for identifying carriers of the X-linked types, and for achieving preclinical and prenatal diagnosis.
3. It has resulted in the recognition of many new types of MD previously consigned to wrong categories or to the unsatisfactory limb-girdle group.
4. It has revealed the molecular basis or cause of many of these disorders for the first time, providing a means not only of identifying but of defining the different types of MD. Incidentally, this also provides a logical direction for the search for a cure.

Advances of the past 13 yr, since the discovery of dystrophin by means of reverse genetics, have been so fundamental that it is now a truism to regard the classification and genetic diagnosis of the MDs as firmly based on molecular biology. No other approach rivals it in precision.

But, crucial as it is, genetic advice is not the only information that patients seek. They (or their families) need to know also the prognosis for progression of the disability and for survival, and here it is plain that clinical information is vital. For example, merosin deficiency has been identified as the molecular basis for the commonest type of CMD in Europe and North America, but a partial deficiency of merosin is the basis of a wide variety of clinical predicaments, ranging from severe CMD, which causes profound weakness from birth and an ever-present risk of early death, to a much less severe LGMD type of proximal weakness, which causes mild to moderate disability in childhood and adult life, and which, only by careful enquiry, is traceable in its onset to early infancy. Other examples of variable clinical problems caused by identical molecular lesions are found in later chapters. Now, and for the foreseeable future, it will be prudent to offer a prognosis based, not upon a molecular genetics laboratory report alone (though that is essential), but also upon the evidence of serum enzyme activity and an experienced clinical opinion. A period of observation at follow-up, during at least the initial progressive stage of the disease, gives added confirmation of the prognosis, as well as providing an opportunity to support and guide patients and families.

They will need support. Having reviewed the general principles of diagnosis, one should here return to prognosis, telling the patient about the future, or, in the case of the early-onset forms, telling the parents (whenever possible, both parents together). The disease will have such an all-pervading influence on patient and family for the rest of their lives that the moment at which the news is broken will be remembered forever, and the content and atmosphere of the consultation will, to a great extent, determine their subsequent attitude to the disease and to medical care. The news must be broken with sensitivity and without haste, by a physician who knows the patient personally and has a full understanding of the disease and its many implications. Enough information must be given to allow the family to plan effectively for the future, and to have confidence that no further unexpected bad news remains to be discovered. The news should be accompanied by an offer of support and a constructive plan for management.

Precision in prognosis is important also in trials of treatment. Here the need to compare outcomes in treated patients and controls, using the smallest effective numbers and the shortest effective period of follow-up, makes an understanding of the natural history of the untreated disease, in all of the subjects in the trial, very important. A preceding period of repeated careful functional measurement makes it much easier to match cases and controls properly. With this in mind, many muscle clinics make regular measurements of their patients' speed of walking or running, of climbing stairs, and of rising from the floor or from a standard chair. More elaborate functional testing, including the use of multiple standard tasks or the direct measurement of the power of individual muscles, are rarely used, except during the course of treatment trials.

References

1. Erb, W. H. (1891) Dystrophia muscularis progressiva: Klinische und pathologischanatomische Studien. *Deutsche Zeittschrift fur Nervenheilkunde* **1,** 13.
2. Bell, J. (1943) On pseudohypertrophic and allied types of progressive muscular dystrophy, in *Treasury of Human Inheritance, vol. 4,* Cambridge University Press, London, pp.
3. Walton, J. N. and Nattrass, F. J. (1954) On the classification, natural history and treatment of the myopathies. *Brain* **77,** 169.
4. Walton, J., Karpati, G., and Hilton-Jones, D. (eds.) (1994) *Disorders of Voluntary Muscle.* 6th ed. Churchill Livingstone, Edinburgh.
5. Duchenne, G. B. (1872) *De l'Electrisation Localisee et de son Application a la Pathologie et a la therapeutique.* 3rd ed. Bailliere, Paris.
6. Gowers, W. R. (1886–1888) *Manual of Diseases of the Nervous System*, vols. 1 and 2 Churchill, London.

3

Histopathological Diagnosis of Muscular Dystrophies

Margaret A. Johnson

1. Introduction

Muscle biopsies from patients with a muscular dystrophy (MD) often arrive at the histopathology laboratory accompanied by information indicating a definite and accurate clinical diagnosis, but, just as frequently, they do not. It is therefore inadvisable to omit conventional histological and histochemical (HC) examination in favor of proceeding directly to protein analysis via immunocytochemistry (ICC) and immunoblotting. Preliminary histopathological screening provides useful information in three major areas ***(1,2)***. First, the application of comprehensive histological and HC protocols ensures that a wide range of analytical techniques is applied to individual biopsies, and this is the most reliable way of excluding disorders such as congenital myopathies, metabolic myopathies, or atypical spinal muscular atrophies from the differential diagnosis. Second, it provides information on current severity, which may have implications for prognosis, and on the presence or absence of complicating factors, such as secondary inflammatory components, which may respond to treatment. Third, it gives useful correlative data for subsequent immunolabeling studies, e.g., information on the degree of replacement of muscle by fat and fibrous connective tissue, which may prompt the adjustment of gel loading for immunoblotting, or the identification of regenerating fibers, whose presence may influence levels of protein expression in ICC analysis.

Modern diagnostic practice dictates that muscle histopathology utilizes frozen tissue samples almost exclusively. This optimizes the correlation of histological and ICC findings, and means that the same tissue blocks can also be used for immunoblotting or for DNA analysis. However, many histopathology laboratories, particularly those in long-established institutions, may have access

From: *Methods in Molecular Medicine, vol. 43: Muscular Dystrophy: Methods and Protocols*
Edited by: K. M. D. Bushby and L. V. B. Anderson © Humana Press Inc., Totowa, NJ

to archives of formalin-fixed, paraffin-embedded material, which is proving to be a valuable resource for retrospective DNA analysis. In addition, techniques of antigen retrieval for ICC studies are constantly improving, so that stored material, which is currently of limited value, may be usable in the future. Conservation of biopsied tissue is always advisable, with emphasis on optimal conditions of storage. Where possible, frozen material should be stored in liquid nitrogen Dewar containers, where it will remain suitable for HC and immunolabeling studies for periods of more than 20 yr. Maintaining an archive of frozen material can prevent the need for rebiopsy, and, as new probes become available, retrospective diagnostic surveys are facilitated.

2. Histological and HC Methods

In most neuromuscular disease laboratories, a routine histopathological screening protocol of 10–15 histological and HC methods is in general use. Not all of these techniques will provide information of specific relevance to the MDs, so this subsection concentrates on those that do, with only passing reference to those techniques used primarily to exclude other disorders.

2.1. Hematoxylin and Eosin

Histological examination of frozen sections relies heavily on hematoxylin and eosin (HE) staining, but hematoxylin–Van Gieson is particularly useful when differential demonstration of muscle fibers and fibrous connective tissue is needed. When reading muscle biopsies from patients with putative MDs the incidence of the following features should be assessed.

1. Variation in muscle fiber diameter. Normal muscle fibers show a 2–3-fold variation; anything greater than this is abnormal, and, in some chronic MDs, a 20-fold variation is possible.
2. Distribution of atrophied and hypertrophied fibers. Primary myopathies are characterized by random variation in fiber size. If the distribution of atrophied fibers is markedly grouped, the biopsy should be examined for other evidence of a neurogenic disorder.
3. Incidence of acute necrosis and phagocytosis. Acutely necrotic fibers are less eosinophilic (paler) in H&E-stained sections, and soon become invaded by phagocytic macrophages. To distinguish definitively between macrophage nuclei and muscle nuclei, a HC or ICC marker (*see* **Subheading 2.3.**) should be used.
4. Hyaline fibers (opaque fibers). These rounded, densely staining fibers represent an early stage in muscle fiber degeneration in many forms of MD, and appear intensely eosinophilic, because of overcontraction brought about by abnormal influx of calcium ions.
5. Regenerating muscle fibers. Necrotic muscle fibers liberate activated satellite cells, which proliferate and fuse to form multinucleate myotubes. These are

Table 1
Histochemical Characteristics of Human Muscle Fiber Types

	Type 1	Type 2A	Type 2B	Type 2C
Myofibrillar ATPase				
pH 10.2 preincubation	+	++	+++	+(+)
pH 4.6 preincubation	+++	+	++	+(+)
pH 4.3 preincubation	+++	–	–	+(+)
Succinate dehydrogenase	+++	++	+	+(+)
Sudan Black B	+++	++	+	+(+)
Myophosphorylase	+	++	+++	+(+)
Periodic acid-Schiff	+	++	+++	+(+)

characterized by their small diameter (less than 20 µm), intensely basophilic cytoplasm, and large vesicular nuclei with prominent nucleoli.

6. Connective tissue increase. Normal muscle shows very little fibrous connective tissue around individual fibers (endomysial), with perifascicular (perimysial) sites showing a more substantial fibrous component. Fat is virtually absent from endomysial sites in normal individuals, with variable amounts in perimysial sites, according to physical build. The degree of replacement of muscle fibers by fat and fibrous connective tissue varies greatly between the different MDs but in general gives an indication of chronicity and severity of the disorder.
7. Internal muscle nucleation. Normal muscle nuclei are peripherally situated, except during muscle development. In myopathic biopsies, central nucleation may persist for a long time in postregenerative fibers. Multiple internal nuclei are seen commonly in hypertrophied fibers.
8. Muscle fiber splitting. Muscle fiber hypertrophy cannot continue indefinitely, and fiber splitting occurs, to limit muscle fiber size. Splitting and fragmentation also occur in smaller-diameter fibers, probably as a response to functional stress in a muscle weakened by myopathy.

HC screening is an important adjunct to histological examination, and should include methods to allow the discrimination of metabolic fiber types, the detection of abnormalities of mitochondrial distribution, and the localization and characterization of phagocytic and inflammatory cell infiltrates.

2.2. Myofibrillar Enzyme Techniques

The demonstration of myofibrillar adenosine triphosphatase (ATPase) activity enables the clear identification of type 1 (slow-twitch, oxidative), type 2A (fast-twitch, oxidative/glycolytic), and type 2B (fast-twitchglycolytic) fibers (*see* **Table 1**). Although the myofibrillar ATPase (mATPase) reactions, after alkaline preincubation, most closely reflect those in vivo in the individual fiber types, the acid preincubation procedures (at pH 4.3 and 4.6) are routinely used,

Table 2
Fiber Type Constitution of Human Skeletal Muscles (range of type 1 fiber% based on 95% confidence limits)

	Type 1 (%)
Biceps	34–51
Detoid	43–63
Gastronemius	37–50
Tibialis anterior	62–84
Triceps	16–48
Quadriceps	37–50

because they provide a very clearcut, if empirical, differentiation of fiber types *(3)*. Major uses of the mATPase techniques include the following:

1. Assessment of the normality or abnormality of the fiber type constitution of the biopsied muscle. This should be done with reference to normal data for the particular muscle under examination (**Table 2**).
2. Identification of type-specific processes, such as selective atrophy or hypertrophy of a particular fiber type or association of degenerative abnormalities with a specific fiber type.
3. Detection of abnormalities of spatial distribution of fiber types. Instead of the normal random fiber type distribution, the myopathic processes operative in many MDs lead to clustering of fibers of uniform type. However, large-scale uniform fiber type grouping, of the sort seen in chronic spinal muscular atrophies is not present.
4. Identification of regenerating fibers. These fibers show the 2C characteristics after pH 4.3 preincubation (*see* **Table 1**), which are common to all fibers during development. Full differentiation under neural influence leads to the expression of either slow (type 1) or fast (types 2A and 2B) myosin, but, during development, fetal myosins are transiently expressed.
5. Detection of fiber type interconversion. Normal diameter (nonregenerating) fibers may show 2C HC characteristics, because of functional transformation from one fiber type to another. In the context of the MDs (and most other chronic neuromuscular disorders), this usually means type 2 to type 1 conversion, and is accompanied by the transient co-expression of both fast and slow myosins.

2.3. Lysosomal Enzyme Techniques

Lysosomes, whether in phagocytic cells or in muscle fibers, contain acid hydrolases, whose activity can be demonstrated histochemically *(4)*. Commonly used lysosomal marker enzymes are acid phosphatase and acid esterase:

Both classes of acid hydrolase can be localized in tissue sections, using synthetic substrates (naphthol phosphate and naphthol acetate, respectively), and either diazonium or hexazonium salts as coupling agents. These generate highly colored azo dyes on reaction with the naphthol moieties liberated from the substrate (simultaneous coupling azo dye techniques). Applications of these techniques include:

1. Identification of macrophages, and discrimination of this cell type from lymphocytes within mixed cell infiltrates, and, within degenerating muscle fibers, of macrophage nuclei from intrinsic muscle fiber nuclei. The technique is therefore a useful screening method for the accurate assessment of the amount of acute necrosis and phagocytosis present in a biopsy.
2. Assessment of the activity of muscle lysosomes. Skeletal muscle has a poorly developed lysosomal system, and, in normal muscle, a few discrete organelles are seen at the fiber periphery, often adjacent to muscle nuclei. In MDs, lysosomal proliferation often occurs; in relatively indolent disorders, lysosomes are still discrete, but disruption of lysosomal membranes, with liberation of acid hydrolases into the cytosol, is an indication of more acute muscle fiber degeneration, and is an autolytic process, as opposed to the dissolution of muscle fibers through phagocytic activity.

2.4. Mitochondrial Enzyme Techniques

Characteristic abnormalities of mitochondrial distribution occur in many MDs and are readily detectable using HC techniques. Succinate dehydrogenase (SDH) is a recommended mitochondrial marker technique, but reduced nicotinaide adenine dinucleotide (NADH) dehydrogenase (NADH-tetrazolium reductase [TR]) is often used as an alternative, although some extramitochondrial enzyme activity contributes to this reaction ***(5)***. The techniques are useful in identifying the presence of:

1. Floccular or lobulated fibers, in which the abnormal distribution of clusters of mitochondria gives affected fibers this distinctive appearance. The abnormality is prevalent in type 1 muscle fibers, in which the peripheral mitochondrial clusters give a scallop-edged aspect to the fibers in mATPase sections. Floccular fibers are particularly common in facioscapulohumeral muscular dystrophy (FSHD) and autosomal dominant (AD) limb-girdle muscular dystrophy (LGMD) (*see* histopathological profiles, **Subheadings 3.4.** and **3.5.**).
2. Moth-eaten fibers show a disordered, patchy distribution of mitochondria, seen in many chronic LGMDs and adult Becker muscular dystrophy (BMD).
3. Central core disease, multicore (minicore) myopathy, and myotubular (centronuclear) myopathy can be excluded from the differential diagnosis, as a result of their detection in SDH/NADH-TR reacted material.

2.5. Glycogen and Lipid Techniques

Some metabolic myopathies and MDs share presentational features, such as exercise intolerance, with muscle pain or cramps. Thus, techniques for the demonstration of intracellular lipid in muscle fibers (Sudan Black, Oil Red O) or the presence of excess glycogen (periodic acid-Schiff [PAS]) are important for the exclusion of lipidoses and glycogenoses *(6)*, as are enzyme HC techniques, such as those for myophosphorylase and phosphofructokinase, which can rule out specific glycogenoses.

3. Histopathological Profiles of Individual MDs

Definitive histopathological diagnosis of individual forms of MD was severely limited in the era before probes for the immunolabeling of dystrophin, sarcoglycans, and laminins became available. Applications of these immunolabeling techniques to tissue sections will be dealt with in Chapter 21, so a major aim of the current chapter is to give some assessment of the degree of diagnostic precision possible prior to the use of specific probes.

3.1. Duchenne Muscular Dystrophy

It is well recognized that, although none of the histopathological features of Duchenne muscular dystrophy (DMD) is specific to that disorder, the pattern, distribution, and configuration of those features are virtually unique *(7)*. Thus in the predystrophin era, histopathologists learned to distinguish DMD's salient features, and to give a diagnosis based on pattern recognition (*see* **Notes 1** and **2**).

DMD is characterized by numerous foci of acutely necrotic muscle fibers, with phagocytosis and evidence of regenerative activity (**Fig. 1A,B**). The prevalence of these features will be at a peak at 3–5 yr of age, (the usual time of diagnosis), compared with the preclinical period and with later stages, when replacement of muscle fibers by fat and fibrous connective tissue is well advanced. Hyaline fibers are more common in DMD than in any other form of MD. The distribution of all these acute features, although referred to as focal, rarely involves more than 5–10 contiguous muscle fibers. The regenerating fibers, which attempt to replace the necrotic parent fibers, are detectable by immunolabeling for vimentin or fetal myosin, or by their 2C HC reaction in mATPase sections. Type 2B fibers become progressively rarer as a result of a degree of preferential susceptibility to necrosis. In later stages, a type 1 predominance develops, linked to the greater capacity for survival of this fiber type, and also to interconversion of type 2 fibers to type 1. This is a common feature of chronic neuromuscular diseases, in which the ability to undertake phasic muscle activity is severely compromised, and in which the maintenance of posture and other restricted activity involving slow-twitch muscle contraction is predominant.

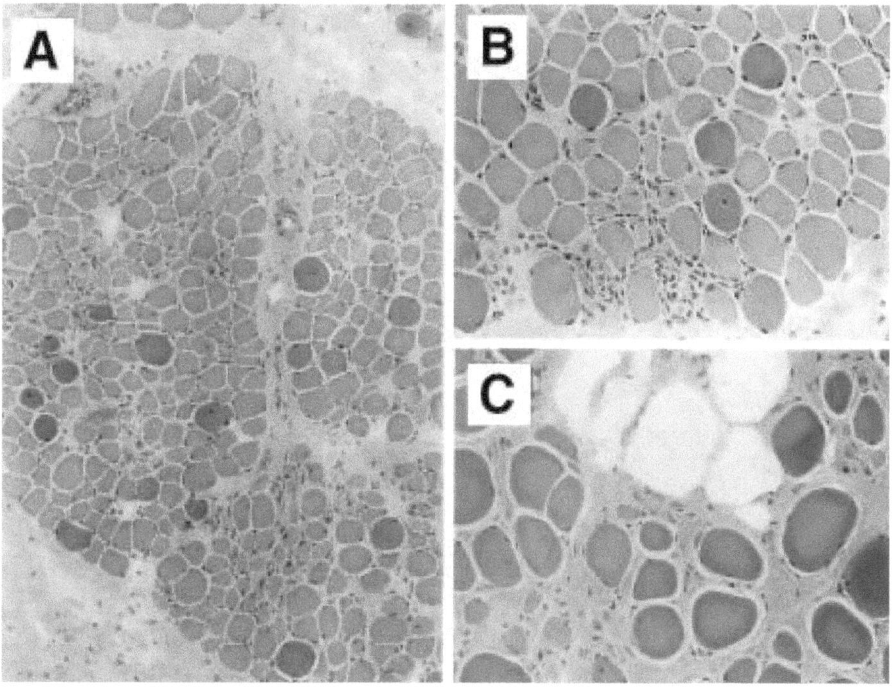

Fig. 1. (**A**) DMD: biopsy from patient aged 4 yr showing increase in interstitial fibrous connective tissue. H&E ×75. (**B**) DMD: detail of Fig A showing hyaline fibers and foci of necrosis, phagocytosis, and regeneration. H&E ×125. (**C**) DMD: biopsy from patient aged 9 yr with severely disrupted muscle architecture caused by increased fat and fibrous connective tissue. H&E ×125.

Increase in perimysial fibrous connective tissue and fat begins at an early age, but, until this process also involves endomysial sites, the overall fascicular architecture of the muscle is preserved. As endomysial fibrous connective tissue increases, the usual polygonal fiber profile is lost, since muscle fibers are no longer in contact with each other, and most fibers appear rounded in outline. Preservation of the normal polygonal fiber shape correlates with milder fibrous connective tissue increase and less severe disease. Muscle fiber size shows increasingly wide random variation because of the constant presence of atrophied fibers, a variable population of regenerating fibers, and increasing hypertrophy and fiber splitting.

3.2. Becker Muscular Dystrophy

In contrast to the diagnosis of DMD, which is straightforward because of its unique histopathological pattern, supported by a relatively clear-cut clinical

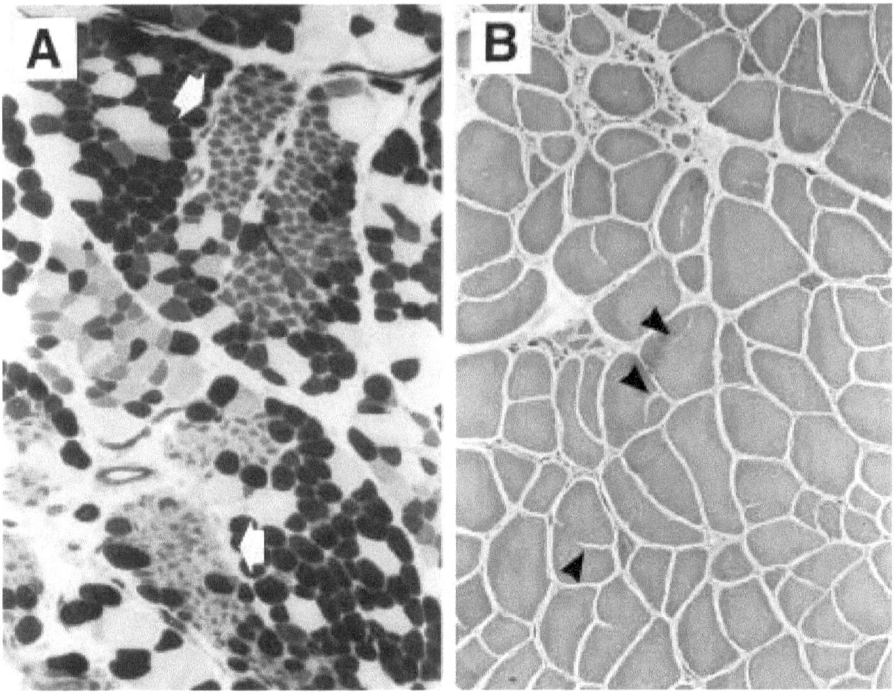

Fig. 2. (**A**) BMD: biopsy from patient aged 5 yr showing grouped degeneration and regeneration typical of juvenile BMD. mATPase ×75. (**B**) BMD: biopsy from patient aged 43 yr showing wide variation in fiber size with splitting in some hypertrophied fibers. H&E ×100.

picture, the diagnosis of BMD in the predystrophin era was fraught with all manner of difficulties. It is only since the use of dystrophin immunolabeling has become routine that full ascertainment of BMD has become possible, and, with this, the realization of the imperfections of the previous situation.

At a histopathological level, both early- and late-presenting forms of BMD can be confused with various other forms of MD. The histological pattern of early BMD has features in common with some severe childhood autosomal recessive muscular dystrophies (SCARMDs) now classified as LGMD2C or LGMD2D (gamma or alpha-sarcogly-canopathy), and later-onset BMD can be indistinguishable from adult limb-girdle syndromes.

Early-presenting BMD shows fewer hyaline fibers than DMD, and a lower overall incidence of acutely necrotic fibers. However, many early BMD biopsies show a strikingly grouped distribution of necrotic fibers and/or of the regenerating fibers that replace them (*1*; **Fig. 2A**). It is this feature in particular that occurs also in LGMD2C and 2D. Early BMD biopsies tend, however, to show a greater range of muscle fiber size, with greater residual atrophy, as well as more hypertrophy.

Late-presenting BMD biopsies can vary immensely in severity. At one end of the spectrum are near-normal biopsies, with an mildly increased range of fiber size, little acute necrosis, and virtually no increase in interstitial fat or fibrous connective tissue. At the other extreme are biopsies showing a wide range of fiber size, with atrophied fibers less than 10 μm in diameter and hypertrophied fibers up to 200 μm in size. In a small proportion of BMD biopsies (verified by dystrophin analysis), the distribution of atrophied fibers may be markedly grouped, prompting previous misdiagnosis as neurogenic disorders with secondary myopathic features.

Hyaline fibers are much less common than in DMD, and the incidence of acute muscle fiber necrosis may be very low. However, features classically associated with chronic late-onset MDs are prevalent. Fibre splitting and fragmentation are common (**Fig. 2B**), as is the presence of fibers with multiple internal nuclei. Coiled and ring fibers, formed by displacement of myofibrils in corkscrew fashion within the muscle fibers, are seen particularly clearly in PAS-reacted sections (**Fig. 3A**), and, as with fiber splitting, appear to be characteristic of disease-weakened muscle fibers subjected to excessive workload. BMD biopsies show no consistent abnormalities of fiber type constitution, and a normal complement of type 2 fibers, including type 2B (fast-twitch glycolytic) fibers, may be preserved. Although some BMD biopsies show a tendency for atrophied fibers to be type 1 and hypertrophied fibers type 2, this is not a consistent finding. The extent of interstitial connective tissue increase is variable and linked to net muscle fiber loss, but endomysial connective tissue rarely obliterates fascicular architecture.

3.3. Emery-Dreifuss Muscular Dystrophy

Few histopathologists have first-hand experience of more than a handful of presumptive Emery-Dreifuss muscular dystrophy (EDMD) *(8)* biopsies, and the advent of emerin labeling has consigned some of these to an Emery-Dreifuss-like category, when they have been found to be emerin-positive. EDMD is typically a mild MD *(1)*, with a very low incidence of acute fiber necrosis, a fiber size spectrum that is only moderately increased, and with little, if any, fibrous connective tissue proliferation. Split and moth-eaten fibers are sometimes encountered, and a high proportion of muscle fibers may contain multiple internal nuclei.

EDMD should not pose any problems of clinical or histopathological differentiation from other X-linked MDs, but a clinical picture of selective upper arm and peroneal muscle weakness, possibly also with mild facial weakness, may prompt a provisional diagnosis of a scapuloperoneal syndrome, or even of

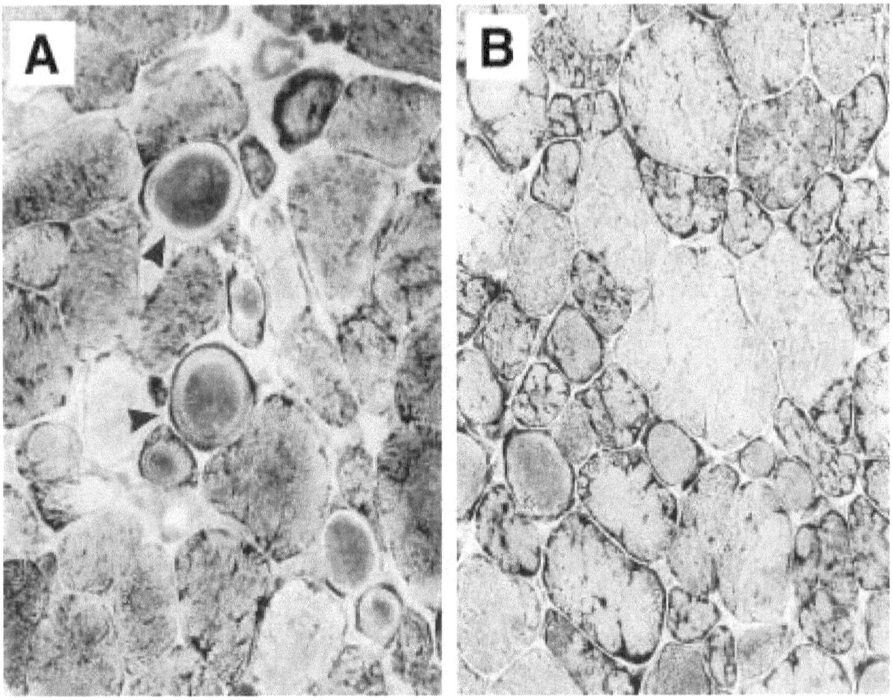

Fig. 3. (**A**) Ring fibers with displacement of peripheral myofibrils in a biopsy from a BMD patient aged 30 yr. PAS ×200. (**B**) Floccular fibers with abnormal mitochondrial distribution in a biopsy from a patient aged 60 yr with an AD LGMD. NADH-TR ×200.

FSHD, in the absence of evidence of X-linkage; because none of these conditions has consistent pathognomonic features, differential histopathological diagnosis may be difficult. EDMD may show type 1 predominance, a feature that has also been noted in a female EDMD carrier. The skeletal myopathy in EDMD is such that most patients remain ambulant into the third decade and beyond, but the cardiomyopathy can prove fatal at an early age, unless heart block is alleviated by insertion of a pacemaker; autopsy findings include severe cardiac fibrosis.

3.4. Limb-Girdle Muscular Dystrophies

The autosomal recessively inherited LGMDs have previously been grouped according to clinical presentation and age of onset. Thus a category of SCARMD was regarded as distinct from later-onset, clinically milder forms. It is now known that many of the sarcoglycanopathies or calpain 3-linked abnormalities, which underlie the various forms of LGMD, may be associated either with severe childhood disease or with milder adult-onset presentation *(9)*. Nevertheless, just as BMD tends to show different histopathological patterns characteristic of severe childhood or later-onset BMD, so LGMDs display distinct histological pictures that seem to be primarily influenced by severity and age of presentation, rather than by the precise nature of the underlying defect.

At their most severe, the childhood autosomal recessive (AR) MDs may produce a DMD-like clinical picture, and prove fatal in the patients' early twenties. The histopathological correlates of this type of LGMD can be defined as follows. Foci of acute muscle necrosis and phagocytosis are common and may involve groups of 20–50 adjacent fibers. Groups of regenerating fibers are seen even more frequently, probably because the process of regeneration takes longer than that of necrosis, and such regenerative foci are striking features of mATPase-reacted sections, where they are clearly delineated as groups of small-diameter 2C fibers. Hyaline fibers are not as common as in DMD, and interstitial fibrous connective tissue increase is more restricted.

Many children with this histological picture have been shown subsequently to have defects of α- or γ-sarcoglycan, and thus to have LGMD2D or LGMD2C, respectively. Other children show a milder histopathological picture, with less variation in fiber diameter and virtually no fibrous connective tissue increase, in which the distinctive foci of acutely degenerating fibers or regenerating fibers may be the only significant abnormality (**Fig. 4A**). Deficiency of calpain 3 has been recorded in association with this type of early-onset LGMD, classifiable as LGMD2A.

Late-onset AR LGMD biopsies show a histological profile characterized by variation in fiber size, which may reach 20-fold, as in severe late-onset BMD biopsies, but may be more restricted. Ring fibers and coiled fibers are common findings, and the distribution of mitochondria and other intermyofibrillar elements demonstrable in NADH-TR-reacted sections often shows a moth-eaten or whorled appearance. The incidence of fiber splitting and of fibrous connective tissue increase is variable. Acute necrosis, phagocytosis, and regeneration are less frequent than in childhood LGMD biopsies, and may be virtually absent from mild cases. Changes in HC fiber type constitution are characteristic of chronic neuromuscular disease, and include moderate type 1 fiber predominance and a decreased proportion of type 2B fibers.

AD LGMDs (chromosome 5q-linked LGMD1A, 1q-linked 1B, and 3p-linked 1C associated with defects in caveolin-3 expression) appear to manifest with varying severity, but are typically milder, later-onset MDs. Histopathologically, the AD LGMDs show few definitive features distinguishing them from AR LGMD biopsies, but hyaline fibers are sparse, and there is often a high incidence of floccular fibers detectable in SDH or NADH-TR sections (**Fig. 3B**), with preferential involvement of type 1 fibers, which are often atrophied.

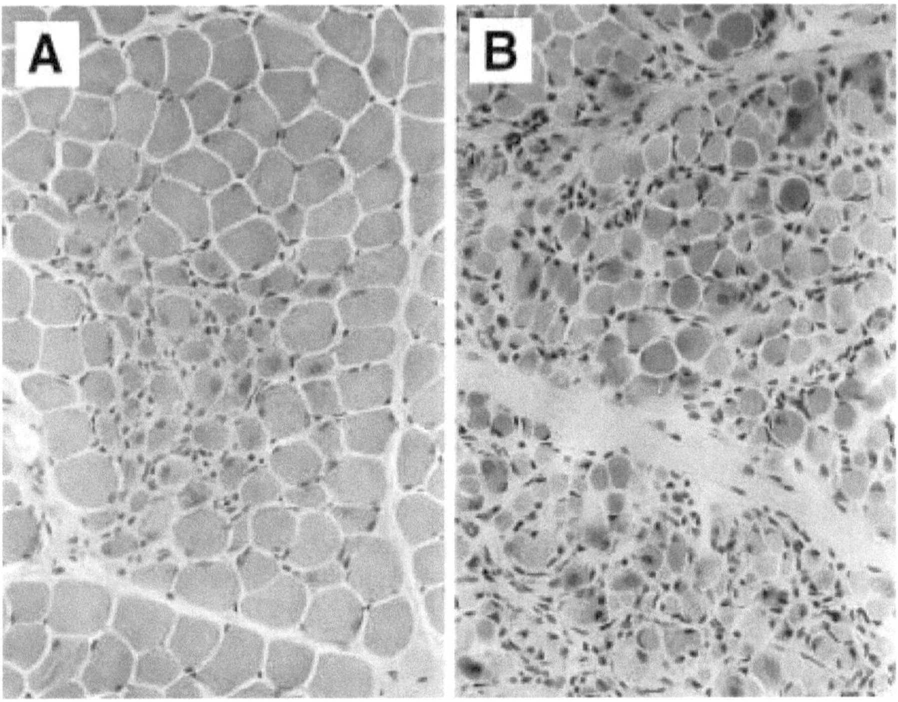

Fig. 4. (**A**) LGMD: biopsy from a patient aged 5 yr with LGMD2A showing grouped distribution of regenerating muscle fibers. H&E ×200 (**B**) CMD: biopsy from patient aged 2 mo, showing severe active degenerative changes. H&E ×200.

3.5. Facioscapulohumeral Muscular Dystrophy

This dominantly inherited MD can present in childhood, as well as later in life. In contrast to biopsies from childhood BMD or childhood LGMD, biopsies from patients under 10 yr of age with FSHD are not characterized by abundant acute muscle fiber necrosis, and often show minimal histological changes of any description. There are, however, exceptions to this general rule (*see* below). Later on, FSHD may give rise to marked variation in muscle fiber size, with hypertrophy often predominating *(1)*. Type 1 fiber atrophy is common, and floccular fibers similar to those seen in AD LGMD are found in at least 30% of biopsies. Marked predominance of type 1 fibers (over 95%) or of type 2 fibers (over 95%) can be encountered, as well as a more normal fiber type constitution.

Although the incidence of acute muscle fiber necrosis in FSHD is typically low, this form of MD is remarkable for a high incidence of inflammatory cell infiltrates (**Fig. 5A**). Both discrete and diffuse infiltrates can be found: the

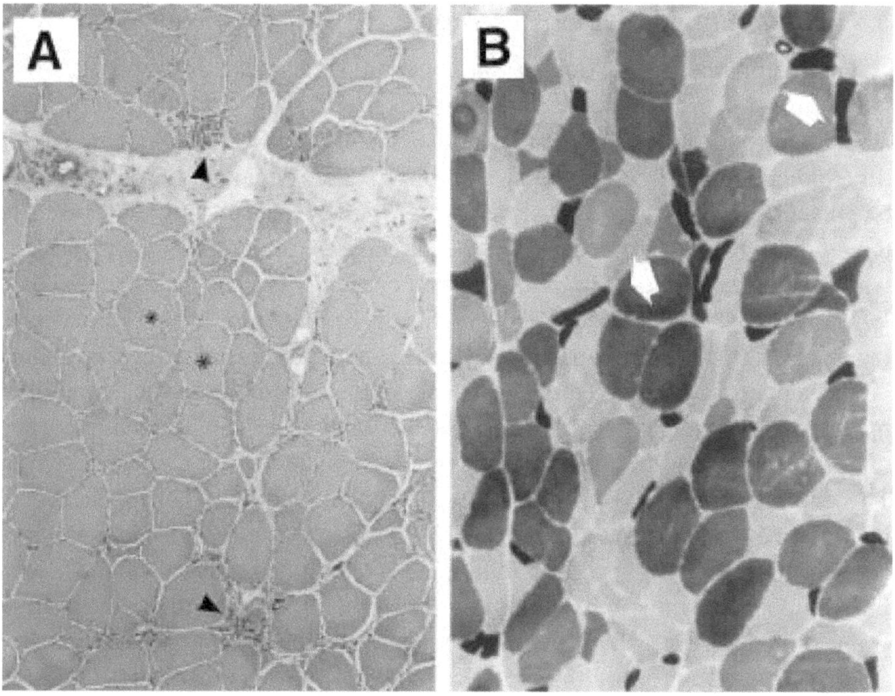

Fig. 5. (**A**) FSHD: biopsy from patient aged 50 yr showing inflammatory cell foci in perimysial areas. H&E ×75. (**B**) DM: biopsy from DM patient aged 38 yr showing selective atrophy of type 1 muscle fibers. mATPase ×100.

former contain mostly $T4^+$-lymphocytes; $T8^+$-lymphocytes predominate in the diffuse infiltrates seen in endomysial sites. In the vicinity of the inflammatory cell infiltrates, major histocompatibility complex type I (MHC-I) antigen may be upregulated on the surface of muscle fibers; normal expression is confined to the endothelial cells of capillaries and larger vessels. Generalized MHC-I upregulation with antigen expression on all muscle fibers in a biopsy is virtually diagnostic of true inflammatory myopathy (polymyositis or dermatomyositis), and is not seen in FSHD. At least one-third of all cases of FSHD biopsied show a significant inflammatory component. Occasionally, this occurs in childhood FSHD, and these biopsies also show other severe histopathological features, including marked atrophy and hypertrophy *(1)*. The hypertrophy present in FSHD is not a feature of true inflammatory muscle disease, and this, together with the restricted MHC-I expression, serves to differentiate the conditions. Identification of an inflammatory component in FSHD is important, regarding treatment of the patient, although response to conventional immunosuppression by steroid therapy is variable.

3.6. Congenital Muscular Dystrophy

The histopathological findings in congenital muscular dystrophy (CMD), including the form associated with merosin deficiency (chromosome 6q2-associated) and the Fukuyama variant (FCMD; chromosome 9q31), provide little indication of disease severity. Although severe degenerative changes may be present, CMD may be only slowly progressive, or even static, in contrast to the other MDs with early onset, and the histological picture is often at variance with the degree of motor impairment seen clinically ***(10)***.

Many CMD biopsies show severe fibrous connective tissue increase; in many cases, this is largely perimysial rather than endomysial. Other individual biopsies may show replacement of muscle fibers by adipose tissue, sometimes making up as much as 50% of the cross-sectional area. The frequent presence of contractures at birth (arthrogryposis) may be linked to the incidence of type 1 fiber predominance, but this is not a constant finding. The prevalence of hyaline fibers and of acute muscle necrosis is also variable, and some biopsies give the impression of having undergone monophasic muscle damage, with little evidence of ongoing degeneration. Regenerative activity can be seen in some biopsies (**Fig. 4B**), but many basophilic fibers show bizarre nuclear abnormalities, suggesting that some regeneration may be abortive. In CMD, most residual fibers appear to retain the capacity for hypertrophy, and this may be considerable, with biopsies from 3-yr-old CMD patients showing fibers up to 100 μm in diameter. Such hypertrophy must be vital to the gradual improvement in muscle strength displayed by some patients, who may have lost up to 50% of muscle fibers.

3.7. Myotonic Dystrophy

Even before the advent of modern genetic analysis, which can define the extent of trinucleotide (CTG) repeats within the gene, and provides the most meaningful indication of disease severity, muscle biopsy was undertaken only rarely for diagnostic purposes, because of the particularly clear-cut clinical picture shown by classical adult cases ***(11)***. Ironically, the histopathological diagnosis of myotonic dystrophy (DM) is also a good deal more straightforward and unequivocal than is the case in most other forms of MD.

The histological features of DM include almost invariable type 1 fiber atrophy, which may be very severe and lead to an overall type 2 fiber predominance (**Fig. 5B**). Ring fibers are found in DM in greater numbers than in any other MD, and are frequently associated with sarcoplasmic masses, which are zones devoid of myofibrils, lying outside the abnormal ring fiber myofibrillar displacement. Internal muscle fiber nuclei are very common, and, in longitudinal section, may be seen to occur in rows of 20–30 contiguous nuclei. The incidence of acute necrosis is typically low, but appears to increase according to disease severity, as does the amount of interstitial fibrous connective tissue.

The biopsy findings in infants and children with congenital DM may be unremarkable, though eventually they will manifest more severe disease than their mothers, who may be mildly affected. However, type 1 atrophy is a common feature, as in adult DM, and there may be a deficiency of type 2B fibers. Internal nuclei are rarely seen in infants with DM, but appear to proliferate throughout the patient's lifetime, so that, in adulthood, 10 or more internally placed nuclei may be seen in a single fiber in cross-section.

4. Notes

1. It will be apparent from histopathological profiles of the various MDs that few show sufficient specific features or combinations of features to enable a definite diagnosis to be made without recourse to additional clues from clinical presentation, creatine kinase levels, or electromyography. Into this select group would fall DMD, although, even here, preclinical biopsies, or those from late DMD, might prove problematical. Classic adult DM, and typical FSHD with an inflammatory component, may also be added to this very short list. All too often, biopsies from patients with a MD can only be reported as just that.
2. The unsatisfactory phrase "consistent with a particular clinical diagnosis" has persisted for decades. Now, the development of molecular probes for individual gene products has revolutionized diagnostic practice, and has enabled the histopathologist to begin to replace conjecture and opinion with certainty.

References

1. Dubowitz, V. (1985) *Muscle Biopsy: A Practical Approach.* 2nd ed. Bailliere Tindall, London.
2. Johnson, M. A. (1990) Skeletal muscle, in *Histochemistry in Pathology* (Filipe, M. I. and Lake, B. D.), 2nd ed. Churchill-Livingstone, Edinburgh, pp. 129–158.
3. Brooke, M. H. and Kaiser, K. K. (1970). Muscle fiber types: how many and what kind? *Arch. Neurol.* **23,** 369–379.
4. Borgers, M., Firth, J. A., Stoward, P. J., and Verheyen, A. (1991) Phosphatases, in *Histochemistry, Theoretical and Applied,* vol. 2 (Stoward, P. J. and Pearse, A. G. E.) 4th ed. Churchill-Livingstone, Edinburgh, pp. 187–218.
5. Stoward, P. J., Meijer, A. E. F. H., Seidler, E., and Wohlrab, F. (1991) Dehydrogenases, in *Histochemistry, Theoretical and Applied,* vol. 3 (Stoward, P. J. and Pearse, A. G. E.) 4th ed. Churchill-Livingstone, Edinburgh, pp. 27–71.
6. Bancroft, J. D. and Stevens, A. (1990). *Theory and Practice of Histological Techniques,* 3rd ed. Churchill-Livingstone, Edinburgh.
7. Schmalbruch, H. (1992) The muscular dystrophies, in *Skeletal Muscle Pathology,* 2nd ed. (Mastaglia, F. L. and Lord Walton of Detchant. Churchill-Livingstone, Edinburgh, pp. 283–318.
8. Emery, A. E. H. and Dreifuss, F. E. (1966) Unusual type of benign X-linked muscular dystrophy. *J. Neurol. Neurosurg. Psychiat.* **29,** 338–342.

9. Zatz, M., Vainzof, M., Passos Bueno, M. R., Akiyama, J., and Marie, S. K. N. (1996) Autosomal recessive limb-girdle muscular dystrophies, in *Handbook of Muscle Disease* (Lane, R. J. M.) Marcel Dekker, New York, pp. 245–255.
10. Banker, B. Q. (1986) Congenital muscular dystrophy, in *Myology* (Engel, A. G. and Banker, B. Q.) McGraw-Hill, New York, pp. 1367–1382.
11. Lane, R. J. M., Shelbourne, P., and Johnson, K. J. (1996) Myotonic dystrophy, in *Handbook of Muscle Disease* (Lane, R. J. M.) Marcel Dekker, New York, pp. 311–328.

4

Serum Creatine Kinase in Progressive Muscular Dystrophies

Mayana Zatz, Mariz Vainzof, and Maria Rita Passos-Bueno

1. Introduction

Several enzymes originating in muscle show increased activity in the serum of patients affected with different forms of muscular dystrophy (MD). These enzymes include creatine kinase (CK), aldolase, transaminase, and pyruvate kinase (PK), among others (reviewed in **ref. *1***). In the premolecular era, determination of serum enzymes represented the only noninvasive method for diagnosis of neuromuscular disorders and estimation of heterozygosity risks in females at risk for Duchenne and Becker muscular dystrophies (DMD/BMD). During many years, the authors' laboratory measured both serum CK (SCK) and PK in patients affected by different forms of muscular dystrophy (MD) as well as in DMD/BMD potential carriers, compared to normal controls ***(2–9)***. Assessment of serum PK activity was an important adjunct test to improve the sensitivity of serum CK, in particular, for carrier detection. However, after the introduction of molecular analysis, determinations of serum PK activity became of little practical use for this purpose.

Even in the molecular era, it is generally accepted that measurement of SCK is the most sensitive and specific screening test for muscle disease, and is often the first test used in cases of suspected muscle disease. In addition, the fact that erythrocytes contain very little CK confers an additional advantage, because assays in samples are not vitiated by hemolysis, an important practical point (*see* **Note 1**). However, since SCK may be assessed through different methods, and may vary in different ethnic groups ***(10)***, as well as during pregnancy ***(11,12)***, it is necessary for each laboratory to establish its own range of normal SCK activities. On the other hand, in order to compare values obtained in different laboratories, through different methods, results of SCK are classified as

From: *Methods in Molecular Medicine, vol. 43: Muscular Dystrophy: Methods and Protocols*
Edited by: K. M. D. Bushby and L. V. B. Anderson © Humana Press Inc., Totowa, NJ

normal (when in the normal range for age and ethnic group), and, when above the upper normal limit, as "fold-increased" above the normal upper limit.

CK transfers a phosphate group from creatine phosphate to adenosine diphoshate, (ADP), forming creatine and adenosine triphosphate (ATP). The rate of ATP and creatine formation may be determined either by colorimetric measurement of creatine or by measuring ATP by means of a coupled enzyme reaction, resulting in the reduction of a pyridine nucleotide, which is measured by a change in ultraviolet absorbance. The colorimetric method used in the laboratory described in this chapter, is performed with Sigma diagnostic kits (code 520-C), according to the following procedure:

$$\text{ADP} + \text{Phosphocreatine} \xrightarrow{\text{CK}} \text{ATP} + \text{Creatine}$$

$$\text{Creatine} + \alpha\text{-Naphtol} + \text{Diacetyl} \longrightarrow \text{Colored complex}$$

The amount of color formed (= absorbance at 520 nm) is proportional to CK activity.

This chapter provides reference data for CK levels in patients and carriers. This represents the results of SCK analysis in 1815 individuals, which includes 663 normal controls (from both sexes and different racial groups) and 1152 individuals belonging to families with neuromuscular disorders. In order to assess the value of SCK activity for differential diagnosis and carrier detection, the authors have compared the enzyme levels in 937 affected patients with different forms of neuromuscular disorders (MDs and spinal muscular atrophy) and 215 DMD/BMD carriers, with those observed in normal controls.

2. Materials

The following items of equipment are required, in addition to the Sigma 520-C assay kit:

1. Spectrophotometer capable of reading at 500–540 nm.
2. Reaction tubes (15-mL centrifuge tubes) and racks.
3. Cuvets (19 × 100 mm).
4. Water bath at 37°C.
5. 20, 200, and 1000 µL, plus 10-mL Pipet.
6. Centrifuge.

3. Methods

3.1. Assays

3.1.1. Calibration Curve

The calibration curve is constructed with known preweighed amounts of creatine ***(13)*** as described in **Table 1**. It is carried out at room temperature (18–26°C);

Table 1
CK Calibration Curve

1 Tube	2 Creatine standard solution (mL)	3 Water (mL)	4 Serum CK (SU/mL)	5 Absorbance at 520 nm
1	0	1.0	0	
2	0.2	0.8	32	
3	0.4	0.6	64	
4	0.6	0.4	96	
5	0.8	0.2	128	
6	1.0	0	160	

color development for the CK test on clinical samples is performed at 37°C. The higher temperature is required to overcome the inhibitory effect of test reagents to color formation.

1. Pipet into test tubes (or cuvets) the solutions indicated in columns 2 and 3, of Table 1.
2. To each tube, add 1.0 mL α-naphthol solution, 1.0 mL diacetyl solution, and 7.0 mL water. Mix contents of tubes immediately after each reagent addition. Allow to remain at room temperature (18–26°C).
3. After 15 min (*see* **Note 2**), read absorbance of tubes 2–6 at 500–540 nm, using tube 1 as the reference.
4. Record absorbance for tubes 2–6 in column 5, and plot a calibration curve of the absorbance vs the corresponding Sigma units (SU) of CK activity.

3.1.2. Clinical Samples

1. According to the number of samples, label tubes as Blank, 1, 2, 3, and so on. Pipet 0.5 mL phosphocreatine solution into each tube.
2. Into sample tubes only, pipet 0.1 mL 10-fold dilution of serum or plasma in water (1 part serum + 9 parts water) (*see* **Note 3**). Mix by gentle tapping. Into Blank tube only, pipet 0.1 mL water. Mix by gentle tapping.
3. Place tubes in 37°C water bath for several minutes. Add 0.2 mL ADP–glutathione solution to each tube to start reaction. Mix by tapping immediately after each addition. Incubate exactly 30 min.
4. Following incubation, add to each tube 0.2 mL p-hydroxymercuribenzoate solution to stop the reaction. Mix thoroughly.
5. To each tube, add 1.0 mL α-naphthol solution, 1.0 mL diacetyl solution, and 7.0 mL water. Mix contents of tubes immediately after each reagent addition.
6. Place tubes in 37°C water bath again for 15–20 min for color development.
7. Centrifuge tubes about 5 min (3000*g*).

Table 2
Serum CK Activities in 663 Normal Brazilian Individuals

Category	Number	Mean age	CK (SU/mL) Mean ± SD
Newborns			
Males	68		15.17 ± 8.38
Females	57		13.92 ± 7.67
Children < 15 yr old			
Boys	100	6.4 ± 3.8	8.3 ± 5.4
Girls	101	6.1 ± 3.7	7.0 ± 6.6
Adults			
Males	74	37.0 ± 5.5	9.6 ± 5.5
Females	263	28.6 ± 7.3	5.1 ± 3.3

8. Transfer supernatants to cuvets, read (or, according to the model of spectrophotometer, read direct from tubes), and record absorbance of Test vs Blank as reference (*see* **Note 2**).
9. Determine CK activity in SU/mL from the calibration curve.

3.2. Results of Serum CK Activity Analysis

3.2.1. Normal Controls

It has been reported that several factors may increase SCK activity in normal controls: alcoholism, strenuous or prolonged physical exercise, hypothyroidism, myocardial infarction, acute cerebrovascular accidents, acute psychiatric disorders, and stroke, among others ***(14–21)***. Therefore, these parameters must be taken into account when analyzing results of SCK. Furthermore, the authors have observed that SCK activity is influenced in normal healthy individuals by age, sex, ethnic background, and pregnancy ***(9,11,12,22–24)***. Therefore, each laboratory must generate its own normal control range, as outlined below.

3.2.1.1. Age and Sex

In order to assess the effect of age and sex, SCK was determined in 663 healthy individuals (242 males and 421 females, who had no known relatives with neuromuscular disorders), with ages ranging from newborn to 59 yr old. Blood from newborns was collected, soon after the umbilical cord was severed, in a sterile dry tube. Normal children were less than 15 yr old, and came to the pediatrician for routine examinations. All girls were premenarchal. The results, partially reported previously ***(22,23)***, are summarized in **Table 2**, which shows that, in normal individuals, SCK decreases with age in both sexes. Among females, SCK in newborns is significantly higher (on average, two-

Table 3
Serum CK and Age in 263 Normal Females from Different Racial Subgroups

Racial group	*n*	Age Mean ± SD	Serum CK (SU/mL) Mean ± SD
Caucasion	40	29.2 ± 7.9	3.7 ± 2.6
Negroid			
Light mulattos	40	28.9 ± 6.4	4.2 ± 1.8
Medium mulattos	47	29.2 ± 6.4	5.9 ± 4.5
Dark mulattos	45	30.2 ± 8.2	6.0 ± 2.9
Black	41	32.2 ± 8.8	6.8 ± 5.7
Orientals	50	23.1 ± 5.9	4.2 ± 2.5

fold) than in young girls and in the adult group (2.7-fold). Among males, SCK is significantly higher in newborns than in young boys (about 1.8-fold higher), but it remains stable afterwards. Comparison between sexes showed no statistically significant difference in newborns and children, but was significantly higher in adult men than women ($P < 0.05$), which is probably the result of the greater muscle mass in adult males than females ***(25)***.

3.2.1.2. Racial Effect

In order to assess the effect of race on SCK, a total of 263 healthy females were analyzed, as reported previously ***(24)***. The results are summarized in **Table 3**. The mean SCK activity in the group of Caucasion females did not differ from light mulattos or Orientals ($P > 0.05$). However, the mean CK among Caucasoids is significantly lower than in the groups of medium mulattos, dark mulattos, and black females ($P < 0.05$), but not significantly different from light mulattos ($P > 0.05$). In addition, a gradual increase in the mean CK activity, according to the degree of black admixture, is observed.

Therefore, it is important that the racial background is taken into consideration when analyzing SCK in at-risk DMD/BMD females. For example, a value of 18 SU/mL, which is about a twofold increased above normal in a Caucasoid or Oriental woman, may be in the normal upper range for an African-Brazilian female.

3.2.2. Duchenne and Becker Muscular Dystrophies

DMD and BMD are allelic conditions, caused by defects in the gigantic Xp21-linked gene, which codes for the protein dystrophin (which is essentially absent in DMD, and qualitatively or quantitatively abnormal in BMD) (***26–28***; *see* Chapters 5 and 6). It is well known that all DMD and BMD patients have grossly elevated SCK from birth (i.e., before the onset of clinical signs), and that CK activity in serum decreases with the progression of the dystrophic process ***(1,4,7,29,30)***.

Table 4
Comparison of Mean Serum CK in Patients with Different Diagnoses

	Mean serum CK ± SD (SU/mL)			
Age range (yr)	DMD	BMD	Sarcoglycanopathy	Nonsarcoglycanopathy LGMD
0–5	1240.1 ± 613.5 $n = 43$	845.0 ± 35.4 $n = 4$	–	440.0 ± 0 $n = 2$
5–10	856.3 ± 657.8 $n = 155$	605.3 ± 322.0 $n = 18$	532.9 ± 313.5 $n = 10$	349.4 ± 235.7 $n = 15$
10–15	459.9 ± 372.2 $n = 72$	568.0 ± 452.6 $n = 19$	200.5 ± 143.5 $n = 13$	731.8 ± 552.9 $n = 30$
15–20	164.2 ± 109.3 $n = 15$	428.5 ± 250.4 $n = 26$	161.7 ± 100.9 $n = 11$	182.8 ± 137.0 $n = 18$
20–25	88.8 ± 59.7 $n = 6$	140.0 ± 56.6 $n = 10$	135.6 ± 95.4 $n = 8$	262.8 ± 293.2 n =25
25–30	–	308.8 ± 215.0 $n = 8$	167.5 ± 17.7 $n = 3$	221.0 ± 211.6 $n = 31$
> 30	–	160.8 ± 130.2 $n = 11$	–	165.0 ± 140.8 $n = 39$
Total	485.9 ± 497.7 $n = 456$	432.7 ± 130.2 $n = 96$	250.4 ± 229.7 $n = 45$	278.7 ± 330.8 $n = 171$

With the aim of assessing the variability and rate of decrease of SCK as a function of age, the authors studied SCK activity in 456 DMD and 96 BMD patients, as shown in **Table 4**. Some of these results have been reported previously ***(31)***. In the total sample, the mean SCK was 485.9 ± 497.7 SU/mL for DMD and 432.7 ± 130.2 SU/mL for BMD, with the upper limit about 2.1-fold higher in DMD than in BMD. The maximum values were found between 0 and 5 yr of age for DMD (up to 130-fold above normal) and between 10 and 15 yr of age for BMD (up to 77-fold above normal). On the other hand, as seen in **Figs. 1** and **2**, the decline in SCK activity as a function of age is about 4.4× greater in DMD than in BMD.

The authors also compared CK levels in patients with and without molecular deletions in the dystrophin gene. **Table 5** summarizes the results for 340 DMD (up to 15 yr of age) and 96 BMD patients who submitted to muscle biopsies, and also had their diagnosis confirmed through dystrophin analysis. The mean SCK was not significantly different in patients with DNA deletions, as compared to those without DNA deletions ($P > 0.05$).

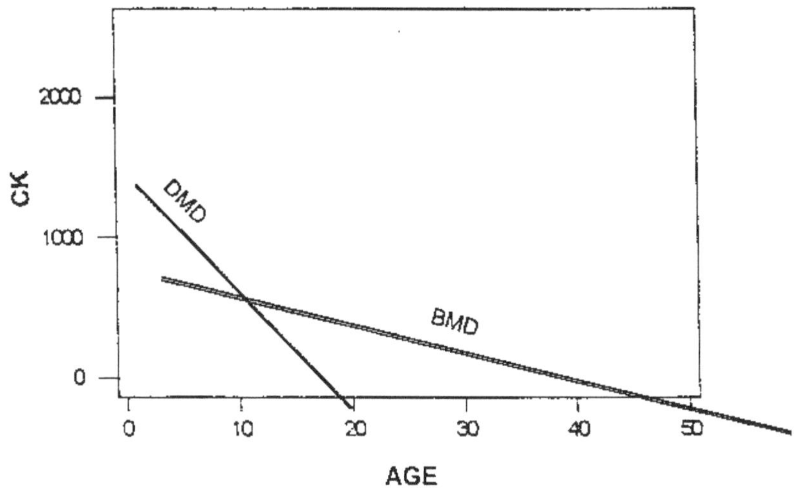

Fig. 1. Decrease of serum CK activity as a function of age in DMD, compared to BMD.

Table 5
Results of serum CK (Sigma units/mL) and DNA Analysis in 340 DMD and 96 BMD Patients Who Had Diagnosis Confirmed also Through Dystrophin Analysis

	N	Mean CK ± SD	Mean age ± SD
Duchenne patients			
With deletions			
3' region	50	725.5 ± 370.0	7.5 ± 1.3
Central region	160	800.8 ± 408.6	7.9 ± 2.1
Subtotal	210	782.8 ± 401.6	7.8 ± 2.0
No deletion	130	806.0 ± 404.2	8.1 ± 2.3
Total	340	791.6 ± 402.7	7.9 ± 2.1
Becker patients			
With deletions			
3' region	20	338.4 ± 241.3	20.1 ± 6.0
Central region	29	452.5 ± 339.3	18.0 ± 9.1
Subtotal	49	424.0 ± 314.8	19.0 ± 8.0
No deletion	47	484.2 ± 146.8	19.0 ± 6.5
Total	96	445.4 ± 257.1	19.0 ± 7.5

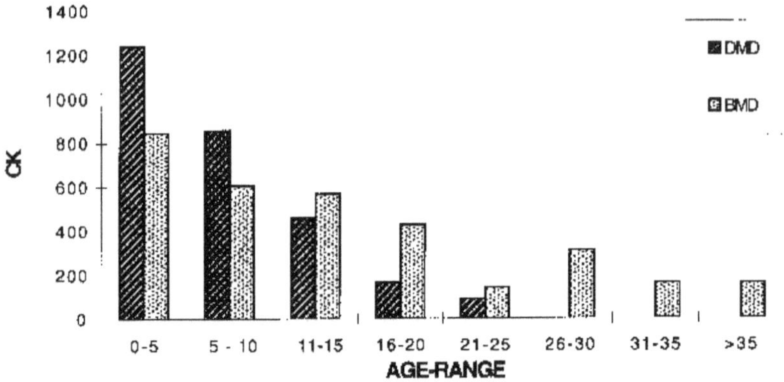

Fig. 2. Mean CK Distribution according to age in DMD vs BMD.

3.2.3. Limb-Girdle Muscular Dystrophies

The limb-girdle muscular dystrophies (LGMDs) are a heterogeneous group of inherited neuromuscular disorders characterized by proximal muscular weakness of the pelvic and shoulder girdles, and by a variable progression, with symptoms ranging from very severe to mild *(32)*. Currently, 14 genes responsible for these conditions have been identified, 6 of them autosomal dominant (AD) and the remaining displaying autosomal recessive (AR) inheritance *(33–36)*. Among the eight mapped recessive forms, four are classified as sarcoglycanopathies: *LGMD2C, LGMD2D, LGMD2E*, and *LGMD2F* (the genes coding for γ-, α-, β- and δ-sarcoglycan, respectively), and pathogenic mutations in any of these genes disrupt the dystrophin-associated sarcoglycan subcomplex. The *LGMD2A* gene codes for a muscle-specific proteolytic enzyme, calpain 3 *(37)*; the protein product for *LGMD2B* gene is the protein dysferlin and for the *LGMD2G* gene is the protein telethonin *(36,38)*. LGMD types 2A, 2B, and 2G are associated with milder phenotypes (comparable with BMD); the sarcoglycanopathies are often associated with a more severe clinical course (generally comparable to DMD) (*see* Chapters 13–17).

In order to compare serum enzyme activities in the different AR LGMDs, the authors determined SCK levels in 216 patients, subdividing them into those with sarcoglycanopathies and those with nonsarcoglycanopathic LGMD. The results from patients of different ages were also compared with the results previously described for the DMD/BMD patients. As seen in **Table 4** and **Figs. 3** and **4**, although the mean SCK may be higher in some groups compared to others, there is a great overlap between SCK values in patients with different diagnosis (*see also* **Notes 4** and **5**).

In addition, the authors compared SCK in the LGMD2A to LGMD2F subgroups (**Table 6**). In the sacroglycanopathies (SG) group of 45 patients (mean

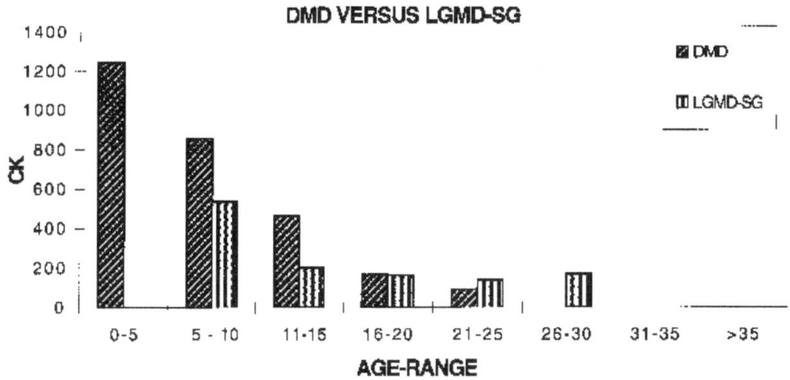

Fig. 3. Mean CK distribution according to age in DMD vs LGMD-SG.

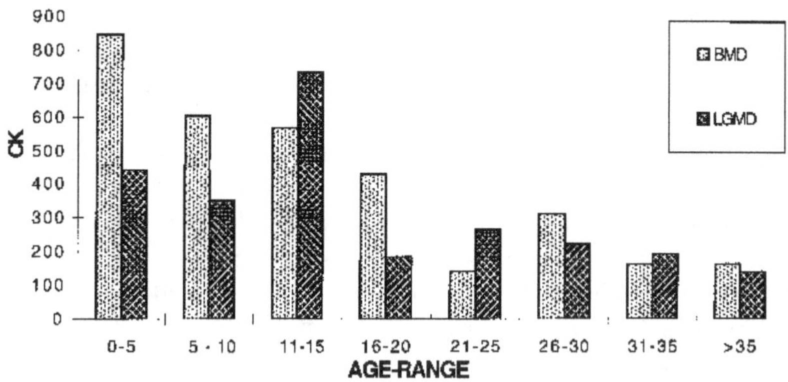

Fig. 4. Mean CK distribution according to age in BMD vs LGMD.

age 15.7 ± 7.9 yr), SCK was 250.4 ± 229.7 SU/mL (up to 37-fold increased). Among the 171 non-SG patients (mean age 23.3 ± 10.4 yr), the mean sCK was 278.7 ± 330.8 SU/mL (up to 80-fold increased), although values more than 100-fold increased may occasionally be found in preclinical patients *(34)*. As seen in **Table 6**, statistical analysis showed that the mean SCK did not differ between SG and non-SG groups (despite the difference in clinical severity) or among the four sarcoglycanopathies ($P > 0.05$).

3.2.4. Facioscapulohumeral MD

Facioscapulohumeral MD (FSHD1) is an AD neuromuscular condition that characteristically affects the facial and shoulder girdle muscles, although there is marked intra- and interfamilial variability in expression. The rate of progression may vary considerably. About 10% of gene carriers may become wheel-

Table 6
Mean Serum CK (SU/mL) in Six AR LGMDs

	N	Mean CK ± SD	Mean age ± SD
Sarcoglycanopathies	45	250.4 ± 229.7	15.7 ± 6.6
LGMD2C (13q)	11	355.3 ± 360.6	14.5 ± 6.7
LGMD2D (17q)	21	241.3 ± 191.0	17.2 ± 6.5
LGMD2E (4q)	6	137.0 ± 98. 5	15.8 ± 4.4
LGMD 2F (5q)	7	237.3 ± 175.8	13.3 ± 4.9
Nonsarcoglycanopathies	171	278.7 ± 330.8	23.3 ± 10.4
LGMD2A (15q)	31	219.3 ± 250.8	22.5 ± 10.1
LGMD2B (2p)	48	383.4 ± 388.0	28. 2 ± 9.4
Total	216	265.8 ± 302.2	21.9 ± 10.3

chair-dependent, and one-third of them have no complaints, but have minor signs that can only be identified by careful physical and neurological examination. Life expectancy is normal for FSHD1 ***(39,40)***. The gene responsible for FSHD1 was localized to 4q35 by linkage with polymorphic markers ***(41,42)***. Subsequently, it was observed that, in normal individuals, the probe p13E-11 detects a polymorphic *Eco*RI fragment that is usually >35 kb; in FSHD1 families, a specific shorter fragment, usually between 14 and 35 kb, was found to co-segregate with the disease (***42–45***; *see* Chapter 18).

Previous studies have shown that SCK activity has little or no increase among FSHD patients ***(32)***. In the present sample, the mean SCK level in 96 patients (mean age 32.3 ± 13.1 yr) was 16.99 ± 10.38 SU/mL. SCK was normal in 45, and only slightly increased (up to threefold above normal limit) in 51 patients (53% of the sample), in accordance to previous reports, and therefore was of little value for clinical diagnosis ***(32)***.

3.2.5. Spinal Muscular Atrophies

Spinal muscular atrophies (SMA) include a group of motor neuron disorders characterized by degeneration of spinal cord anterior horn cells, leading to muscular wasting and atrophy. According to age at onset, development milestones, and severity of the phenotype-affected patients are classified into three groups: SMA-I, SMA-II, and SMA-III ***(46)***. SMA-I or Werdnig-Hoffmann disease, the most severe form, starts at birth or within 6 mo of age. In SMA-II, the intermediate form, affected children are able to sit unassisted and may be able to walk for a short time. SMA-III, or Kugelberg-Welander disease, is the mildest form.

The locus for all three forms of SMA was mapped to chromosome 5q11.2–13.3 by linkage analysis ***(47–49)***. In 1995, two candidate genes were mapped

Table 7
Serum CK (SU/mL) in 73 SMA Patients with Deletions (*n* = 48) and Without Deletion (*n* = 25) in Exons 7 and 8 of the *SMN* Gene

	N	Mean CK ± SD	Mean age ± SD
SMA-I			
With deletion	13	6.3 ± 2.6	3.9 ± 3.1
Without deletions	3	8.0 ± 5.6	2.0 ± 0
Subtotal	16	6.7 ± 3.2	3.5 ± 2.8
SMA-II			
With deletion	17	14.2 ± 11.2	5.8 ± 3.5
Without deletions	3	8.7 ± 3.2	5.7 ± 5.5
Subtotal	20	13.4 ± 10.5	5.8 ± 3.7
SMA-III			
With deletions	18	21.6 ± 17.8	17.9 ± 10.0
Without deletions	19	10.1 ± 6.9	22.7 ± 15.6
Subtotal	37	15.7 ± 14.4	20.4 ± 13.2
TOTAL	73	13.1 ± 12.2	13.5 ± 12.7

in the *SMA* region ***(50,51)***: the survival motor neuron (*SMN*) gene (present in two copies, the *SMN* which is telomeric, and *cBCD54,* which is centromeric) and the neuronal apoptosis inhibitory protein (*NAIP*) gene. Molecular studies have shown that the majority of SMA patients are homozygously deleted for exons 7 and 8 of the SMN telomeric copy, and a proportion of them also are deleted for the *NAIP* gene ***(50,51)***, independently of the severity of the disease.

Because SCK may be raised in SMA, particularly in the adult forms ***(1)***, the authors have analyzed CK levels in 73 SMA patients, as summarized in **Table 7**. Comparison between the three groups showed that the mean CK is significantly higher in SMA-II and SMA-III than in SMA-I ($P < 0.05$), but did not differ between SMA-II and SMA-III ($P > 0.05$). On the other hand, among SMA-III patients, SCK was significantly higher among patients with deletions (and therefore with a confirmed diagnosis of Kugelberg-Welander) than among those without deletions (*see* also **Note 6**).

3.2.6. Carrier Detection of Females at Risk for DMD/BMD

Numerous reports have shown that SCK levels in DMD/BMD carriers (with a normal chromosome constitution) may vary from normal to grossly elevated, because of random inactivation of the X chromosome. In the premolecular era, results of SCK levels in females at risk for DMD/BMD, combined with results from pedigree analysis, were used to estimate the probability of heterozygosity in suspected carriers. The detection rate obtained by numerous investigators is about 60–70% ***(1–6,9)***.

Table 8A
Estimated Risk of Heterozygosity (Not Taking into Account the Possibility of Germinal Mosaicism) in a Mother of Isolated DMD Patient with Normal Serum CK

Probabilities	Carrier	Not a carrier
Genetic	2/3 or 0.66	1/3 or 0.33
Conditional		
Normal serum CK	0.4	0.95
Final	0.66 × 0.4 = 0.26	0.95 × 0.33 = 0.31
Posterior	0.26/0.31 + 0.26 = 0.46	0.31/0.31 + 0.26 = 0.54

Table 8B
Estimated Risk of Heterozygosity (Not Taking into Account the Possibility of Germinal Mosaicism) in a Mother of Isolated DMD Patient with Normal Serum CK and with a Daughter with Normal CK

Probabilities	Carrier	Not a carrier
Genetic	2/3 or 0.66	1/3 or 0.33
Conditional		
Normal serum CK in mother	0.4	0.95
Normal serum CK in daughter	0.5 × 0.4 + 0.5 × 0.95 = 0.48	0.95
Final	0.66 × 0.4 × 0.48 = 0.13	0.95 × 0.95 × 0.33 = 0.3
Posterior	0.13/0.13 + 0.3 = 0.30	0.3/0.3 + 0.13 = 0.70

Here, the authors included results from 215 females (mean age 32.7 ± 28.3 yr) classified as DMD/BMD obligate carriers, based on pedigree or DNA analysis: 105 have molecular deletions in the dystrophin gene; seven have point mutations in the dystrophin gene, and 103 have at least one DMD/BMD brother or maternal uncle and at least one affected DMD/BMD son. The mean SCK in this group was 33.6 ± 33.5 SU/mL. Approximately 60% (n = 125) of DMD/BMD females have SCK levels above the 95% upper-normal limit. Therefore, although an elevated enzyme activity is strong evidence that a female at risk is indeed a DMD/BMD carrier, normal results cannot rule out that she is not a DMD/BMD heterozygote, but may be valuable for estimating heterozygosity risks when DNA analysis is not informative or not available. Some examples are summarized in **Table 8**.

Taking into account that 1/3 of DMD cases arise through new mutations (and not taking into consideration the possibility of germinal mosaicism, which

Table 8C
Estimated Risk of Heterozygosity (Not Taking into Account the Possibility of Germinal Mosaicism) in a Mother of a Deceased DMD Patient, Who Has No Detected DNA Deletion

Probabilities	Carrier	Not a carrier
Genetic	2/3 or 0.66	1/3 or 0.33
Conditional		
No DNA deletion in mother	0.4	1
Final	0.66 × 0.4 =0.26	1 × 0.33 = 0.33
Posterior	0.26/0.26 + 0.33 = 0.44	0.33/0.26 + 0.33 = 0.56

Table 8D
Estimated Risk of Heterozygosity (Not Taking into Account the Possibility of Germinal Mosaicism) in a Mother of a Deceased DMD Patient, Who Has No Detected DNA Deletion and a Normal Serum CK

Probabilities	Carrier	Not a carrier
Genetic	2/3 or 0.66	1/3 or 0.33
Conditional		
No DNA deletion in mother	0.4	1
Normal serum CK in mother	0.4	0.95
Final	0.66 × 0.4 × 0.4 = 0.10	0.95 × 1 × 0.33 = 0.31
Posterior	0.10/0.10 + 0.31 = 0.25	0.31/0.31 + 0.10 = 0.75

will be discussed in Chapter 7), a mother of an isolated DMD boy has a genetic probability of about 2/3, or 66%, to be a DMD carrier. If the patient has no detectable DNA deletion, DNA analysis will not determine if this mother carries the defective *DMD* gene (unless a point mutation or a duplication is detected in the proband). If this mother has a normal SCK level, her estimated risk of being a DMD carrier will be 46% (**Table 8A**). If she has one daughter with normal CK, her estimated risk of heterozygosity will drop to 30% (**Table 8B**) and will decrease progressively according to the number of daughters with normal enzymes, as detailed previously by the authors ***(1,21)***. In opposition, if one of her daughters has increased serum levels, this will be an indication that both the mother and daughter are DMD carriers.

Another common situation in practice is when there is no affected patient alive in the family. For example, a mother who had a deceased son who had

Table 9
Effect of Age on Serum CK (in Sigma Units/mL) in 211 DMD/BMD Carriers

Age range	*N*	Mean serum CK ± SD
0–10	18	130.6 ± 11.8
11–20	25	63.7 ± 68.0
21–30	49	23.2 ± 22.1
31–40	80	20.4 ± 14.7
41–50	27	19.7 ± 15.9
51–70	12	7.0 ± 3.5

DMD (and from whom there is no DNA available). Considering that approx 60% of DMD patients have DNA deletions, if no deletion is detected in this mother, she will still have an estimated chance of 44% of carrying a DMD mutation (**Table 8C**); if she has a normal CK, her estimated risk will drop to 25% **Table 8D**). Therefore, in practice, if DNA results are not informative, or if DNA is not available, it is very important to test SCK in as many females at risk as possible who are related to the affected proband.

In order to assess the effect of age on serum CK levels in DMD/BMD carriers, the authors have compared the mean serum CK levels in 211 females (whose ages were recorded), who were divided into six groups (ranging from newborns to 70 yr old). As seen in **Table 9**, there is a sharp decline on SCK activities from the newborn period to adulthood, and an apparent stabilization afterwards. These observations are in accordance with Emery *(1)*, who did not find any clear relationship between age and CK levels after the late teens. These results also support the authors' previous report, which suggested, in the premolecular era, that the mean SCK was significantly higher in young at risk DMD girls than among adult carriers *(24)*, probably because of the same progressive elimination of dystrophic fibers that occurs in affected DMD/BMD patients.

Although the introduction of molecular methods has greatly improved the diagnosis of MDs, as well as the identification of DMD/BMD carriers, determinations of SCK should be the first screening test when a muscle disease is suspected. In addition, repeated serial determinations of SCK may prove to be important in evaluating the effect of any therapeutic trial in affected patients.

4. Notes

1. CK activity can be measured in plasma or serum. Blood can be collected in a tube containing ethylenediamine tetraacetic acid, or in a plain tube, and allowed to clot. The plasma or serum is obtained by centrifugation (5 min, 3000*g*).

2. It is important to complete the readings within 10 min, because the color fades slowly thereafter.
3. In samples with high SCK activity (that occurs very often in young Duchenne patients) the amount of creatine which is formed goes off the spectrophotometer scale. In these cases, the serum (or plasma) should be diluted 100-fold (add 0.01 mL serum to 0.9 mL water). In order to obtain the final SCK activity, the result is multiplied by 10.
4. In the absence of a family history, differential diagnosis may be difficult between Xp21 and AR LGMD for isolated male patients, or between manifesting DMD/BMD carrier state and AR LGMD for isolated female patients. The differential diagnosis will depend on DNA and muscle protein analysis ***(52–60)***.
5. In some situations, although serum CK values may be comparable, the severity of the clinical course allows a differential diagnosis, e.g., for DMD vs BMD in patients who are older than 10 yr. On the other hand, a very high serum CK in a young patient is more suggestive of Xp21 MD than AR LGMD (although, as outlined previously, very high serum CK levels have been observed by the authors in preclinical LGMD).
6. Serum CK levels are also important for discriminating between adult forms of SMA and LGMD, since although some SMA patients may have CK levels up to fivefold above normal, they are significantly lower than the ones observed for LGMD.

Acknowledgments

The collaboration of the following persons, without whom the writing of this chapter would not be possible, is gratefully acknowledged: Marta Canovas, Simone Campiotto, Denilce Sumita, Antonia Cerqueira, Reinaldo Takata, Dr. Rita de Cassia M. Pavanello, Dr. Suely K. Marie, and Constancia Urbani. This work was supported with grants from FAPESP, CNPq, FINEP, ABDIM, and PRONEX.

References

1. Emery, A. E. H. (1993) *Duchenne Muscular Dystrophy,* Oxford University Press.
2. Zatz, M., Frota-Pessoa, O., and Peres, C. (1975) Use of normal daughters CPK levels in the estimation of heterozygosity risks in X-linked muscular dystrophies. *Human Heredity* **25,** 354–359.
3. Zatz, M., Frota-Pessoa, O., Levy, J. A., and Peres, C. A. (1976) Creatine-phosphokinase (CPK) activity in relatives of patients with X-linked muscular dystrophies: a Brazilian study. *J. Genet. Hum.* **24,** 153–168.
4. Zatz, M., Shapiro, L. J., Campion, D. S., Oda, E., and Kaback, M. M. (1978) Serum pyruvate-kinase (PK) and creatine-phosphokinase in progressive muscular dystrophies. *J. Neurol. Sci.* **36,** 349–362.
5. Zatz, M. and Otto, P. A. (1980) Effect of age on the detection rate in Duchenne muscular dystrophy. *J. Neurol. Sci.* **47,** 407–410.
6. Zatz, M. and Otto, P. A. (1980) The use of concomitant serum pyruvate-kinase (PK) and creatine-phosphokinase (CPK) for carrier detection in Duchenne's muscular dystrophy through discriminant analysis. *J. Neurol. Sci.* **47,** 411–417.

7. Zatz, M., Shapiro, L. J., Campion, D. S., Kaback, M. M., and Otto, P. A. (1980) Serum pyruvate-kinase (PK) and creatine-phosphokinase (CPK) in females relatives and patients with X-linked muscular dystrophies (Duchenne and Becker). *J. Neurol. Sci.* **46,** 267–279.
8. Zatz, M. and Otto, P. A. (1986) Evaluation of carrier detection rate for Duchenne and Becker muscular dystrophies using serum creatine-kinase (CK) and pyruvate-kinase (PK) through discriminant analysis. *Am. J. Med. Genet.* **25,** 219–231.
9. Zatz, M., Passos, M. R., Rabbi-Bortolini E, Vainzof, M., Rapaport, D., Rocha, J. M. L., and Pavanello, R. C. (1988) Serum creatine (CK) and pyruvate-kinase (PK) levels in females at-risk for Duchenne muscular dystrophy (DMD) from different racial backgrounds. *Rev Bras de Genet* **11,** 761–768.
10. Passos-Bueno, M. R., Rabbi-Bortolini, E. R., Azevedo, E., and Zatz, M. (1989) Racial effect on serum creatine-kinase for females at-risk for Duchenne dystrophy. *Clin. Chim. Acta.* **179,** 153–168.
11. Zatz, M., Karp, L. E., and Rogatko, A. (1982) Pyruvate-kinase (PK) and creatine-phosphokinase (CPK) in normal pregnancy and its implication in genetic counseling of Duchenne muscular dystrophy (DMD). *Am. J. Med. Genet.* **13,** 257–262.
12. Zatz, M., Passos, M. R., and Bortolini, E. R. (1983) Serum pyruvate-kinase (PK) activity during pregnancy in potential carriers for Duchenne muscular dystrophy. *Am. J. Med. Genet.* **15,** 149–151.
13. Sigma Diagnostics (1988). Creatine phosphokinase (CK): quantitative colorimetric determination in serum or plasma at 540–540 nm, No 520.
14. Hess, J. W. and MacDonald, R. P. (1963) Serum creatine phosphokinase activity. A new diagnostic aid in myocardial and skeletal muscle disease. *J. Mich. Med. Soc.* **62,** 1095.
15. Hess, J. W., MacDonald, R. P., Frederick, R. I., Jones, R. N., Neely, J., and Gross, D. (1964) Serum creatine phosphokinase (CPK) activity in disorders of heart and skeletal muscle. *Ann. Intern. Med.* **61,** 1015.
16. Duma, R. J. and Siegel, A. L. (1965) Serum creatine phosphokinase in acute myocardial infarction. *Arch. Intern. Med.* **115,** 443.
17. Herschkowitz, N. and Cummings, J. N. (1964) Creatine kinase in cerebrospinal fluid. *J. Neurosurg. Psychiatry* **27,** 247.
18. Acheson, J., James, D. C., Hutchinson, E. D., and Westhead, R. (1965) Serum creatine-kinase levels in cerebral vascular disease. *Lancet* **2,** 1306.
19. Dubo, H., Park, D. C., Pennington RJT, Kalbag, R. M., and Walton, J. N. (1967) Sewrum creatine-kinase in cases of stroke, head injury and meningitis. *Lancet* **2,** 743.
20. Bengzon, A., Hippius, H., and Kanig, K. (1966) Some changes in the serum during treatment with psychotropic drugs. *J. Nerv. Ment. Dis.* **143,** 369.
21. Meltzer, H. (1968) Creatine kinase and aldolase in serum: abnormality common to acute psychoses. *Science* **159,** 1368.
22. Passos, M. R. and Zatz, M. (1983) Creatine-kinase (CK) and pyruvate-kinase (PK) activities in cord blood of normal neonates; application to Duchenne mular dystrophy screening programmes. *Am. J. Med. Genet.* **16,** 367–372.

23. Passos, M. R., Gonzalez, C. H., and Zatz, M. (1985) Creatine-kinase (CK) and pyruvate-kinase (PK) activities in normal children: implications in Duchenne muscular dystrophy carrier detection. *Am. J. Med. Genet.* **23,** 225–235.
24. Passos-Bueno, M. R., Otto, P. A., and Zatz, M. (1989) Estimates of conditional heterozygosity risks for young females in Duchenne muscular dystrophy. *Human Heredity* **39,** 202–211.
25. Meltzer, H. Y., Belmaker, R. J., Wyatt, W., Pollin, W., and Cohen, S. (1976) Serum creatine phosphokinase (CPK) activity in monozygotic twins discordant for schizophrenia: heritability of serum CK activity. *Comp. Psychiatry* **17,** 469–475.
26. Koenig, M., Hoffmann, E. P., Bertelson, C. J., Monaco, A. P., Feener, C., and and Kunkel, L. M. (1987) Complete cloning of the Duchenne muscular dystrophy (DMD) cDNA and preliminary genomic organization of the DMD gene in normal and affected individuals. *Cell* **50,** 509–517.
27. Hoffman, E. P., Brown, R. H., and Kunkel, L. M. (1987) Dystrophin: the protein product of the Duchenne muscular dystrophy locus. *Cell* **51,** 919–928.
28. Hoffman, E. P., Fischbeck, K. H., Brown, R. H., et al. (1988) Characterization of dystrophin in muscle-biopsy specimens from patients with Duchenne's or Becker's muscular dystrophy. *N. Eng. J. Med.* **318,** 1363–1368.
29. Pennington, R. J. T. (1980) Clinical biochemistry of muscular dystrophy. *Br. Med. Bull.* **36,** 123–126.
30. Rowland, L. P., Willner, J., Cerri, C., DiMauro, S., and Miranda, A. (1980) Approaches to the membrane theory of Duchenne muscular dystrophy, in *Muscular Dystrophy Research* (Angelini, C., Danieli, G. A., and Fontanari, D., eds.), Experta Medica, Amsterdam, pp. 3–13.
31. Zatz, M., Rapaport, D., Vainzof, M., Rocha, J. M. L., Passos-Bueno, M. R., Rabbi-Bortolini, E., Pavanello, R. C. M., and Peres, C. A. (1991) Serum creatine-kinase (CK) and pyruvate-kinase (PK) activity as a function of clinical evolution in Duchenne (DMD) and Becker (BMD) muscular dystrophies. *J. Neurol. Sci.* **102,** 190–196.
32. Walton, J. N. and Gardner-Medwin, D. (1988) The muscular dystrophies, in *Disorders of Voluntary Muscle,* 5th. ed. (J. N. Walton, J. N., ed.), pp. 519–569, Churchill Livingstone, Edinburgh.
33. Bushby, K. M. D. and Beckmann J. S. (1995) Diagnostic criteria for the limb-girdle muscular dystrophies: report of the ENMC workshop on limb-girdle muscular dystrophies. *Neuromusc. Disord.* **5,** 71–74.
34. Passos-Bueno, M. R., Moreira, E. S., Marie, S. K., Bashir, R., Vasquez, L., Love, D. R., et al. (1996) Main clinical features for the three mapped autosomal recessive limb-girdle muscular dystrophies and estimated proportion of each form in 13 Brazilian families. *J. Med. Genet.* **33,** 97–102.
35. Passos-Bueno, M. R., Moreira, E. S., Vainzof, M., Marie, S. K., and Zatz, M. (1996) Linkage analysis in autosomal recessive muscular dystrophy (AR LGMD) maps a sixth form to 5q33-34 (LGMD2F) and indicates that there is at least one more subtype of ARLGMD. *Hum. Mol. Genet.* **5,** 815–820.
36. Moreira, E. S., Wiltshire, T. J., Faulner, G., Nilforoushan, A., Vainzof, M., Suzuki, O. T., et al. (2000) Limb-girdle muscular dystrophy type 2G (LGMD2G) is caused by mutations in the gene encoding the sarcomeric protein telethonin. *Nat. Genet.* **24,** 163–166.

37. Richard, I., Broux, O., Allamand, V., et al. (1995) A novel mechanism leading to muscular dystrophy: mutations in calpain 3 cause limb girdle muscular dystrophy type 2A. *Cell* **81,** 27–40.
38. Bashir, R., Britton, S., Strachan, T., Keers, S., Vafiadaki, E., Lako, M., Richard, I., Marchand, S., et. al. (1998) A gene related to Caenorhabditis elegans spermatogeneiss factor fer-1 is mutated in limb-girdle muscular dystrophy type 2B. *Nat. Genet.* **20,** 37–42.
39. Lunt, P. W., Compston, D. A. S., and Harper, P. S. (1989) Estmation of age dependent penetrance in facioscapulohumeral muscular dystrophy by minimizing ascertainment bias. *J. Med. Genet.* **26,** 755–760.
40. Padberg, G. (1982) Facioscapulohumeral disease. MD thesis. University of Leiden, Leiden, Germany.
41. Wijmenga, C., Padberg, G. W., Moerer, P., Wiegant, J., Liem, L., Brouwer, O. F., et al. (1991) Mapping of facioscapulohumeral muscular dystrophy gene 4q35-qter by multipoint linkage analysis and in situ hybridization. *Genomics* **9,** 570–575.
42. Wijmenga, C., Sandkuijl, L. A., Moerer, P., Van Der Boom, N., Bodbrug, S. E., Ray, P. N., et al. (1992) Genetic-linkage map of facioscapulohumeral muscular dystrophy and 5 polymorphic loci on chromosome 4q35-qter. *Am. J. Hum. Genet.* **51,** 411–415.
43. Wijmenga, C., Wright, T. J., Baan, M. I., Padberg, G. W., Williamson, R., Van Ommen, G. J. B., et al. (1993) Physical mapping and YAC cloning connects a genetically distinct 4qter loci (D45153, D45139, D4F35S, and D4F104S1) in the FSHD gene region. *Hum. Mol. Genet.* **2,** 1667–1672.
44. Passos-Bueno, M. R., Wijmenga, C., Takata, R. E., Marie, S .K. N., Vainzof, M., Pavanello, R. C., et al. (1993) No evidence of genetic heterogeneity in Brazilian facioscapulohumeral muscular dystrophy families (FSHD) with 4q markers. *Hum. Mol. Genet.* **2,** 557–562.
45. Zatz, M., Marie, S. K., Passos-Bueno, M. R., Vainzof, M., Campiotto, S., Cerqueira, A., et al. (1995) High proportion of new mutations and possible anticipation in Brazilian facioscapulohumeral muscular dystrophy families. *Am. J. Hum. Genet.* **56,** 99–105.
46. International SMA Consortium (1992) *Neuromusc. Disord.* **2,** 423–428.
47. Brzustowicz, L. M., Leshner, T., Castilla, L. H. , Penchaszadeh, G. K., Wilhelmsen, K. C., Daniels, R., et al. (1990) Gene mapping of chronic childhood-onset spinal muscular atrophy to chromosome 5q11.2-13.3. *Nature* **344,** 540–541.
48. Davies, K., Thomas, N.H., Daniels, R. J., and Dubowitz, V. (1991) Molecular studies of spinal muscular atrophy. *Neuromusc Disord.* **1,** 83–85.
49. Melki, J., Abdelhak, S., Sheth, P., Bachelot, M. F., Burlet, P., Marcadet, A., et al. (1990) Gene for chronic proximal spinal muscular atrophies maps to chromosome 5q. *Nature* **344,** 767–768.
50. Lefebvre, S., Bürglen, L., Reboullet, S., Clermon, O., Burlet, P., Viollet, L., et al. (1995) Identification and characterization of a spinal muscular atrophy-determining gene. *Cell* **80,** 155–165.

51. Roy, N., Mahadevan, M. S., Mclean, M., Shutler, G., Yaraghi, Z., Farahani, R., et al. (1995) The gene for neuronal apoptosis inhibitory protein is partially deleted in individuals with spinal muscular atrophy. *Cell,* **80,** 167–173.
52. Passos-Bueno, M. R., Rapaport, D., Love, D., Flint, T., Bortolini, E. R., Zatz, M., and Davies, K. (1990) Screening of deletions in the dystrophin gene with the cDNA probes Cf23a, Cf56a and Cf115. *J. Med. Genet.* **27,** 145–150.
53. Passos-Bueno, M. R., Lima, M. A. B. O., and Zatz, M. (1990) Estimate of germinal mosaicism in Duchenne muscular dystrophy. *J. Med. Genet.* **27,** 727–728.
54. Passos-Bueno, M. R., Bakker, E., Kneppers, A. L. J., Takata, R. I., Rapaport, D., den Dunnen, J. T., Zatz, M., and van Ommen, G. J. B. (1992) Mosaicism for Duchenne muscular dystrophy mutations: new recurrence risk estimates based on the deletion site in the gene. *Am. J. Human Genet.* **51,** 1150–1155.
55. Vainzof, M., Pavanello, R. C. M., Pavanello, I., Hoffman, E. P., Passos-Bueno, M. R., Rapaport, D., and Zatz, M. (1990) Dystrophin immunostaining in muscles from patients with different types of muscular dystrophy: a Brazilian study. *J. Neurol. Sci.* **98,** 221–233.
56. Vainzof, M., Pavanello, R. C. M., Pavanello, I., Rapaport, D., Passos-Bueno, M. R., Zubrzycka-Gaarn, E. E., Bulman, D., and Zatz, M. (1991) Screening of male patients with autosomal recessive Duchenne dystrophy through dystrophin and DNA studies. *Am J. Med. Genet.* **39,** 38–41.
57. Vainzof, M., Pavanello, R. C. M., Pavanello, I., Tsanaclis, A. M., Levy, J. A., Passos-Bueno, M. R., Rapaport, D., and Zatz M. (1991) Dystrophin Immunofluorescence pattern in manifesting and asymptomatic carriers of Duchenne's and Becker muscular dystrophy of different ages. *Neuromusc. Disord.* **1,** 177–183.
58. Vainzof, M., Zubrzycka-Gaarn, E. E., Rapaport, D., Passos-Bueno, M. R., Pavanello, R. C. M., Pavanello, I., and Zatz, M. (1991). Immunofluorescence dystrophin study in Duchenne dystrophy through the concomitant use of two antibodies directed against the carboxi-terminal and the amino-terminal region of the protein. *J. Neurol. Sci.* **101,** 141–147.
59. Vainzof, M., Passos-Bueno, M. R., Takata, R. I., Pavanello, R. C. M., and Zatz, M. (1993) Intrafamilial variability in dystrophin abundance correlated with difference in the severity of the phenotype. *J. Neurol. Sci.* **119,** 38.
60. Vainzof, M., Passos-Bueno, M. R., Pavanello RCM, Zatz, M. (1995) Is dystrophin always altered in Becker muscular dystrophy patients? *J. Neurol. Sci.* **131,** 99–104.

II

The Molecular Approach

A. Genetics: *X-Linked Muscular Dystrophy*

5

Deletion and Duplication Analysis in Males Affected with Duchenne or Becker Muscular Dystrophy

Ann Curtis and Daisy Haggerty

1. Introduction

Mutations in the gene that encodes the protein, dystrophin, underlie the allelic disorders, Duchenne and Becker muscular dystrophy (DMD/BMD). Although the complete spectrum of mutations has not been fully defined, the largest category of mutation is one of intragenic deletion *(1,2)*, and this dictates the molecular diagnostic strategies that are employed. Other important factors that influence the approaches adopted in the molecular analysis of both DMD and BMD are the large size of the gene and its X chromosomal location. The dystrophin gene comprises a total of 79 exons, extending over 2.4 Mb of DNA, and is the largest human gene characterized to date *(3,4)*. The exons are of average size, ranging between 30 and 300 bp *(4)*, as shown in **Fig. 1**, and are sparsely distributed, although some of those that code for particular protein domains are clustered. For example, exons 65–67, encoding the cysteine rich domain of the protein, are contained within 6 kb, and exons 68–74 lie within 14 kb, encoding the syntrophin-binding region *(5)*. However, it is the introns that make the greatest contribution to the overall size of the gene. For example, intron 44 is 270 kb, and brain intron 1 extends for 400 kb (the 5' end of the transcript has four alternative first exons, which are expressed in a tissue specific manner *[6]*).

1.1. Mutations in the Dystrophin Gene

Approximately 60–65% of the mutations that cause DMD are large deletions and 5–10% are duplications, each of which include one or more exons *(1,2)*. The majority of the remainder are point mutations (either nonsense or located at splice sites) or small rearrangements (reviewed in **ref.** *7,* and *see*

From: *Methods in Molecular Medicine, vol. 43: Muscular Dystrophy: Methods and Protocols*
Edited by: K. M. D. Bushby and L. V. B. Anderson © Humana Press Inc., Totowa, NJ

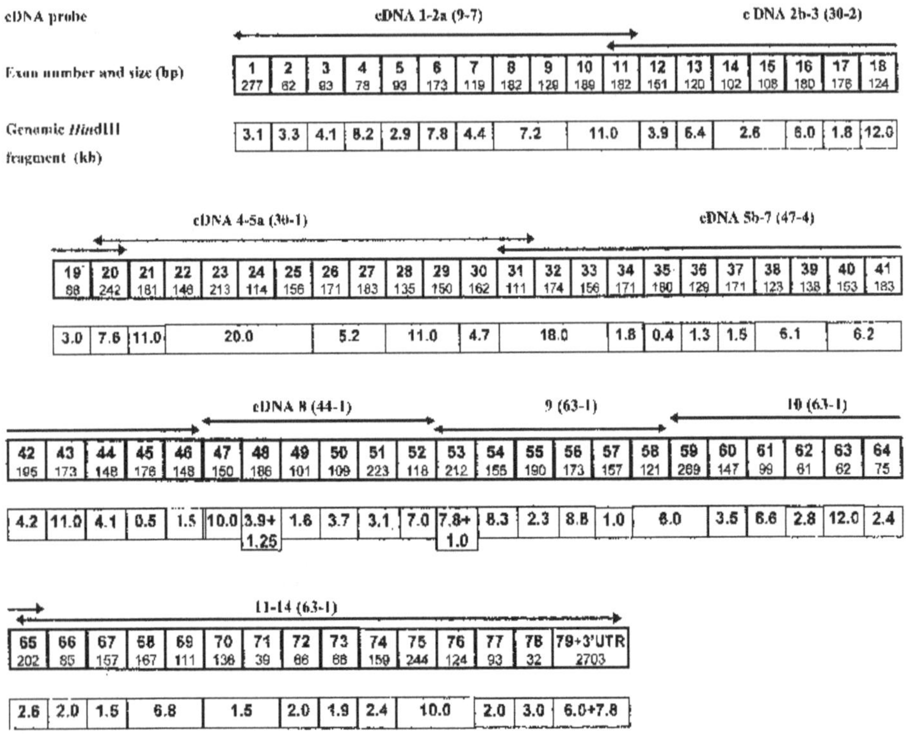

Fig. 1. Dystrophin gene exons and the corresponding nine cDNA probes. The genomic *Hind*III fragments detected by each cDNA probe are shown below each corresponding exon. Bolded exon boxes are those which are included in the multiplex PCR sets.

Chapter 6). In BMD, the proportion of mutations that are large deletions and duplications is higher (85%). The remainder are missense and splice-site mutations. In agreement with the relative severity of the two disorders, it is significant that almost all of the pathological mutations in DMD either shift the translational reading frame of the transcript or create a stop codon, both of which lead to premature truncation of the dystrophin protein during translation. In contrast, transcripts with mutations that cause BMD maintain an open reading frame, but are frequently internally deleted. A patient with BMD and an in-frame deletion of 46% of his dystrophin transcript has been described *(8)*; single-exon deletions are known to cause DMD, thus confirming the lack of correlation between phenotype and deletion size. Overall, in 92% of patients, the phenotype correlates with genotype and the frame shift hypothesis *(9)*.

1.2. Location of Deletions and Duplications in Dystrophin Gene

Both the size and distribution of deletions and duplications are variable, but are also clearly nonrandom. The same distribution has been demonstrated in many populations and ethnic groups. There are two commonly deleted regions involving exons 2–20 at the proximal end and exons 45–53 in the midportion of the gene, with the larger proportion of deletions located within the latter hot spot. The two hot spots may be explained by the observation that most deletion breakpoints occur in the large introns, 1, 7, and 44. The distribution of duplications differs from that of deletions, in that most locate to the 5' end of the gene, overlapping with the proximal deletion hot spot.

1.3. Detection of Deletions and Duplications

1.3.1. Purpose and Strategy

When samples are available from affected males, scanning for the presence of a deletion is generally the first step in the molecular analysis of both DMD and BMD families. Identification of a deletion as the disease-causative mutation will then allow subsequent, highly accurate, carrier detection and prenatal diagnosis to be carried out, if appropriate. In the case of BMD, the detection of a deletion in an isolated case will confirm the diagnosis of the condition, and thus exclude the recessively inherited forms of MD, with which there can be some diagnostic confusion. Scanning for duplications is less straightforward, and, also because of their reduced abundance, compared with deletions, are not generally tested for as part of the initial strategy. When DNA from an affected male is not available, it may be possible to detect the presence of a deletion using an indirect approach, which involves tracking the inheritance of intragenic polymorphic markers through female members of the family. Failure of a woman to inherit a maternal allele would indicate that she has a deletion at that locus. The limitations of this approach are that polymorphic markers are often uninformative and do not exist for all potentially deleted regions of the gene.

1.3.2. Laboratory Approaches

1.3.2.1. Multiplex PCR

Rapid and efficient scanning for deletions in males affected with DMD or BMD is performed using the multiplex polymerase chain reaction (PCR) method described by Chamberlain et al. ***(10)***, which was modified by Beggs et al. ***(11)***. A further modification is presented in this chapter. In four separate reactions, 36 exons, located in regions that are particularly prone to deletion, can be amplified to give products that are discriminated by size following an appropriate form of gel electrophoresis. Deleted exons are identified as missing bands, when compared with a nondeleted control after staining with ethidium bromide (EfBr) or silver (Ag). This simple approach has a detection rate of greater than 98% of all deletions. The four reaction mixes are designed to amplify specific clusters of exons, but each mix contains at least one primer pair that will amplify an exon that is located at a distance from the cluster. This acts as an important amplification control in the case of very large deletions that extend over the whole cluster.

The identification of duplications is technically more demanding by the multiplex PCR and conventional gel electrophoresis approach. The final judgement of a double dose of an exon is based on a comparison of the intensity of the relevant band with one that is known to be present in single dose only. To be able to judge this by eye, or by using a densitometer, it is necessary to optimize the PCR conditions with extreme precision.

More recently, with the development of automated DNA analysis, multiplex PCR, using fluorescently labeled primers, has become established as an efficient procedure for the detection of deletions and duplications ***(12)***. Once again, absolute precision in the PCR conditions is required. Following PCR, electrophoresis is performed, and the gel is automatically scanned. A series of peaks each corresponding to an amplification product, is generated, and the peak height is indicative of the amount of product present. A missing peak, therefore, indicates a deleted exon, and a peak of double height would suggest a duplicated exon. This form of analysis is particularly powerful in duplication detection.

1.3.2.2. cDNA Hybridization to Conventional Southern Blots

For the 2% of cases in whom a deletion is present, but is not detected by the multiplex PCR approach, Southern blot analysis is performed. For cost and time-effectiveness, it is best to batch samples that require this second level of deletion scanning. The digested and blotted DNA is sequentially hybridized with nine cDNA probes, which cover the complete 14-kb transcript (*see* **Fig. 1**). When the DNA is digested with *Hin*dIII or *Eco*R1, a single band on the blot approximates to a single exon, and thus deletions are again identified as missing bands when compared with a nondeleted control.

cDNA hybridization complements the multiplex PCR method in three other important areas. First, because a full complement of exon primers is not present in the PCR mixes, often the end points of a deletion are not established. Subsequent cDNA analysis is able to fully define the extent of a deletion. Second, this approach has the advantage of being able to detect novel fragments of altered size, which are generated at deletion junctions. Third, false-positive results, indicating the apparent deletion of a single exon, can arise as a result of the technical failure of a single pair of primers in one of the PCR mixes. Such a finding should always be confirmed by a second procedure, such as cDNA hybridization. Differences in the intensity of bands on Southern blots may indicate the presence of a duplication, but, to achieve this level of discrimination, the loading of DNA onto the gels must be extremely precise.

1.3.2.3. cDNA Hybridization to Pulsed Field Gel Electrophoresis Southern Blots

Because of the large size of both the dystrophin gene itself and the deletions that occur within it, pulse-field gel electrophoresis (PFGE) is also a powerful technique for deletion scanning. The principle of PFGE is that high-mol-wt DNA is digested with a rare-cutting restriction enzyme, such as *Sfi*1, to generate large DNA fragments of between 50 and 2000 kb. Standard Southern blotting and hybridization with the battery of cDNA probes is then carried out. Deletions are detected as bands of altered size compared to nondeleted controls. The technology involved is fairly specialized, and therefore is not applicable to all laboratories. However, the power of PFGE lies in its ability to detect dystrophin gene duplications in a qualitative manner, and to unambiguously identify carriers of either a deletion or a duplication caused by the separation of the normal and mutant allele by size.

1.3.2.4. Reverse Transcription-PCR of Dystrophin Gene Transcripts

Reverse transcription PCR (RT-PCR) of dystrophin mRNA has been developed for deletion and duplication scanning by specialized research laboratories, when amplification products of increased or decreased size, compared to controls, would suggest the presence of a deletion or duplication ***(13,14)***. However, this has not been adopted as a routine procedure because of the inconsistent yield of ectopic dystrophin gene transcripts from lymphocytes.

2. Materials

2.1. Deletion Screening by Multiplex PCR

1. *Taq* polymerase: The authors use *Taq* polymerase purchased from Promega (Madison, WI) at a concentration of 5 U/µL, which is stored at –20°C (*see* **Note 1**).
2. 10X PCR amplification buffer, containing 166 m*M* ammonium sulphate, 670 m*M* Tris-HCl, pH 8.8, 67 m*M* magnesium chloride (MgCl), 100 m*M* β-mercaptoethanol, 1.7 mg/mL bovine serum albumin (BSA), and 68 µ*M* ethylenediamine tetraacetic acid (EDTA). Store at –20°C.
3. Deoxynucleoside triphosphates (dNTPs): Prepare a working stock containing a mixture of deoxyadenosine triphosphate (dATP), deoxycytidine triphosphate (dCTP), deoxyguanosine triphosphate (dGTP), and (deoxythymidine triphosphate (dTTP), each at 5 m*M*, in sterile dH_2O. These can be purchased individually as 100 m*M* stocks from Boehringer Mannheim. Both 100 and 5 m*M* stocks should be stored at –20°C.

4. Oligonucleotide primers (sequences shown in **Table 1**): Prepare each of these at a concentration of 10 μ*M* in sterile dH_2O.
5. Sterile dH_2O.
6. Control DNA (*see* **Note 2**).
7. 10X sucrose loading buffer containing the following: 0.25% bromophenol blue, 0.25% xylene cyanole, 65% w/v sucrose, dissolved in dH_2O.
8. pBR322 digested with *Msp*1 (*see* **Note 3**), prepared at 0.5 μg/10 μL in 1X sucrose loading buffer.
9. EtBr solution prepared at 2.5 mg/mL in dH_2O (*see* **Note 4**).
10. (TAE) electrophoresis buffer: Dilute to 1X concentration from a 10X stock solution containing 48.4 g Tris base, 5.7 mL glacial acetic acid, and 10 mL 0.5 *M* EDTA, pH 8.0., per L.
11. 4.5% agarose gel prepared with three parts NuSieve GT agarose to 1 part SeaKem LE agarose (both supplied by Flowgen, Sittingbourne, UK), approximate dimensions 12 × 13 cm, prepared in 1X TAE electrophoresis buffer, and containing 5 μL of a solution of 10 mg/mL EtBr.

2.2. Quantitative PCR for Detection of Dystrophin Gene Duplications by Dosage Analysis

1. Amplitaq Gold *Taq* polymerase supplied by Applied Biosystems Division of Perkin-Elmer (Norwalk, CT) (*see* **Note 5**).
2. Items 2–8 detailed in **Subheading 2.1.** above.
3. 40% w/v Acrylogel solution (19:1 ratio of acylamide to *bis*-acrylamide) supplied by BDH (London).
4. 10% ammonium persulphate (APS): Prepare in dH_2O and store at –20°C in 1-mL aliquots. Once thawed, use within 48 h.
5. *N,N,N',N'*-Tetramethylethylenediamine (TEMED [Sigma]).
6. (TBE) electrophoresis buffer: Dilute to 0.6X concentration from a 10X stock solution containing 108 g Tris base, 55 g orthoboric acid, 40 mL 0.5*M* EDTA, pH 8.0., per L.
7. Midi Atto-type gel apparatus (GRI,) approximate dimensions 15 × 15 cm, gel thickness 0.75 mm. Glass plates should be cleaned with ethanol before assembling the cassette. Prepare 20 mL 5% nondenaturing acrylamide gel solution as follows: Mix 2.5 mL Acrylogel solution, 1.0 mL 10X TBE, 0.3 mL 10% APS, 15 μL TEMED, and dH_2O to a volume of 20 mL. Pour into the gel cassette and allow to polymerize overnight covered with Clingfilm.
8. Ag staining solution 1 (fixer): 10% ethanol, 0.5% acetic acid, prepared in dH_2O.
9. Ag staining solution 2 (stain): 0.1% silver nitrate, dissolved in dH_2O.
10. Ag staining solution 3 (developer): 1.5% sodium hydroxide (NaOH), 1.5% formaldehyde, freshly prepared before use in dH_2O.
11. Ag staining solution 4 (neutralizer): 0.75% Na carbonate in dH_2O.
12. Hot air gel drier (Bio-Rad, Hercules, CA).
13. Cellophane sheets for drying gels (Bio-Rad).

2.3. Fluorescent PCR for Detection of Deletions and Duplications

1. Genomic DNA from a normal control male and test samples (*see* **Note 2**).
2. 26 pairs of oligonucleotide primers in two multiplex sets (*see* **Note 6** and **Tables 1** and **2**). The forward primer of each pair should be labeled with the fluorescent dye phosphoramadite 6-FAM (Applied Biosystems Division of Perkin-Elmer, ABI) (*see* **Note 7**). Primer stocks should be stored at –20°C. Prepare 10 m*M* working solutions of each primer in dH_2O, and store at 4°C.
3. 10X PCR amplification buffer (*see* **Subheading 2.1., item 2**).
4. 5 m*M* dNTPs (*see* **Subheading 2.1., item 3**).
5. *Taq* polymerase (Amplitaq Gold supplied by ABI) (*see* **Note 5**).
6. 0.2 mL thin-walled PCR tubes.
7. Size standard 1: Genescan-500 ROX (ABI).
8. Size standard 2 (*see* **Note 8**): Prepare a 547 bp PCR fragment of exon 45 using a ROX-labeled forward primer (5' AAA CAT GGA ACA TCC TTG TGG GGA C 3') with the exon 45 reverse primer shown in **Table 1**. PCR should be performed under the same conditions as described in **Subheading 3.1.1.**
9. Formamide loading buffer: 95% formamide in 1X TBE (*see* **Subheading 2.2., item 6**) with 5 mg/mL dextran blue.
10. ABI 377 automated DNA sequencer.
11. 1X TBE (*see* **Subheading 2.2., item 6**).
12. 5% denaturing polyacrylamide gel (PAG) prepared in 1X TBE for use in the ABI automated sequencer.
13. Excel software (Microsoft).

2.4. Southern Blot Analysis in the Detection of Dystrophin Gene Deletions and Duplications

2.4.1. Restriction Enzyme Digestion

1. *Hin*dIII restriction endonuclease. Most manufacturers supply restriction enzymes at a concentration of 10 U/µL, and require that they are stored at –20°C. Always incubate on ice when the stock is removed from the freezer for use at the bench.
2. 10X *Hin*dIII digestion buffer. This is supplied by most enzyme manufacturers, optimized for use with the particular batch of enzyme.
3. 10X sucrose loading buffer prepared as in **Subheading 2.1., item 7**.
4. Spermidine (Sigma) prepared at a concentration of 10 mg/mL in sterile dH_2O. Store in aliquots at –20°C.
5. 0.8% agarose gel (SeaKem LE), approximate dimensions 12 × 13 cm, prepared in 1X TAE electrophoresis buffer (*see* **Subheading 2.1., item 10**), and containing 5 µL of a solution of 2.5 mg/mL EtBr (*see* **Subheading 2.1., item 9**).
6. Horizontal electrophoresis tank appropriate for the prepared gel.

2.4.2. Electrophoresis and Southern Transfer

1. 20 × 20 cm 0.8% agarose (SeaKem LE) transfer gel. Thoroughly dissolve 1.6 g agarose in 200 mL 1X TAE buffer (*see* **Subheading 2.1., item 10**) by boiling in

Table 1
Sequences of Primers Used for Amplification of Dystrophin Gene Exons in Multiplex PCR

Exon no.	Fragment size (bp)	Forward primer	Reverse primer	Ref.
Pm + 1	535	gaa gat cta gac agt gga tac ata aca aat gca tg	ttc tcc gaa ggt aat tgc ctc cca gat ctg agt cc	*11,15*
2	174	aga tga aag aga aga tgt tca aaa g	aat gac act atg aga gaa ata aaa cgg	*20*
3	410	tca tcc atc atc ttc ggc aga tta a	cag gcg gta gag tat gcc aaa tga aaa tca	*11,15*
4	196	ttg tcg gtc tcc tgc tgg tca gtg	caa agc cct cac tca aac atg aag c	*10,15*
5	93	gtt gat tta gtg aat att gga agt ac	ctg cca gtg gag gat tat att cca aa	*20*
	202	cca cat gta gGT CAA AAA TGT AAT GAA	gtc tca gta atc ttc tta cCT ATG ACT ATG G	*11,15*
7	111	tat ttg act gga gtg tgg ttt gc	ctt cag gat cga ata gtt tct cta	*20*
8	360	ggc ctc att ctc atg ttc taa tta g	gtc ctt tac aca ctt tac CTG TTG AG	*10,15*
9	125	atc acg gtc agt cta gca ca	tga agg aaa tgg gct ccg tgt a	*1*
12	331	gat agt ggg ctt tac tta cat cct tc	gaa agc acg caa cat aag ata cac ct	*10*
13	238	aat agg agt acc tga gat gta gca gaa at	ctg acC TTA AGT TGT TCT TCC AAA GCAG	*11,15*
17	416	gac ttt cga tgt tga gat tac ttt ccc	aag ctt gag atg ctc tca cCT TTT CC	*10*
19	459	ttc tac cac atc cca ttt tct tcc a	gat ggc aaa agt gtt gag aaa aag tc	*10,15*
20	239	gtg tta atg cag ata gca tca aac	aca aat ttt taa ctg act ttt aat tg	*18*
21	178	gat gaa gtcaac cgg cta tc	gtc tgt agc tct ttc tct c	*19*
22	140	ttg aca ctt tgc cac caa tgc gct atc	caa ttc ccc gag tct ctg ctc cat g	*18*
34	100	gaa att gtc ccg taa gat gcg	agg cat tcc ttc aac tgc tg	*19*
37	314	ctt tct cac tct tct cgc tca c	ttc gca aga gac cat tta gca c	*22*
42	155	CAC ACT GTC CGT GAA GAA ACG ATG ATG	TTA GCA CAG AGG TCA GGA GCA TTG AG	*15*
43	357	gaa cat gtc aaa gtc act gga ctt cat gg	ata tat gtg tta cct acC CTT GTC GGT CC	*11,15*

44	426	gtt gtg tgt aca tgc tag gtg tgt a	tcc atc acc ctt cag aac ctg atc t	***15***
45	307	ctt tct ttg cca gta caa ctg cat gtg	cat tcc tat tag atc tgt cgc cct ac	***15***
46	148	GCT AGA AGA ACA AAA GAAC TAT CTT GTC	CTT GAC TTG CTC AAG CTT TTC TTT TAG	***10***
47	181	cgt tgt tgc att tgt ctg ttt cag TTA C	gtc taa cCT TTA TCC ACT GGA GAT TTG	***11,15***
48	506	ttg aat aca ttg gtt aaa tcc caa cat g	cct gaa taa agt ctt cct tac cac ac	***10***
49	439	gtg ccc tta tgt acc agg cag aaa ttg	gca atg act cgt taa tag cct taa gat c	***11***
50	271	cac caa atg gat taa gat gtt cat gaa t	tct ctc tca ccc agt cat cac ttc ata g	***11,15***
51	388	gaa att ggc tct tta gct tgt gtt tc	gga gag taa agt gat tgg tgg aaa atc	***10,15***
52	113	AAT GCA GGA TTT GGA ACA GAG GCG TCC	TTC GAT CCG TAA TGA TTG TTC TAG CCT C	***11,15***
53	212	TTG AAA GAA TTC AGA ATC AGT GGG ATG	CTT GGT TTC TGT GAT TTT CTT TTG GAT TG	***15***
54	450	gtt tgt cct gaa agg tgg gtt ac	tta tcg tct tga acc ctc cca ag	***1***
55	119	ggc tgc ttt gga aga aac tc	tta cgg gta gca tcc tgt agg a	***19***
60	139	AGG AGA AAT TGC GCC TCT GAA AGA GAA CG	CTG CAG AAG CTT CCA TCT GGT GTT CAG G	***11,15***
62	191	gtc ttt cct gtt tgc gat gaa ttt gac c	ctc act tgt gaa tat aca ggt tag tca c	***12***
65	347	tat gag aga gtc cta gct agg	taa gcc tcc tgt gac aga gc	***22***
66	70	cag gga gga tcc gtg tcc tg	gtc ttc caa atg tgc ttt ac	***21***

Lower case-letters represent intronic sequences and upper-case letters represent exonic sequences. PCR is performed in four multiplex reactions, each with nine pairs of primers, as detailed in Table 3.

Table 2
Sequences of 5'F set of Primers Used in Fluorescence Multiplex PCR

Exon no.	Fragment size (bp)	Forward primer	Reverse primer
Pm + 1	535	tag aca gtg gat aca taa caa atg cat g	As in **Table 1**
2	253	taa ttt gga tgc ccc aaa cca gct	gta aca aac cat tct tac ctt aga
3	410	As in **Table 1**	As in **Table 1**
4	196	As in **Table 1**	cca ttc atc agg att ctt acc tgc c
5	167	As in **Table 1**	ctg cca gtg gag gat tat att cca aa
6	202	As in **Table 1**	As in **Table 1**
8	360	gtc ctt tac aca ctt tac ctg ttg ag	ggc ctc att ctc atg ttc taa tta g
9	278	tct atc cac tcc cga acc tct ctg cag	aac aaa cca gct ctt cac gag gag a
13	238	As in **Table 1**	As in **Table 1**
17	326	gct att ttg atc tga agg tca atc tac c	as in **Table 1**
19	459	As in **Table 1**	As in **Table 1**
30	175	agg ctg taa gga ggc aaa agt tgc	gat gta ctt gcc tgg gct tcc tga ggc

Sequences of the 3'F set of primers used in fluorescence multiplex (exons 42, 43, 44, 45, 46, 47, 48, 49, 50, 51, 52, 53, 60, and 62) PCR are identical to those presented in **Table 1**.

a microwave. Replace evaporated liquid with dH_2O and allow to cool to approx 60°C. Pour the agarose into the gel plate, insert a comb with 14–15 wells, and allow to set.

2. Horizontal electrophoresis tank appropriate for the prepared gel.
3. λ DNA digested with *Hin*dIII prepared at 1 μg/30 μL in 1X sucrose loading buffer (*see* **Subheading 2.1., item 7**), to act as a mol-wt marker (*see* **Note 9**).
4. 10 mg/mL EtBr solution (*see* **Subheading 2.1., item 9**).
5. Plastic trays suitable for immersing and agitating a 20 × 20 cm gel in approx 500 mL buffer solution.
6. Denaturing solution: 0.5 *M* NaOH, 1.5 *M* NaCl, in dH_2O. Store at room temperature (RT).
7. Neutralizing solution: 0.4 *M* Tris-base, 0.25 *M* trisodium citrate, pH 5.5, prepared in dH_2O. Store at RT.
8. 20X standard sodium citrate (SSC): 3 *M* sodium chloride, 0.3 *M* trisodium citrate, prepared in dH_2O, and stored at RT.
9. 10X SSC diluted from a 20X SSC stock (*see* **item 8** above).
10. 2X SSC diluted from a 20X SSC stock (*see* **item 8** above).
11. Rectangular glass plate slightly larger than the transfer gel (20 × 20 cm) which will suspend on top of a tray (*see* **item 5** above and **Fig 2**), leaving a gap on either side.
12. 17 Chroma paper (Whatman).
13. 20 × 20 cm sheets of 3MM paper (Whatman).
14. Nylon nucleic acid blotting membrane, such as Hybond N^+ (Amersham Pharmacia Biotech).
15. Absorbent paper towels.
16. 0.4 *M* NaOH solution prepared in dH_2O and stored at RT.

2.4.3. Labeling and Hybridization of Radiolabeled cDNA Probes to Southern Filters

1. Hybridization bottles suitable for use in a rotisserie style hybridization oven, or good quality thick polythene, which can be securely sealed to contain a radioactive 20 × 20 cm blotting membrane.
2. 2X SSC diluted from a 20X SSC stock (*see* **Subheading 2.4.2., item 8**).
3. 50X Denhardt's solution: 0.5% Ficoll, 0.5% polyvinylpyrrolidone, 0.5% BSA fraction V (all reagents from Sigma). Prepare in dH_2O, filter sterilize, and store at –20°C.
4. Denatured salmon sperm DNA: Prepare a solution of salmon sperm DNA (Sigma) at 10 mg/mL in dH_2O. Autoclave to denature. Store in 5-mL aliquots at –20°C.
5. Hybridization solution: Prepare sufficient solution for 10 hybridizations by mixing 40 mL 20X SSC (*see* **Subheading 2.4.2., item 8**), 20 mL 50X Denhardt's solution, 20 g dextran sulphate (Amersham Pharmacia Biotech), 2.5 mL 10% Na pyrophosphate solution, 18.8 mL 10% sodium dodecyl sulfate (SDS) solution, and 2.5 mL 10 mg/mL denatured salmon sperm DNA. Make up to 200 mL in distilled water, filter-sterilize, and store in 20 mL aliquots at –20°C.
6. cDNA probes (*see* **Table 5** and **Fig. 1**) at 10–100 ng/μL.

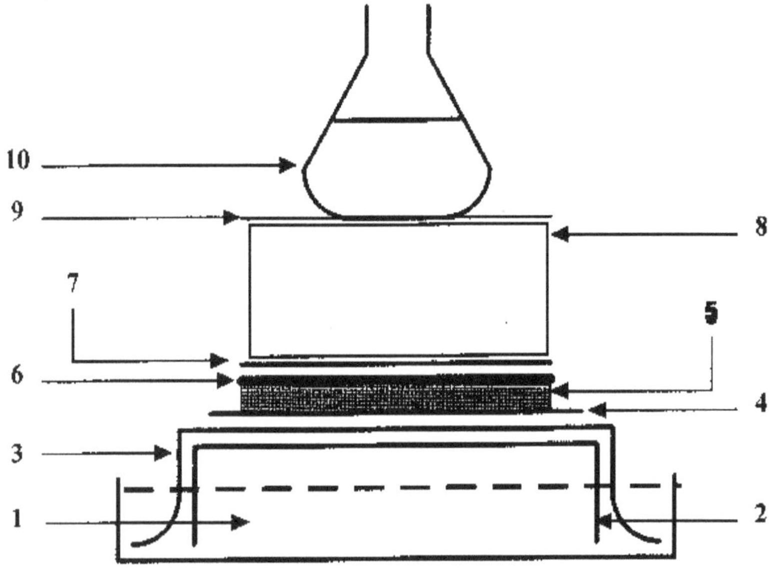

Fig. 2. Preparation of Southern blotting tray. 1. Tray containing 20X SSC. 2. Suspended glass plate or tray. 3. Wick of 17 Chroma paper. 4. Two sheets 3MM paper. 5. Agarose gel. 6. Nylon membrane. 7. Two sheets 3MM paper. 8. Stack of paper towels. 9. Glass plate. 10. Weight, such as flask containing 500 mL water.

7. 10X labeling buffer: 500 m*M* Tris-HCl, pH 8.0, 50 m*M* MgCl, 0.2 m*M* dATP, 0.2 m*M* dGTP, 0.2 m*M* dTTP, 100 m*M* 2-mercaptoethanol, 100 µg/mL BSA. Prepare in sterile distilled water, and store in aliquots at –20°C.
8. Random hexanucleotides (pd $[N]_6$, Amersham Pharmacia Biotech) adjusted to 90 optical density units with sterile dH_2O. Store in aliquots at –20°C.
9. [α-^{32}P]dCTP at 10 µCi/µL.
10. Klenow fragment of DNA polymerase (NBL Gene Sciences,).
11. Glass fiber disks: GF/B 21 mm (Whatman).
12. 5% solution of trichloroacetic acid (TCA).
13. Tris-EDTA (TE) buffer: 10 m*M* Tris-HCl pH 7.5, 1 m*M* EDTA, pH 8.0. Autoclave, and store at 4°C.
14. Nick columns (Amersham Pharmacia Biotech).
15. 1.5-mL microcentrifuge tubes with screw caps.
16. Radioactively labeled λ DNA (*see* **Note 10**).
17. Wash solution 1: 1X SSC diluted form 20X stock (*see* **Subheading 2.4.2., item 8**), 0.1% SDS, 0.1% Na_2HPO_4.
18. Wash solution 2: 0.5X SSC, 0.1% SDS, 0.1% Na_2HPO_4.
19. Further wash solutions, as required, containing decreasing concentrations of SSC (0.25X, 0.1X) and 0.1% SDS, 0.1% Na_2HPO_4.
20. X-ray film such as Kodak X-OMAT AR (Sigma).

3. Methods

3.1. Deletion Screening by Multiplex PCR

The dystrophin gene can be screened for the presence of deletions in an affected male in a total of four amplification reactions, each containing primers for nine exons (*see* **Note 11**). The combinations of primers that have been optimized for use in the same reaction are shown in **Table 3** (*see* **Note 12**).

3.1.1. Multiplex PCR and Electrophoresis

1. In a 1.5-mL microcentrifuge tube, cooled on ice, prepare a master mix of the components of the amplification reaction (*see* **Note 13**). For each DNA sample to be amplified (*see* **Note 2**), mix the following: 5 µL 10X PCR amplification buffer, 5 µL 5 m*M* dNTPs, 2 µL each forward primer at 10 µ*M* (up to 10 per reaction), 2 µL each reverse primer at 10 µ*M* (up to 10 per reaction), 1 µL *Taq* polymerase (0.5 U per primer set), and water, to allow a total reaction volume of 49 µL per sample.
2. Aliquot 49 µL master reaction mix into thin-walled, 0.5-mL PCR tubes. Add 100–250 ng DNA to each tube in a volume of 1 µL. Substitute with 1 µL sterile dH_2O in a no-DNA control tube. Mix well by flicking the base of the tube.
3. With some thermal cycling machines, it is necessary to overlay with one drop of light mineral oil to prevent evaporation.
4. Perform the PCR under the following cycling conditions: one cycle of 94°C for 5 min; 30 cycles of 94°C for 1 min, 59°C for 1 min, 72°C for 2 min; one cycle of 72°C for 10 min.
5. Electrophorese 30 µL each PCR product in 1X sucrose loading buffer (*see* **Note 14**) through a 4.5% 3:1 agarose gel, together with a suitable mol-wt marker, such as pBR322 digested with *Msp*1 (*see* **Note 3**), at 10 V/cm for 2 h.
6. View the bands under UV illumination, and photograph.

3.1.2. Interpretation of Multiplex PCR Gels

Deletions are observed as missing bands in the patient sample lanes, compared with the positive control lane (*see* **Note 15**). Examples are shown in **Fig. 3**.

3.2. Quantitative PCR for Detection of Dystrophin Gene Duplications by Dosage Analysis

This is a variation of the multiplex PCR protocol described by Abbs and Bobrow ***(15)***.

3.2.1. Multiplex PCR and electrophoresis

1. Prepare the amplification reactions as described for multiplex deletion screening in **Subheading 3.1.1., steps 1–3**, using Amplitaq Gold *Taq* polymerase in

Table 3
Combinations of Exons Included in Each of Four Multiplex Amplification Reactions, 5'M, BM, DM, and 3'M.

5'M (5' exons)		DM		BM		3'M (3' exons)	
Exon no.	PCR fragment size (bp)	Exon no.	PCR fragment size (bp)	Exon no.	PCR fragment size (bp)	Exon no.	PCR fragment size (bp)
Prm + 1	535	19	459	48	506	49	439
54	450	17	416	44	426	51	388
3	410	37	314	43	357	65	347
8	360	53	212	45	307	50	271
12	331	21	178	20	239	13	238
4	196	22	140	6	202	62	191
2	174	7	111	47	181	60	139
46	148	5	93	42	155	55	119
9	125	66	70	52	113	34	100

The exons are listed in order of decreasing PCR fragment size, as they appear on the gel from top to bottom.

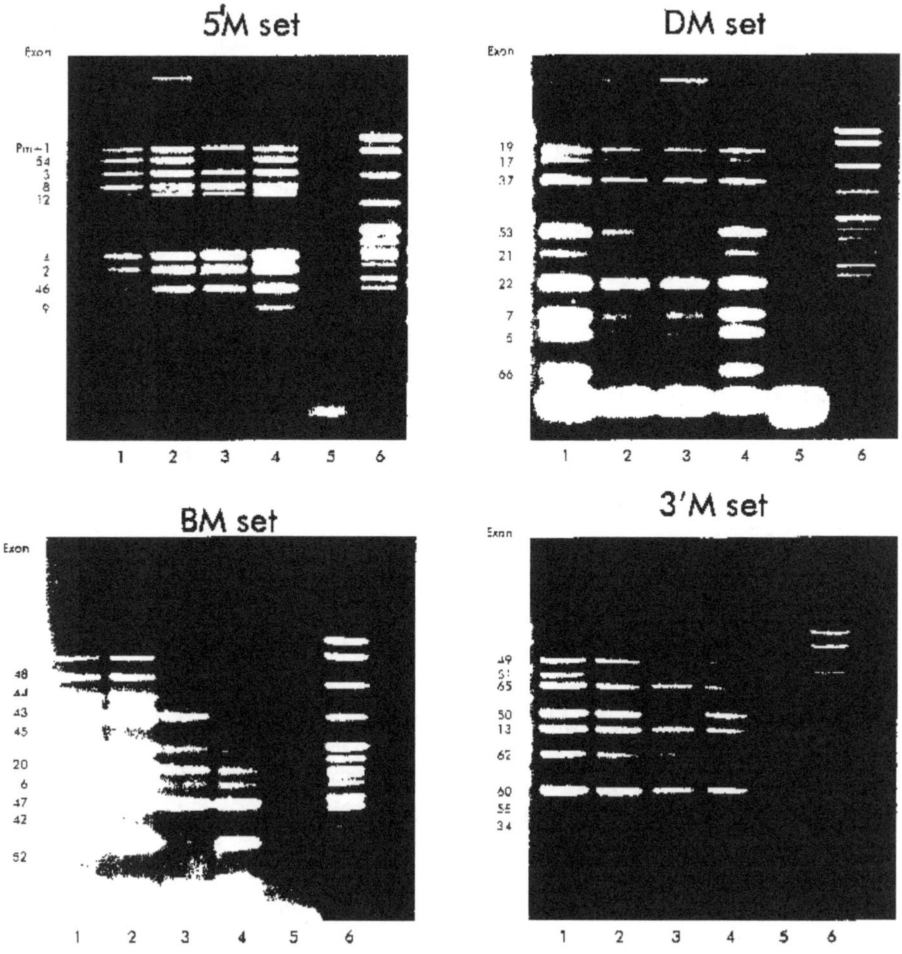

Fig. 3. Electrophoresis of the PCR products from the four multiplex reactions, each containing 9 pairs of primers. The amplified exons are listed on the left of each photograph against the corresponding PCR product. In all four gels, lanes 1 and 4 represent normal male controls, lane 5 is a no-DNA control and lane 6 is the molecular weight ladder, pBR322 digested with *Msp*1. Lane 2 in each set contains amplification products from a patient with a single deletion (exon 51 in the 3'M set). Lane 3 in each set is the result of the analysis of a patient with a deletion of exons 48 to 54. Deleted bands are evident in all four reactions. The normal male sample in lane 6 of the BM set illustrates a problem which can arise due to degradation of the DNA sample or degradation of the primer sets with age, where the high molecular weight fragments, representing exons 43, 44, 45, and 48 have not amplified efficiently.

step 1 (*see* **Note 5**) and 150–200 ng sample DNA per tube in **step 2** (*see* **Notes 2** and **16**).

2. Perform the PCR under the same conditions as described in **Subheading 3.1.1., step 4**, but reduce the number of cycles to 21 (*see* **Note 16**).
3. Separate 10 µL of the PCR products in 1X sucrose loading buffer on a 6% neutral PAG (*see* **Note 17**).
4. Electrophorese at 1 mA/cm for 2 h, until the bromophenol blue tracking dye reaches the bottom of the gel. Use 0.5X TBE as the electrophoresis buffer.
5. Dismantle the apparatus, leaving the gel adhered to one of the plates (*see* **Note 18**), and stain as follows:
6. Pour 500 mL Ag stain solution 1 (fixer) on to gel, and agitate gently for 5 min (*see* **Note 19**). Pour away the fixing solution. Cover with 500 mL Ag stain solution 2 (stain), and agitate gently for 15 min. Pour off solution 2 (*see* **Note 20**), and rinse the gels briefly in dH_2O. Cover with 500 mL Ag stain solution 3 (developer), and agitate gently for 20–30 min, during which time the bands will appear. Discard solution 3, and replace with 500 mL Ag stain solution 4 (neutralizer). Shake gently for 10 min.
7. Discard solution 4, and cover the gel with dH_2O. It can be photographed to obtain a permanent record.
8. If possible, the gel should be dried between cellophane sheets, using a hot air gel drier, because interpretation is simpler if reference can be made to the original gel.

3.2.2. Interpretation of Multiplex PCR Dosage Gels

1. Duplications are recognized as intensity differences of the bands, compared both with other bands in the same lane and with bands in the control lane. An example is shown in **Fig. 4**.
2. The human eye is very sensitive to recognizing intensity differences between bands. However, this can be achieved in a more quantitative manner by densitometric scanning of each lane.

   The following comparison should be made:

   Patient sample band A/ : Control sample band A/
   Patient sample band B   Control sample band B

   If this gives a ratio of 1:1, then neither band is duplicated in the patient. A ratio of 2:1 suggests that band A is duplicated, and a ratio of 1:2 suggests that band B is duplicated. In the first instance, band B should represent the control exon from another part of the gene. Single exon duplications should be confirmed by a second procedure (*see* **Note 15**).

3.3. Fluorescent Multiplex PCR for Detection of Deletions and Duplications

This protocol is based on that described by Yau et al. *(12)*, using two multiplex sets of primers, referred to as the 5'F and 3'F sets (*see* **Note 6**).

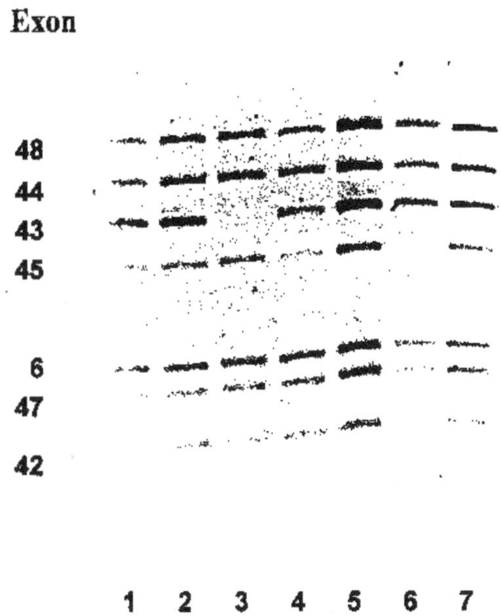

Fig. 4. Multiplex PCR was performed under optimized conditions to demonstrate the detection of duplications by dosage analysis. All lanes contain male samples. Lanes 4, 5, and 7 are nonduplicated contols. Lanes 3 and 6 contain samples from patients with single deletions of exons 43 and 45 respectively. A comparison of band intensities, both within a lane and between lanes, allows identification of a duplication of exon 43 in lane 1 and of exons 42 and 43 in lane 2.

3.3.1. Multiplex PCR and Electrophoresis

1. Dilute genomic DNA 1:1–1:9 with sterile dH_2O, and heat at 55°C for 2 h, or at 37°C overnight, on a rotary mixer. Use an aliquot of this to obtain concentration readings, and use the rest to dilute to a working concentration of 25 ng/µL.
2. In a 1.5-mL microcentrifuge tube, cooled on ice, prepare a master mix of the components of the amplification reaction (*see* **Note 13**). For each DNA sample to be amplified (*see* **Note 2**), mix the following: 2.5 µL 10X PCR amplification buffer, 2.5 µL 5 m*M* dNTPs, 0.5 µL each forward primer at 10 µ*M* (either 5'F or 3'F multiplex reaction), 0.5 µL each reverse primer at 10 µ*M* (either 5'F or 3'F multiplex reaction), 1.5 U Amplitaq Gold *Taq* polymerase, and water, to allow a total reaction volume of 20 µL per sample.
3. Aliquot 20 µL master reaction mix into thin walled PCR tubes, and mix well with 5 µL diluted sample DNA. Substitute the DNA with 5 µL sterile dH_2O in a no-DNA control tube. If necessary, overlay the reaction mix with oil. This will depend on the thermal cycler that is to be used.
4. Initial denaturation is performed at 96°C for 10 min, during which time sufficient *Taq* polymerase is activated to initiate the PCR (*see* **Note 5**). This is followed by

18 cycles of denaturation for 48 s at 95°C, 48 s annealing at 61°C (5' assay), or 58°C (3' assay), and extension for 3 min at 70°C, with a final extension for 7 min at 70°C, and finally a holding temperature of 4°C.

5. Mix a 3-µL aliquot of the PCR product with 0.5 µL of each size standard (547-bp fragment of exon 45 and Genescan-500 ROX standard). Add an equal volume of formamide loading buffer, and mix well.
6. Denature the mixture for 7 min at 96°C, and electrophorese using an ABI 377 automated sequencer through a 5% denaturing PAG, at a constant 30 W for 4 h.

3.3.2. Interpretation of Fluorescent Multiplex PCR Data

1. The data are analyzed automatically using the Model 672 Genescan and Genotyper Analysis Software (ABI). An electrophoretogram is produced for each sample, with peaks showing the size of each amplification product present (*see* **Fig. 5A,B**). The areas under the peaks represent the amount of fluorescence signal incorporated into each of the products (*see* **Note 21**).
2. Deletions are observed as missing peaks in the trace from the patient sample, when compared with the positive control sample (*see* **Note 15**). An example is shown in **Fig. 5A**.
3. In order to determine the dosage of every exon amplified in the multiplex reaction, the peak areas from the test sample are compared against each other and against those from the nondeleted, nonduplicated, control ***(12)***. This generates a series of dosage quotients (DQ), which can be calculated as follows:

   $$DQ = \frac{\text{peak area exon A in test sample/peak area exon B in test sample}}{\text{peak area exon A in control sample/peak area exon B in control sample}}$$

   This is most simply done by transferring the peak area data from the Genotyper program into an Excel (Microsoft) spreadsheet to produce a gridded array, on which the DQ values for each pair of exon peak areas is recorded, as shown in **Table 4**.
4. When an exon is present in single copy in a male sample, the theoretical DQ value is 1.0. The theoretical DQ value for a duplication in a male sample is 0.5 or 2.0, depending on whether the duplicated peak area is the denominator or the numerator in the above equation. An example of a gridded array of DQ values demonstrating a duplication is shown in **Table 4**. The corresponding electrophoretogram is in **Fig. 5B**.

Fig. 5. *(opposite page)* **(A)** Electrophoretogram of deletion analysis by fluorescent multiplex PCR using the 5' set of pimers. The upper trace shows a non-deleted control patient and the lower trace is that of a patient with a deletion of exons 13, 17, 19, and 30. **(B)** Electrophoretogram of duplication analysis by fluorescent multiplex PCR using the 3' set of pimers. The upper trace shows a non-duplicated control patient and the lower trace is that of a patient with a duplication of of exon 43. The corresponding DQ values are shown in **Table 4**.

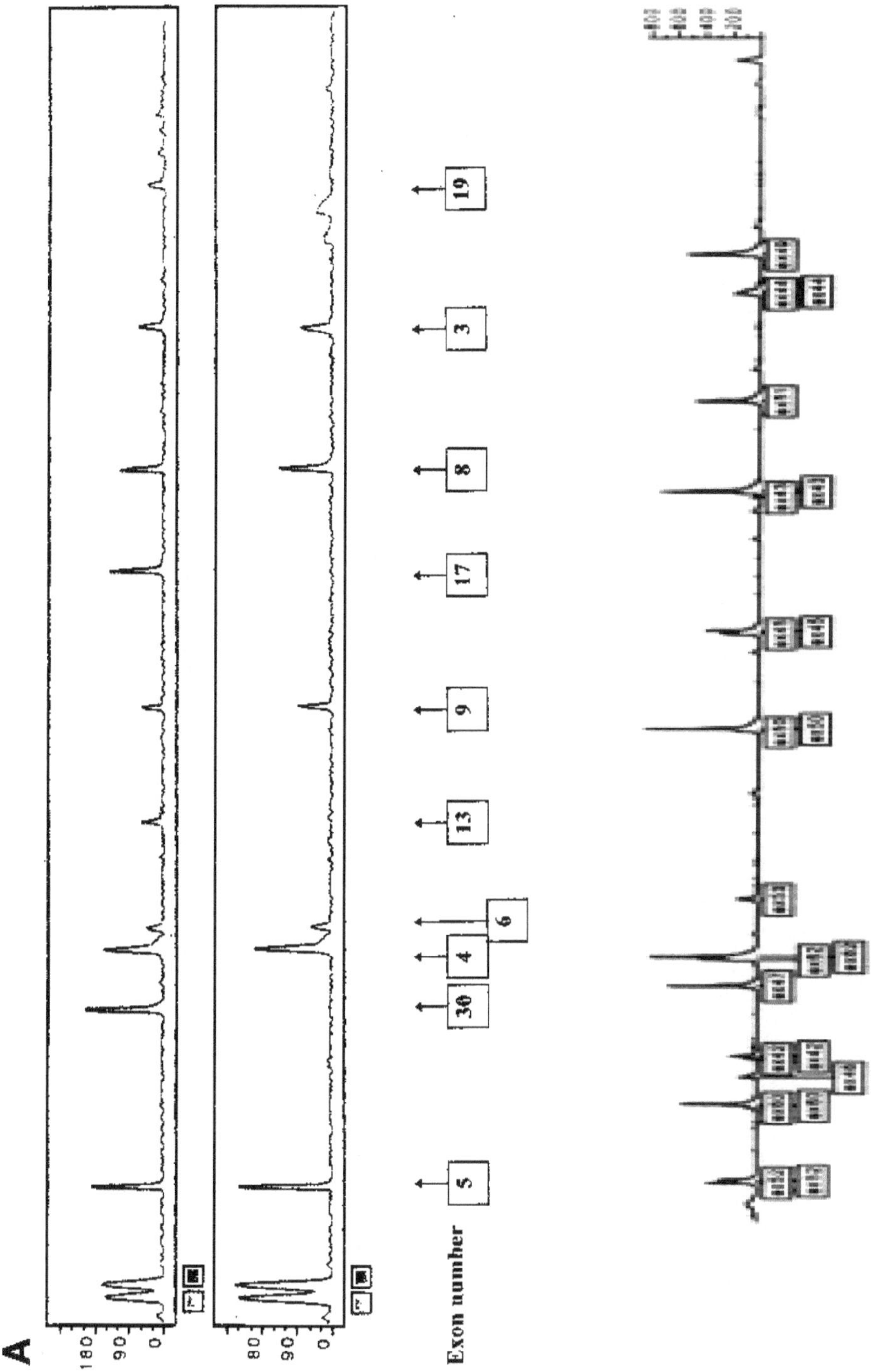
A
180
90
0
80
90
0
Exon number
5
30
4
6
13
9
17
8
3
19

Table 4
Gridded Array of Dosage Quotient (DQ) Values Compiled on Microsoft Excel SpreadSheet for Fluorescent Multiplex PCR Using 3'F Set of Primers.

	Peak area		Exon												
Exon	Control	Sample	42	43	44	45	46	47	49	50	51	52	53	60	62
42	642	2040	1.00	0.60	1.04	1.01	1.36	0.98	0.98	0.89	1.02	1.11	1.03	1.15	0.95
43	1733	9186	1.67	1.00	1.75	1.69	2.26	1.63	1.63	1.48	1.69	1.85	1.72	1.92	1.59
44	1192	3646	0.96	0.58	1.00	0.98	1.31	0.94	0.94	0.86	0.98	1.07	0.99	1.11	0.92
45	1949	6102	0.99	0.59	1.02	1.00	1.34	0.96	0.96	0.88	1.00	1.09	1.02	1.14	0.94
46	482	1129	0.74	0.44	0.77	0.75	1.00	0.72	0.72	0.66	0.75	0.82	0.76	0.85	0.70
47	1693	5507	1.02	0.61	1.06	1.04	1.39	1.00	1.00	0.91	1.04	1.14	1.06	1.18	0.98
49	2463	7998	1.02	0.61	1.06	1.04	1.39	1.00	1.00	0.91	1.04	1.14	1.05	1.18	0.98
50	2747	9819	1.12	0.67	1.17	1.14	1.53	1.10	1.10	1.00	1.14	1.25	1.16	1.30	1.07
51	1778	5566	0.99	0.59	1.02	1.00	1.34	0.96	0.96	0.88	1.00	1.09	1.02	1.14	0.94
52	1567	4482	0.90	0.54	0.94	0.91	1.22	0.88	0.88	0.80	0.91	1.00	0.93	1.04	0.86
53	533	1641	0.97	0.58	1.01	0.98	1.31	0.95	0.95	0.86	0.98	1.08	1.00	1.12	0.92
60	1766	4867	0.87	0.52	0.90	0.88	1.18	0.85	0.85	0.77	0.88	0.96	0.90	1.00	0.83
62	3283	10931	1.05	0.63	1.09	1.06	1.42	1.02	1.03	0.93	1.06	1.16	1.08	1.21	1.00

The corresponding electrophoretogram is shown in Fig. 7B. A duplication of exon 43 is evident as the DQ values approximate to 0.5 and 2.0, from the expected value of 1.0. Note that exon 48 failed to amplify.

3.4. Southern Blot Analysis in Detection of Dystrophin Gene Deletions and Duplications

3.4.1. Restriction Enzyme Digestion

The restriction Endonucleases *Hin*dIII, *EcoR*1, *Pst*1, and *Bgl*II cut within the introns of the dystrophin gene, but not within the majority of exons. Following digestion with any of these enzymes, therefore, the majority of exons are contained within a single DNA fragment. The sizes of the fragments generated following digestion with *Hin*dIII have been fully characterized, and are shown in **Fig. 1** and **Table 5**.

1. In 1.5-mL microcentrifuge tubes, prepare restriction endonuclease digested DNA samples as follows: 10–12 µg genomic DNA, 40–50 U *Hin*dIII, 4 µL 10X *Hin*dIII digestion buffer, sterile dH_2O, to give a total volume of 40 µL. Incubate at 37°C for 16 h, or overnight.
2. Check that the digestion is complete by taking 4 µL from the digest mix. Add 1 µL 10X sucrose loading buffer and 5 µL dH_2O. Electrophorese this aliquot through a 0.8% agarose gel, using 1X TAE as the electrophoresis buffer, at 10 V/cm for 2 h. View under UV light (*see* **Note 22**).
3. If the digestion is incomplete, add a further 10–20 U of *Hin*dIII and 4 µL spermidine (Sigma) at 10 mg/mL. Incubate for a further 4 h at 37°C, and check progress as in **step 2** above.

3.4.2. Electrophoresis and Southern Transfer

1. Add 4 µL 10X sucrose loading buffer to each fully digested sample. The EDTA content of the loading buffer will stop the enzyme reaction (*see* **Note 23**). Load the samples into the wells of a 20 × 20 cm 0.8% transfer gel (*see* **Note 24**). One well should be loaded with 30 µL λ DNA digested with *Hin*dIII (1 µg/30 µL) as a mol-wt marker (*see* **Note 9**). By loading the mol-wt marker in either the first or last well, orientation of the gel and the final autoradiograph can easily be achieved.
2. Electrophorese the samples at 1.5 V/cm for 16 h or overnight (*see* **Note 25**).
3. Using a tray that is just larger than the gel, stain the gel with gentle agitation for 20 min in 1X TAE buffer (can use the electrophoresis buffer from the tank) containing one drop 10 mg/mL EtBr solution. Rinse in dH_2O. View and photograph the gel under UV light.
4. Using a similar tray, denature the DNA by submerging the gel in approx 500 mL denaturing solution. Agitate gently for 30 min.
5. Rinse the gel in dH_2O, and then cover with approx 500 mL neutralizing solution. Agitate gently for a minimum of 30 min.
6. Set up a blotting tray as follows: Place a glass plate over a trough containing 20X SSC. Cut a sheet of 17 Chroma paper, soak briefly in 10X SSC, and place it on top of the plate, with both ends dipping into the 20X SSC to act as wicks. Ensure that there are no air bubbles trapped between the paper and the glass plate. These can be rolled out using a glass rod. Wet two pieces of 20 × 20 cm 3MM paper with 10X SSC, and place on the 17 Chroma paper (**Fig. 2**).

Table 5
Size and Corresponding Exon Mumber of Dystrophin Gene *Hind*III Fragments Identified by cDNA Hybridization

	cDNA probe															
Band no.	1–2a (9–7)		2b–3 (30–2)		4–5a (30–1)		5b–7 (47–4)		8 (44–1)		9 (63–1)		10 (63–1)		11–14 (63–1)	
from top of gel	Size (kb)	Exon no.	Size (kb)	Exon no.	Size (kb)	Exon no.	Size (kb)	Exon no.	Size (kb)	Exon no.	Size (kb)	Exon no.	Size (kb)	Exon no.	Size (kb)	Exon no.
1	11.0	10 + 11	12.0	18	20.0	22–25	18.0	31–33	10.0	47	8.8	56	12.0	63	10.0	75 + 76
2	8.2	4	11.0	10 + 11	18.0	31	11.0	43	7.0	52	8.3	54	6.6	61	7.8	79
3	7.8	6	7.6	20	11.0	21	6.2	40 + 41	3.9	48	7.8	53	6.0	58 + 59	6.8	68 + 69
4	7.2	8 + 9	6.4	13	11.0	28 + 29	6.1	38 + 39	3.7	50	6.0	58 + 59	3.5	60	6.0	79
5	4.4	7	6.0	16	7.6	20	4.2	42	3.1	51	2.3	55	2.8	62	3.0	78
6	4.1	3	3.9	12	5.2	26 + 27	4.1	44	1.6	49	1.0	57	2.6	65	2.4	74
7	3.3	2	3.0	19	4.7	30	1.8	34	1.25	48	1.0	53	2.4	64	2.0	72
8	3.1	1	2.6	14 + 15			1.5	37							2.0	77
9	2.9	5	1.8	17			1.5	46							1.9	73
10							1.3	36							1.5	67
11							0.5	45							1.5	70 + 71
12							0.4	35								

Following digestion of genomic DNA with *Hind*III, the majority of dystrophin gene exons are contained within a single DNA fragment. These can be detected by Southern blotting and sequential hybridization with nine cDNA probes. This table shows the size (kb) of each DNA fragment and its corresponding exon number detected by each of the cDNA probes.

7. Rinse the gel in 10X SSC, and gently slide onto the 20 × 20 cm Whatman 3MM paper on the blotting tray. Ensure that there is good contact and no air bubbles between the gel and the paper, because this will disrupt the capillary flow. In order to prevent short-circuiting of the buffer around the sides of the gel, a layer of cling film should be applied to all four sides of the gel. This also prevents distortion of the lanes at the edges.
8. Place a sheet of positively charged nylon membrane carefully on top of the gel, ensuring that no bubbles are trapped (*see* **Notes 26** and **27**).
9. Place two more layers of wetted 3MM paper on top of the transfer membrane, followed by a 5–10 cm stack of paper towels. Cover the towels with a glass plate, and put a weight of approx 1 kg on top.
10. Allow blotting to proceed for 3–5 h. Dismantle the blotting tray, and treat the membrane according to the manufacturer's instructions. In the case of Hybond N$^+$, presoak a sheet of 3MM paper in 0.4 *M* NaOH, and place the membrane on top, DNA side uppermost. Allow the NaOH to coat the surface of the membrane without allowing it to become submerged. Leave for 20 min, then quickly rinse in 2X SSC. The membrane can then be taken directly into the hybridization procedure, or air-dried and stored sealed in a plastic bag.

3.4.3. Labeling and Hybridization of Radiolabeled cDNA Probes to Southern Filters

Nine cDNA probes are required to identify all of the dystrophin exons by Southern hybridization, as shown in **Fig. 1** and **Table 5** (*see* **Note 28**). The following random primed labeling and hybridization protocols should be conducted in a laboratory suitable for the use of radioisotopes, under the local regulations that apply to that laboratory.

1. Soak the nylon membrane in 2X SSC, and place in a hybridization bottle, so that the filter adheres to the inner surface of the bottle with the DNA bound side facing inward (*see* **Note 29**). Fill the bottle with 2X SSC to allow any trapped air bubbles to rise to the surface, then empty completely.
2. Add 20 mL hybridization solution to the bottle, seal the lid, and incubate at 65°C on the rotisserie in the hybridization oven for at least 30 min.
3. While the filter is prehybridizing, take 10–100 ng cDNA probe to be labeled in a total volume of 20 µL made up with sterile dH_2O. If the cDNA is an excised insert contained within an agarose gel fragment, then no more than 10 µL of the total volume should be agarose (*see* **Note 30**). Denature the probe by boiling in a water bath or heating at 100°C in a hot block for 3 min.
4. If the solution does not contain agarose, snap cool on ice, then centrifuge very briefly in a microcentrifuge before adding the components of the labeling reaction. If agarose is contained in the solution, then cool it for a few seconds, centrifuge briefly, and add the labeling components quickly. It is important that the agarose does not set.
5. Add the following to the denatured probe: 3 µL 10X labeling buffer, 3 µL random hexanucleotides, 3 µL (30 µCi) [α-^{32}P]dCTP, and, lastly, 2 U Klenow fragment of DNA polymerase.

6. Incubate at 37°C for 1–4 h.
7. An arbitrary assessment of the radioactive incorporation can be made as follows: Place 1 μL probe mixture onto a Whatman GF/B filter disk, and position the head of a Geiger counter above it, at a point where the Geiger counter registers 100 counts. Clamp the Geiger tube in this position.
8. Place the disk on the sintered glass platform of a filtration tower (Millipore, Bedford, MA) and wash with 5–10 mL 5% TCA to remove unincorporated deoxynucleotide precursors.
9. Return the disk to the original position beneath the Geiger tube, and note the number of counts registered. This can be roughly taken as an estimate of the percentage incorporation into the probe (*see* **Note 31**).
10. Steps 10 and 11 are optional (*see* **Note 32**). Add 100 μL sterile TE buffer to the labeled probe mix, and purify using a Nick column (Amersham Pharmacia Biotech).
11. Wash the Nick column with 3 mL TE buffer, then apply the 100 μL probe solution directly to the resin bed of the column. Allow the probe to enter the resin, then apply and elute 3 × 400-μL aliquots of TE buffer into separate 1.5-mL microcentrifuge tubes with screw caps (*see* **Note 33**). The second fraction should contain the purified probe. Use the Geiger counter to confirm that this contains the highest amount of radioactivity.
12. Add 1–10 μL radioactively labelled λ DNA (*see* **Note 10**) to the probe solution, and denature by boiling in a water bath, or heating to 100°C in a hot block, for 5 min. Cool rapidly by plunging into wet ice.
13. Add the radioactive probe to the hybridization solution in the bottle, without allowing the temperature to fall unduly. Ensure that the top is sealed, and replace in the hybridization oven for a minimum of 16 h or overnight.

3.4.4. Washing of Nylon Membranes and Autoradiography

The following protocol should be conducted in a laboratory suitable for the use of radioisotopes under the local regulations that apply to that laboratory.

1. Discard the radioactive hybridization solution safely, according to local regulations. Briefly rinse the membrane in 2X SSC at RT.
2. Preheat 1 L wash solution 1 to 65°C, and pour into a plastic box that is just larger than the filter. Submerge the filter in the wash solution, and secure the lid of the box. Agitate gently for 20 min at 65°C. Monitor the surface of the filter with the Geiger counter, and, if this registers more that 5 cpm, then more stringent washing is required.
3. Repeat **step 2** above, using wash solution 2. If the Geiger counter continues to register greater than 5 cpm, then continue the washing steps at 65°C in the same way, but halve the SSC concentration of the washing solution each time.
4. Drain the filter of as much liquid as possible, place in a thin polythene bag, exclude all the air from the bag, and seal.
5. Place in a light-tight cassette with intensifying screens, with a sheet of X-ray film pressed against the DNA side of the filter.

6. Leave the cassette at –70°C for a minimum of 4–6 h; however, often an overnight exposure is required, before developing the film.

3.4.5. Interpretation of Autoradiographs

1. Deletions are observed as missing bands in the patient sample lanes, when compared with the positive control lane. Examples are shown in **Fig. 6**.
2. Duplications are recognized as intensity differences of the bands, when compared both with other bands in the same lane and with bands in the control lane. An example of a family in which several female members were identified as deletion carriers, using dosage interpretation, is shown in **Fig 7**.
3. Quantitative differences between the bands can be achieved by scanning each lane in a densitometer and making the comparisons described in **Subheading 3.2.2.**

3.4.6. Striping the Membrane of Previously Hybridized Probe (see ***Note 34***)

1. Boil 1 L 0.5% SDS in dH_2O.
2. Pour into a suitable plastic tray, and submerge the nylon membrane.
3. Allow to cool to RT while agitating gently on a shaking platform.
4. Remove the filter, and allow to air dry. Store sealed in polythene, if not proceeding to a further hybridization immediately.

4. Notes

1. The BM multiplex set (*see* **Table 3**) can give poor results, and this is improved by substituting Amplitaq Gold *Taq* polymerase (ABI).
2. DNA samples to be tested should include the patient sample and a sample from a control male who does not carry a dystrophin gene mutation.
3. pBR322 digested with *Msp*1 produces DNA fragments that are within an ideal size range for comparison with the multiplex PCR products. The sizes are 622, 527, 404, 307, 242, 238, 217, 201, 190, 180, 160 (x2), 147 (x2), 123, 110, 90, 76, and 67 bp. Digested DNA can be purchased from New England Biolabs and diluted to 0.5 µg/10 µL with 1X sucrose loading buffer, and used directly. Alternatively, a stock can be prepared as follows: Mix 10 µg native pBR322 DNA with 10 U *Msp*I and 5 µL 10x *Msp*I digestion buffer. Make up to a total volume of 50 µL, and incubate at 37°C for 4 h. Remove 2 µL and add 8 µL sucrose loading buffer. Check that digestion is complete by electrophoresing this aliquot through a 2% agarose gel. Make the stock digest mix up to 300 µL (1 µg/30 µL) with 1X sucrose loading buffer.
4. **CAUTION:** Take extreme care when preparing EtBr solution, because it is highly carcinogenic. Handle the stock EtBr powder in a fume cupboard while wearing a mask, or use tablets (Sigma). Store the solution in a well-labeled brown glass bottle, and treat with care.
5. Amplitaq Gold *Taq* polymerase is only activated when heated to 95°C for 10 min. Additional enzyme is activated as the PCR progresses through repeated denaturation cycles at this high temperature. In the authors experience, this property improves the results of quantitative PCR.

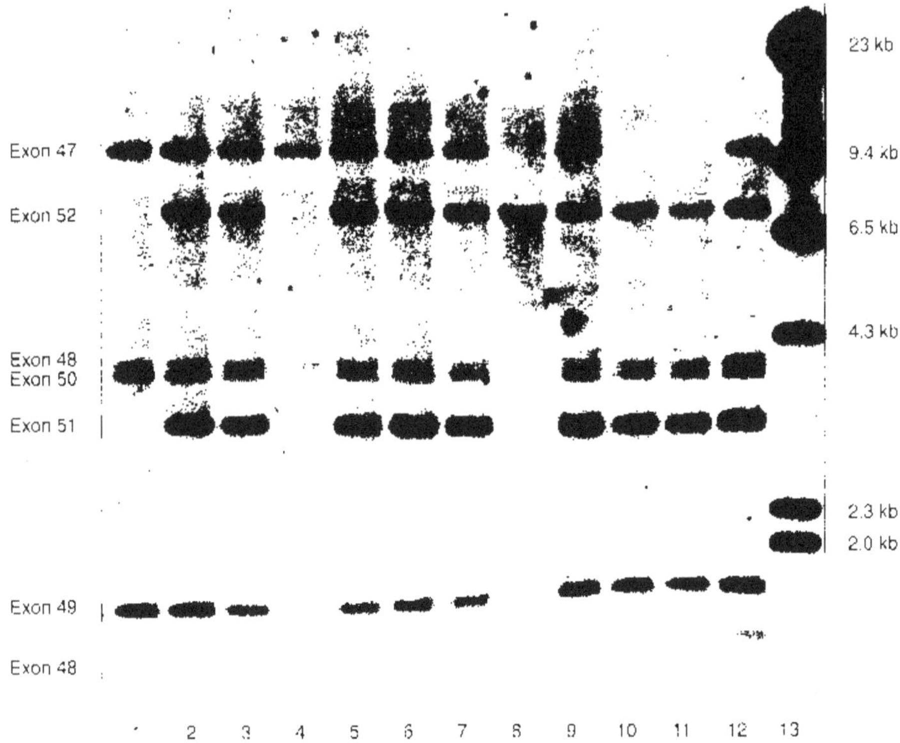

Fig. 6. Southern blot probed with cDNA 8 (44-1) showing dystrophin gene deletions. Lanes 1 to 11 contain *Hin*dIII digested DNA samples from males affected with DMD Lane 12 contains DNA from a control female and lane 13 contains λ DNA digested with *Hin*dIII as a molecular weight marker. Deletions are recognized as missing bands when the patient samples are compared with the control female. Deletions are present in the samples in lanes 1 (exons 51, 52), 4 (exons 49, 50, 51, 52), 8 (exons 47, 48, 49. 50. 51), 10 (exon 47) and 11 (exon 47).

Fig. 7. *(opposite page)* **(A)** shows an autoradiograph of a Southern blot probed with cDNA 1-2a (9-7). A corresponding pedigree is shown above the autoradiograph. Dosage comparisons have been used to identify a dystrophin gene deletion in female members of a family with no living affected male. A photograph of the corresponding ethidium bromide stained gel prior to Southern transfer is shown in **B** and demonstrates approximate equivalent loading of DNA in each lane. Lanes 3, 6 and 9 contain *Hin*dIII digested DNA from unaffected males and therefore represent single copies of the dystrophin gene. Comparison of band intensities, both within and between lanes indicate that the female samples in lanes 1 and 5 have two copies of the gene and the female samples in lanes 2, 4, 7 and 8 have a deletion involving exons 3 to 11. Note that the hybridization signal is weak for exons 2, 4 and 5. **(B)** shows the ethidium bromide stained gel prior to Southern transfer which was used to generate the autoradiograph

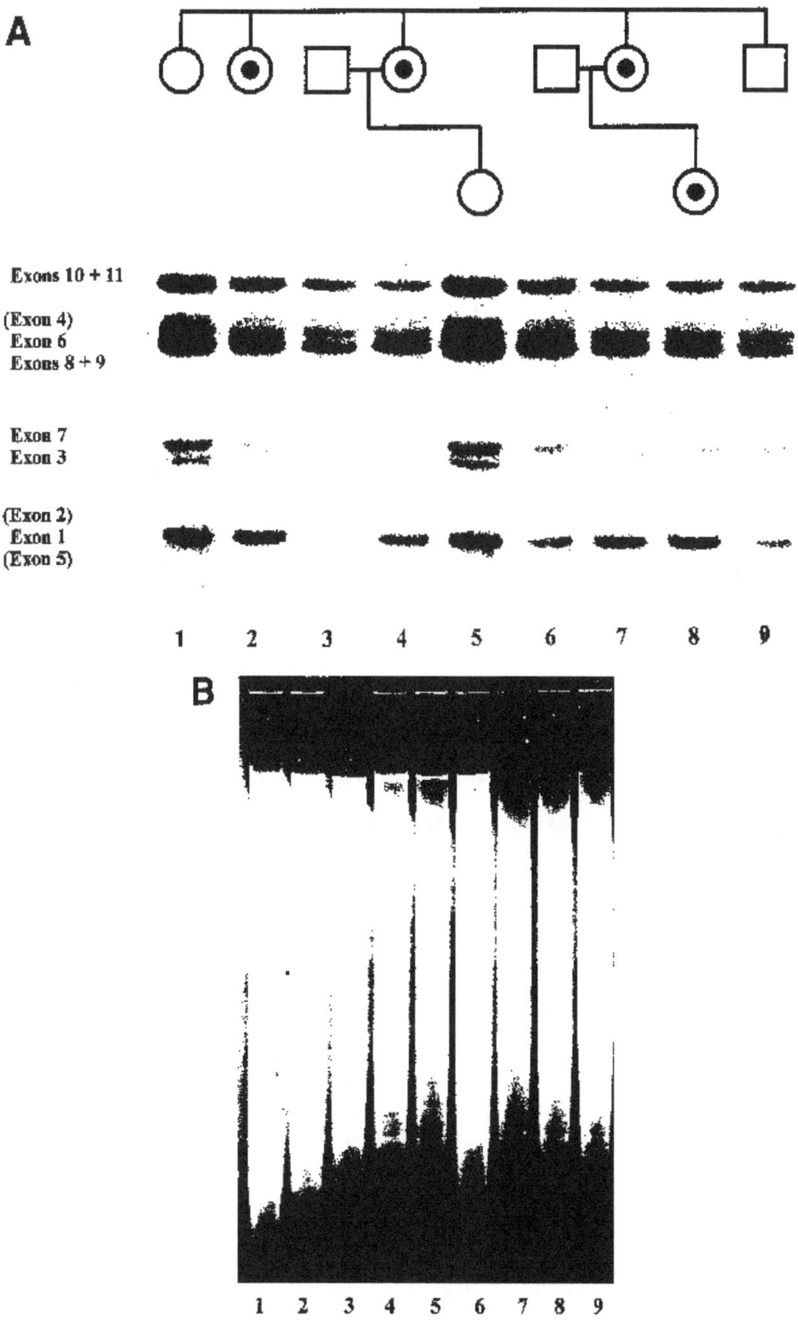

shown in **A**. This demonstrates an approximately equivalent loading of DNA in each lane, thus allowing dosage comparisons to be made.

6. The 5' multiplex set of fluorescent primers (5'F) amplifies 12 exons (muscle specific promotor + 1, 2, 3, 4, 5, 6, 8, 9, 13, 17, 19, and 30) from the 5' deletion hot spot, and the 3'F fluorescent set (3'F) amplifies 14 exons (42, 43, 44, 45, 46, 47, 48, 49, 50, 51, 52, 53, 60, and 62) from the central deletion hot spot of the dystrophin gene. Sequences for the 3' set are as shown in **Table 1**. Some of the sequences for the 5'set differ from those in Table 1, and these are shown in **Table 2**.
7. Yau et al. *(12)* originally recommended that the 3' set of forward primers should be labeled with the fluorescent dye HEX. However, this has since been shown to be less efficient than 6-FAM.
8. Because both PCR assays generate fragments that are larger than the longest fragment in the Genescan-500 ROX size standards (i.e., 500 bp), preparation of an additional standard of 547 bp is recommended.
9. λ DNA digested with *Hin*dIII gives fragments of 23.13, 9.42, 6.56, 4.36, 2.32, 2.02, 0.57, and 0.13 kb and can be purchased from several biotechnology companies, then diluted to the required concentration of 1 µg/30 µL with 1X sucrose loading buffer. Alternatively, native λ DNA can be digested with *Hin*dIII according to the protocol detailed in **Note 3**. Check that digestion is complete, by electrophoresing an aliquot through a 0.8% agarose gel, before making the stock digest mix up to 300 µL (1 µg/30 µL) with 1X sucrose loading buffer.
10. 100 ng bacteriophage λ DNA can be radioactively labeled as described in **Subheading 3.4.3., steps 3–11**. This can be stored in a lead-lined pot at –20°C for about 8 wk. It will be necessary to proportionally increase the amount used in the hybridization reaction over this period, because of decay of the isotope. A volume between 1 and 20 µL, which registers 100 cpm when held close to a Geiger counter, is sufficient.
11. If required, an additional pair of primers can be added to any of the four multiplex sets, to allow 10 exons to be amplified. The only restriction on this is that it must be possible to resolve the additional amplified fragment from all others.
12. Exons to be amplified in multiplex have been grouped into four sets, according to their position within the gene. However, at least one pair of primers is included in each set, which will amplify an exon that lies at a distance from the main set. This will act as a positive control in the event of a large deletion that encompasses all of the exons from the region being tested.
13. In order to avoid contamination of a PCR mix with products of previous amplifications, it is recommended that two sets of pipets are available, one set for preparing reaction mixes, and a second set for analysis of the products.
14. Sucrose loading buffer contains both xylene cyanole and bromophenol blue. The migration of these dyes sometimes coincides with that of multiplex PCR fragments. This reduces the intensity of EtBr staining, and, thus, the bands are more difficult to see when viewed under UV light. If this is a problem, it can be resolved by using an alternative loading buffer such as Ficoll orange. 10X Ficoll orange loading buffer: 0.25% orange G (Sigma), 25% Ficoll type 44 (Amersham Pharmacia Biotech). Store at 4°C.
15. It is important to establish that missing bands represent either deleted exons or point mutations arising within the primer binding sites, and are not simply tech-

nical failures. If several bands, representing contiguous exons, are missing, but the control exon from another part of the gene is present, then one can be confident that a deletion has been identified. However, if only a single band is missing, and the flanking exons are shown to be present, then this apparent single exon deletion should be confirmed by another method, such as PCR amplification with alternative primers or Southern blotting and probing with the appropriate cDNA.

16. In order that the intensity of bands can be compared in a quantitative manner, it is essential that the quantity of genomic DNA used in the PCR is accurately measured and falls within a narrow concentration range, and that the amplification reaction remains within the exponential phase of the assay by using a reduced number of cycles in the PCR.
17. Separation and staining of the PCR products on 6% PAGs allows more discriminatory dosage comparisons to be made than when separation is on agarose gels.
18. Take care to avoid touching the gel, even when wearing gloves, because finger marks are easily detected by the Ag stain solution.
19. The gel will float off the plate when covered with fixer. The plate can be removed at this stage without damaging the gel, which is delicate.
20. The Ag stain solution can be reused 3–4X after which the amount of silver becomes depleted for efficient staining.
21. Often, a single PCR fragment is represented by two peaks that differ by 1 bp in size. These peak areas should be added together to give the true peak area representing that particular fragment.
22. When genomic DNA is completely digested with *Hin*dIII, an even smear of stained DNA should be evident on the check gel, running from the origin to the electrophoresis front, as shown in **Fig 7A**. Heavier staining at the top of the gel indicates incomplete digestion.
23. If necessary, digested samples can be stored at this stage at 4°C for 1–2 d, or at –20°C for longer periods.
24. In general, 0.8% agarose gels are adequate for achieving good separation of the dystrophin gene *Hin*dIII fragments. However, exon 45 lies on a small fragment of only 0.5 kb. It is, therefore, important to ensure that this fragment does not electrophorese off the bottom of the gel. If necessary, the fragments can be separated on a higher-percentage gel of 1–1.5%, but this will reduce the resolution of the large fragments.
25. The 0.5 kb λ–*Hin*dIII fragment should be 1–2 cm from the bottom of the gel when the electrophoresis is complete. The gel can be returned to the tank, to be run further, if required.
26. The authors use Hybond N^+ nylon membrane, purchased from Amersham Life Science. Other manufacturers may recommend pretreatment of membranes before blotting. Manufacturers' instructions should always be consulted.
27. Before applying the membrane to the gel, it is recommended that the membrane is marked with the lane positions and other details, such as the experiment date, enzyme digest, and probe to be used.

28. If necessary, a single filter can be prepared and hybridized sequentially with more than one probe, stripping the filter of the previous probe between each hybridization. If it is necessary to hybridize all nine cDNAs, then duplicate filters can be made and hybridized 4–5× each.
29. This assumes use of a hybridization oven in which hybridization bottles are attached to a rotisserie. If this is not available, the hybridizations can be performed in good-quality, thick-gage, sealed polythene bags, incubated in plastic sandwich boxes in a shaking water bath.
30. The authors recommend using cDNA that has been excised as an insert from the host plasmid. 100–200 μg recombinant plasmid should be digested with the appropriate restriction enzyme, to release the cloned insert. Plasmid and insert DNA can be separated on a 1.5% low-melting-point agarose gel, and the insert band carefully cut out with a sterile scalpel. Excess exposure to UV light should be avoided at this stage. The agarose slice should then be melted at 65°C, and diluted with an equal volume of TE buffer. 5–10 μL of this solution is sufficient for a single labeling reaction. The stock can be aliquoted and stored at –20°C.
31. The method described here provides a crude measure of the efficiency of the labeling reaction. However, it will detect a failed reaction. The degree of accuracy depends on the amount of probe DNA used. If this is high, then the percentage of [α-^{32}P]dCTP incorporated may also be high, but the specific activity of the labeled probe will be low because of its high concentration. On the other hand, a small amount of probe may appear to have low levels of incorporation when measured as a proportion of the radioisotope used, but it could be labeled to high specific activity. The figure obtained also varies from probe, to probe and it is only with experience of working with particular probes that acceptable values become apparent. However, in general, percentages of >25% upwards are reasonable.
32. In the authors' experience, the ^{32}P-labeled cDNA probes give very clean signal on Southern blots, without separation from unincorporated nucleotides and hexamers, and therefore the purification steps described in **Subheading 3.4.3., steps 10** and **11**, are rarely carried out. However, these steps are recommended if high background is a problem on the final autoradiograph.
33. Screw-capped tubes are recommended as the safest for boiling radioactive solutions.
34. The recommended procedure for removal of previously hybridized probes from Southern filters may vary from that described here, according to different membrane manufacturers.

References

1. Forest, S., Cross, G. S., Speer, A., Gardner-Medwin, D., Burn, J., and Davies, K. E. (1987) Preferential deletion of exons in Duchenne and Becker muscular dystrophies. *Nature* **329,** 638–640.
2. Den Dunnen, J. T., Grootscholten, P. M., Bakker, E., Blonden, L. A., Ginjaar, H. B., Wapenaar, M. C., et al. (1989) Topography of the DMD gene, FIGE and cDNA analysis of 194 cases reveals 115 deletions and 13 duplications. *Am J. Hum. Genet.* **45,** 835–847.

3. Koenig, M. Monaco, A. P., and Kunkel, L. M. (1988) The complete sequence of dystrophin predicts a rod-shaped cytoskeletal protein. *Cell* **53,** 219–228.
4. Roberts, R. G., Coffey, A. J., Bobrow, M., and Bentley, D. R. (1993) Exon structure of the human dystrophin gene. *Genomics* **16,** 536–538.
5. Roberts, R. G., Coffey, A. J., Bobrow, M., and Bentley, D. R. (1992) Determination of the exon structure of the distal portion of the dystrophin gene by vectorette PCR. *Genomics* **13,** 942–950.
6. Boyce, F. M., Beggs, A. H., Feener, C., and Kunkel, F. M. (1991) Dystrophin is transcribed from a distant upstream promoter. *Proc. Natl. Acad. Sci.* **88,** 1276–1280.
7. Roberts, R. G., Gardner, R. G., and Bobrow, M. (1994) Searching for the 1 in 2,400,000: A review of dystrophin gene point mutations *Human Mutat.* **4,** 1–11.
8. England, S. B., Nicholson, L. V. B., Johnson, M. A., Forrest, S. M., et al. (1990) Very mild muscular dystrophy associated with the deletion of 46% of dystrophin. *Nature* **434,** 180–182.
9. Koenig, M., Begges, A. H., Moyer, M., et al. (1989) The molecular basis for Duchenne and Becker muscular dystrophy: correlation of severity with type of deletion. *Am. J. Hum. Genet.* **45,** 498–506.
10. Chamberlin, J. S., Gibbs, R. A., Rainier, J. E., Nguyen, P. N., and Caskey, C. T. (1988) Deletion screening of the Duchenne muscular dystrophy locus via multiple DNA amplification. *Nucl. Acids Res.* **16,** 11,141–11,156.
11. Beggs, A. H., Koenig, M., Boyce, F. M., and Kunkel, L. M. (1990) Detection of 98% of DMD/BMD deletions by polymerase chain reaction. *Human Genet.* **86,** 45–48.
12. Yau, S. C., Bobrow, M., Mathew, C. G., and Abbs, S. J. (1996) Accurate diagnosis of carriers of deletions and duplications in Duchenne/Becker muscular dystrophy by fluorescent dosage analysis. *J. Med. Genet.* **33,** 550–558.
13. Roberts, R. G., Bentley, D. R., Barby, T. F. M., Manners, E., and Bobrow, M. (1990) Direct diagnosis of carriers of Duchenne and Becker muscular dystrophy by amplification of lymphocyte RNA. *Lancet* **336,** 1523–1526.
14. Roberts, R. G., Barby, T. F. M., Manners, E., Bobrow, M., and Bentley, D. R. (1991) Direct detection of dystrophin gene rearrangements by analysis of dystrophin mRNA in peripheral blood lymphocytes. *Am. J. Hum. Genet* **49,** 298–310.
15. Abbs, S. and Bobrow, M. (1992) Analysis of quantitaive PCR for the diagnosis of deletion and duplication carriers in the dystrophin gene. *J. Med. Genet.* **29,** 191–196.
16. Prior, T. W., Wenger, G. D., Papp, A. C., Snyder, P. J., Sedra, M. S., Bartolo, C., Moore, J. W., and Highsmith, W. E. (1995) Rapid DNA haplotyping using a multiple heteroduplex approach: application to Duchenne muscular dystrophy carrier testing. *Human Mutat.* **5,** 263–268.
17. Prior, T. W., Bartolo, C., Pearl, D. K., Papp, A. C., Snyder, P. J., Sedra, M. S., Burghes, A. H. M., and Mendell, J. R. (1995) Spectrum of small mutations in the dystrophin coding region. *Am J. Hum. Genet.* **57,** 22–33.

18. Covone, A. E., Caroil, F., and Romeo, G. (1992) Screening Duchenne and Becker muscular dystrophy patients for deletions in 30 exons of the dystrophin gene by three-multiplex PCR. *Am J. Hum Genet.* **51,** 675–677.
19. Niemann-Seyde, S., Slomski, R., Rininsland, F., Ellermeyer, U., Kwiatkovska, J., and Reiss, J. (1992) Molecular genetic analysis of 67 patients with Duchenne/Becker muscular dystrophy. *Hum. Genet.* **90,** 65–70.
20. Beggs, A. H., Hoffman, E. P., Snyder, J. R., Arahata, K., Specht, L., Shapiro, F., et al. (1991) Exploring the molecular basis for variability among patients with Becker muscular dystrophy: dystrophin gene and protein studies. *Am. J. Hum. Genet.* **49,** 54–67.
21. Heikoop, J.C , Hogervorst, F. B. L., Meershoek, E. J., Grootscholten, P. M., den Dunnen, J. T., and van Ommen, G.-J. B. (1995) Expression of the human Dp71 (Apo-Dystrophin-1) Gene from a 760-kb DMD-YAC transferred to mouse cells. *Eur. J. Hum Genet.* **3,** 168–179.
22. Internet site for DMD data pages. http://www.dmd.nl/.

6

Point Mutation Detection in the Dystrophin Gene

Johan T. den Dunnen

1. Introduction

Patients with Duchenne and Becker muscular dystrophy (DMD/BMD) carry mutations in the dystrophin gene. To date, the dystrophin gene is the largest gene ever found in a living organism, measuring 2.4 Mb *(1–3)*. The major muscle transcript consists of 79 exons, spliced together in a 14-kb mature RNA *(1,2)*. The protein coding region spans 11,058 bp, and encodes a 3685 amino acid protein with a mol wt of 427 kDa *(2)*. Transcripts have been identified in many nonmuscular tissues, initiated from eight different promoters, some of which are tissue-specific. Extensive alternative splicing, especially toward the 3' end of the gene (i.e., exons 70–78), produces a range of slightly shorter transcripts. The gene thus encodes a very complex set of protein isoforms, of which the major constituents have been designated Dp427m (muscle), Dp427c (cortical), Dp427p (Purkinje cells), Dp260 (retina), Dp140 (central nervous system), Dp116 (peripheral nerve), Dp71, and Dp40 *(4)*.

Because of the size and complexity of the dystrophin gene, detection of mutations is a daunting task. Mutation detection is partly simplified by the fact that DMD/BMD is an X-linked disease. Consequently, in patients, no interfering healthy allele is present. Furthermore, about two-thirds of the patients carry (large) intragenic deletions, which are focused around a minor and a major deletion hot spot (approx exons 3–12 and 45–50, respectively), and can be detected efficiently using a multiplex polymerase chain reaction (PCR) protocol amplifying 18 of the most frequently deleted exons (*5,6*; *see* Chapter 5). Deletions can also be detected efficiently on Southern blots, using a set of dystrophin cDNA probes. High-quality Southern blots also facilitate the identification of patients carrying partial gene duplications (estimated frequency up to 6% of all patients *[3,7]*). Protocols using pulsed-field gel electrophoresis

From: *Methods in Molecular Medicine, vol. 43: Muscular Dystrophy: Methods and Protocols*
Edited by: K. M. D. Bushby and L. V. B. Anderson © Humana Press Inc., Totowa, NJ

have also been reported as an efficient tool for deletion and duplication detection *(3)*, but their application has been limited.

If no deletion or duplication mutation can be identified, current diagnosis is mostly based on dystrophin staining of a muscle biopsy and/or on haplotype analysis, i.e., an Xp21-linked segregation. However, dystrophin staining is not possible when material from a patient is not available (no living patients in the family), and it may be inconclusive in BDM patients, who often have dystrophin of a slightly altered size or with a reduced expression level. Haplotype analysis is complicated by the high intragenic recombination frequency (approx 10% *[8]*), the high new mutation rate (one-third of all cases), and the frequent absence of a suitable family structure. Furthermore, because ultimately only the identification of a causative mutation will give absolute certainty for a diagnosis, efficient techniques to identify the mutation in the remaining one-third of non-deletion/duplication cases are highly desired.

The current belief is that, in DMD, most (probably over 90% of the non-deletion/duplication cases) have mutations that affect only one or a few nucleotides, and that cause premature translation termination (for an overview, see the dystrophin point mutation database at the "Leiden Muscular Dystrophy pages" at http://www.dmd.nl/database.html). Several techniques have been applied to detect these mutations, but all, except RNA-based protocols, failed to yield a high success rate. Even 12 yr after the identification of the gene, not one DNA-based study has been reported that scanned the entire gene for mutations. The most extensive studies were reported by Prior scanning 71 exons using heteroduplex analysis (HA), and by Barbieri and Nigro *(9)*, scanning 40 and 37 exons, respectively, using single-strand conformation analysis (SSCA). Most studies only focused on the 18 exons amplified with the multiplex PCR for deletion detection, using techniques such as SSCA, HA, double-strand conformation analysis (DSCA), chemical mismatch cleavage (CMC), and direct sequencing *(4)*. The overall low efficiency in detecting mutations in the DNA-based studies probably derives from the fact that those affecting RNA-processing are missed, partly because many intronic sequences were not available, and, consequently, intron/exon boundaries could not be analyzed.

The only successful applied strategies that yielded a high success rate in identifying mutations were RNA-based, either using CMC *(10)* or the protein truncation test (PTT) *(11,12)*. Success was mostly because the entire dystrophin coding region was scanned, and because mutations affecting RNA-processing were also revealed. The success of dystrophin PTT results from its specific design to detect mutations, causing premature translation termination, because these are found in over 90% of the patients. The major drawback of the RNA-based techniques lies in the difficulty in amplifying the dystrophin sequences from the only readily available source, i.e., blood-derived RNA.

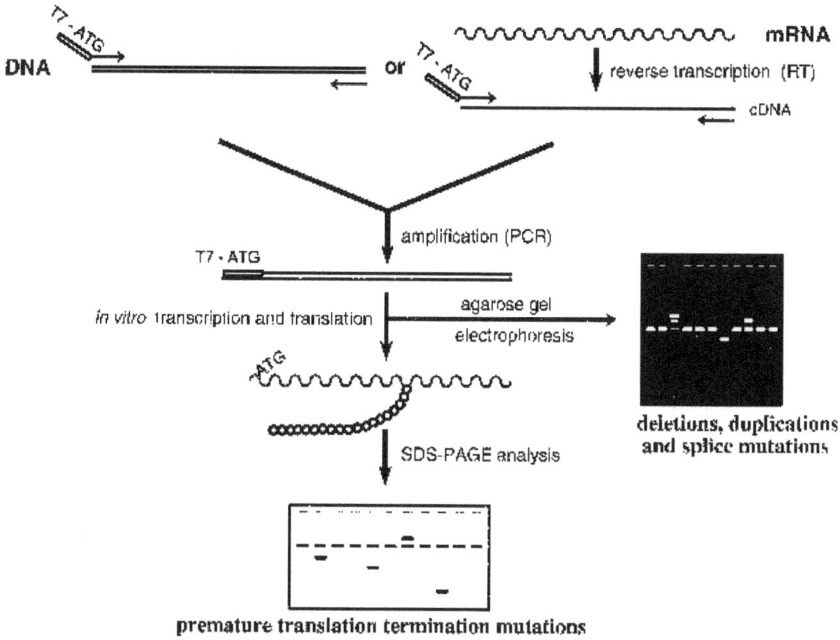

Fig. 1. Principle of the PTT. Schematic presentation of the individual steps of the assay. First, RNA is reverse transcribed (RT), to generate a cDNA copy. Second, the cDNA (or genomic DNA) is amplified using the polymerase chain reaction (PCR), in combination with a specifically tailed forward primer facilitating in vitro transcription by T7-RNA polymerase. Products are analyzed on agarose gel to verify amplification, determine yield, and check size; abnormally migrating products point to mutations (deletions, duplications, or affecting splicing). Finally, in vitro transcription/translation is used to generate peptide fragments, analysed on PAA gel, to detect translation-terminating mutations. T7 symbolizes the T7-RNA polymerase promoter sequence, and ATG, the Kozak translation initiation sequence.

1.1. Protein Truncation Test

The PTT is a rapid and efficient technique that specifically uncovers disease-causing mutations only, i.e., mutations causing premature termination of translation *(11)*. The principle of a PTT analysis is outlined in **Fig. 1**. Using *de novo* protein synthesis from an amplified RNA copy, the coding region of a gene is screened for the presence of mutations truncating protein translation. Three important steps are distinguished: amplification of the target gene-coding sequences from a patient sample, using specifically designed tailed primers in combination with reverse transcription polymerase chain reaction (RT-PCR); the use of the amplification products as template for the synthesis of RNA and,

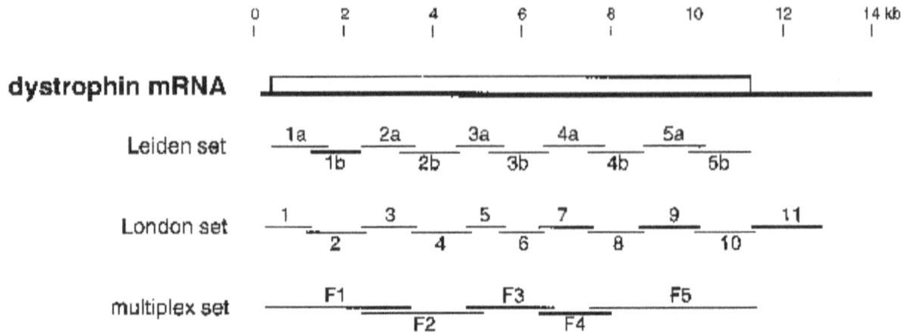

Fig. 2. PTT primer sets covering the dystrophin-coding sequence. Shown are the location and extent of the individual PCR fragments used for in vitro transcription/translation of the Leiden set, the London set, and the Multiplex set (primer sequences from **Tables 1** and **2**).

subsequently, protein; and analysis of synthesized protein using sodium dodecyl sulfate-polyacrylamide gel electrophoresis (SDS-PAGE). Shorter proteins, easily identifiable from fully translated run-off products, represent products derived from mutated alleles with their size pinpointing the site of the mutation.

The key feature of a PTT assay is a specifically designed sense primer. This primer contains four different regions. At the 5' region, a T7 (or SP6/T3) RNA-polymerase promoter sequence facilitates the production of RNA. This sequence is separated, by a spacer of 5–7 bp, from a eukaryotic translation initiation sequence (consensus Kozak sequence). The 3' region contains the target-gene sequence, in frame with the ATG codon from the Kozak sequence. To facilitate cloning of the amplified product, a restriction site is frequently added to the 5' end of the primer.

The dystrophin gene is much too large to enable PTT analysis from one fragment. Consequently, the gene must be split in partly overlapping segments, together spanning the entire coding region (**Fig. 2**). The most convenient lengths for the analysis of the translation products are determined mostly by the possibility of detect small mobility shifts in SDS-PAGE; fragments of 1–2 kb give optimal results.

Dystrophin RNA is the starting template for amplification. Ideally, the RNA source is muscle, which is the tissue in which the target gene is abundantly expressed. However, in most circumstances, muscle tissue is not available, and RNA is isolated from freshly drawn peripheral blood leucocytes or cultured skin fibroblasts. In such cases, a nested PCR is often required to successfully amplify the minute levels of ectopic transcripts present.

2. Materials

1. Acrylamide–*bis*-acrylamide (AA/BA)-mix: 30% acrylamide and 0.8% *N*',*N*'-*bis*-methylene-acrylamide dissolved in an end volume of 500 mL, filtered, and stored

at 4°C in the dark (**CAUTION:** Acrylamide is a neurotoxin; always wear gloves when handling acrylamide, preparing solutions, or pouring gels). Polyacrylamide is not toxic.

2. 1.5% agarose RNA gel: 1.5 g agarose (SeaKam LE) in 100 mL sterile TBE.
3. 10% Ammonium persulfate in H_2O, freshly prepared.
4. Diethylpyrocarbonate (DEPC)-treated solutions: Add 0.05–0.1% v/v DEPC (Sigma), leave overnight, and autoclave.
5. Destaining solution: 10% v/v methanol, 10% v/v acetic acid, and 80% v/v H_2O.
6. Dimethylsulfoxide/platelet peroxidase (DMSO/PPO): 226 g 2,5-diphenyloxazole, dissolved in 1000 mL DMSO.
7. Ethanol-70%: 700 mL pure ethanol, 300 mL H_2O.
8. Ethidium bromide (EtBr): stock solution of 10 mg/mL EtBr in H_2O.
9. 3 *M* NaAc: 408.1 g NaAc·$3H_2O$ dissolved in 1 L H_2O, adjusted to pH 5.6 with HAc.
10. Deoxyribonuleoside triphosphate (dNTP's): 25 m*M* dNTP's = 25 m*M* deoxyadenosine triphosphate, 25 m*M* deoxycytodine triphosphate, 25 m*M* deoxyguanosine triphosphate, and 25 m*M* deoxythiomidine triphosphate (prepared in H_2O from 100 m*M* stock, Pharmacia).
11. Polyacrylamide (PAA) gel mix (per 5 mL): 2 mL AA/BA mix, 1.65 mL dH_2O, 1.25 mL 1.5 *M* Tris-HCl, pH 8.8, 50 µL 10% sodium dodecyl sulfate (SDS).
12. PAA stacking mix (per 4 mL): 0.5 mL AA/BA mix, 3 mL dH_2O, 0.5 mL 0.5 *M* Tris-HCl, pH 6.8, 40 µL 10% SDS.
13. Phosphate-buffered saline (PBS): 144 m*M* NaCl, 10 m*M* KH_2PO_4, adjusted to pH 7.8 with K_2HPO_4.
14. PCR buffer: 166 m*M* $(NH_4)_2SO_4$, 0.67 *M* Tris-HCl, pH 8.8, 67 m*M* $MgCl_2$, 0.1 *M* β-mercaptoethanol.
15. RNA loading mix: 95% formamide, 20 m*M* ethylenediamine tetraacetic acid (EDTA), 0.05% bromophenol blue, 0.05% xylene cyanol.
16. Running buffer: 25 m*M* Tris-base, 200 m*M* glycine, and 0.1% SDS.
17. SDS sample buffer: 100 m*M* Tris-HCl, pH 6.8, 4% SDS, 0.1% (w/v) bromphenol blue, 20% glycerol, and, optional, 200 m*M* dithiothreitol (DTT) or 8% (v/v) β-mercaptol (added immediately before use).
18. Staining solution: 50% methanol, 0.05% Coomassie brilliant blue R, 10% acetic acid, 40% H_2O.
19. TBE buffer: 90 m*M* Tris, 90 m*M* boric acid, 1 m*M* EDTA, pH 8.3.
20. Tris-EDTA (TE)-buffer: 10 m*M* Tris-HCl, 0.1 m*M* EDTA, pH 8.0.

3. Method

3.1. RNA Isolation

3.1.1. Preparation of Blood Sample

RNA is isolated from peripheral blood leucocytes, which is the most readily available RNA source. However, if available, material from a muscle biopsy is highly recommended, to ensure efficient amplification of the dystrophin sequences (usually with a single round of PCR).

1. Collect one tube of 10 mL EDTA blood (Greiner, Solinger, Germany, no. 455036) (*see* **Note 1**).
2. Fill two white cap tubes with 5 mL Histopaque-1077 (Sigma). Slowly add 5 mL blood on top of the Histopaque. Spin at 2000 rpm for 20 min at room temperature (RT) in a swing-out rotor (do not use brakes). Four layers should be visible after centrifugation: The top layer contains serum and thrombocytes; the second, white layer contains leucocytes; the third, colorless layer is the Histopaque; and the fourth layer contains the erythrocytes.
3. Discard most of the first layer and transfer the second layer to a fresh tube.
4. Wash with 10 mL cold and sterile PBS, and spin at 1500 rpm for 10 min at RT; a small, white, sometimes red, pellet should be visible.
5. Remove the supernatant by carefully inverting the tube, resuspend the pellet in the remaining fluid by tapping the tube, and put on ice.

3.1.2. RNA Isolation Using RNAzolB

RNA isolation can be performed using many different protocols. Currently, several manufacturers sell excellent RNA isolation kits, one of which, the RNAzolB system from Campro Scientific, is described here. Recent experiments also indicate that the use of poly(A)$^+$-RNA may be advantageous for increasing RT-PCR yields of genes transcribed at very low levels (*see* **Note 2**).

1. Directly add 1.2 mL RNAzolB. Lyse the cells by passing the lysate several times through the pipet tip. Transfer to a 1.5–2 mL Eppendorf tube (*see* **Note 3**).
2. Add 0.1 mL chloroform per 1 mL homogenate, shake vigorously for 15 s, and incubate 5 min on ice.
3. Centrifuge the suspension at 12,000*g* for 15 min at 4°C (two phases should be formed: an upper, colorless, aqueous phase; and a lower, blue phenol–chloroform phase).
4. Carefully transfer the aqueous phase (0.6–0.7 mL) to a fresh tube, add an equal volume of isopropanol, and incubate 15 min on ice. After this step, the solution can be stored at 4°C until further use.
5. Centrifuge 15 min at 12,000*g* and 4°C; an RNA precipitate should be visible at the bottom of the tube.
6. Remove the supernatant, wash the pellet with 200 µL 70% ethanol, and centrifuge 10 min at 12,000*g*. Carefully remove all supernatant. Air-dry the pellet (do not dry too long, otherwise the pellet will not dissolve).
7. Dissolve the pellet in 50 µL TE (*see* **Note 4**).
8. Precipitate the RNA by adding 5 µL 3 *M* NaAc (pH 5.6) and 145 µL ethanol. Store at –20 or –70°C.

3.1.3. RNA Analysis

To check the quality and yield of the isolated RNA, it is analyzed on gel.

1. Carefully clean an electrophoresis tank, the gel tray, and comb, to remove any residual RNase activity. Incubate for 1 h with 1 *M* NaOH, and wash extensively with sterile water.
2. Pour a 1.5% agarose RNA gel (SeaKam-LE) in sterile TBE. Add EtBr to 0.2 µg/mL.
3. Take an aliqout of the RNA sample (i.e., 5–10%), and add an equal volume of RNA loading mix. Incubate for 5 min at 65°C. Load on the gel, together with a standard, facilitating determination of size and yield.
4. Run the gel and analyze the RNA on a UV transilluminator (*see* **Note 5**).

3.2. Amplification of Target Sequences

Because dystrophin transcripts are present at very low levels in blood-derived RNA samples, a nested PCR reaction is required to amplify sufficient PCR product for the in vitro transcription/translation. Several RT-PCR kits are commercially available, of which especially those directed at the amplification of large targets can be highly recommended, e.g., Expand High Fidelity PCR System (Boehringer Mannheim) and the Gene Amp XL RNA PCR Kit (Perkin-Elmer, Norwalk, CT).

3.2.1. cDNA Synthesis by Reverse Transcription

1. Transfer 50 µL ethanol-stored RNA (i.e., 1–3 µg total RNA) to a fresh Eppendorf tube, and centrifuge 10 min at 12,000 rpm and 4°C.
2. Remove the ethanol using a sterile pipet, and air-dry the pellet (do not dry too long; otherwise, the pellet will not dissolve).
3. Make a premix containing 2 µL random primer (0.5 µg/µL, Promega, Madison, WI) and 30 µL TE, and add it to the RNA pellet. Mix, incubate for 10 min at 65°C, and put directly on ice (*see* **Note 6**).
4. Add directly (or make a premix containing 12 µL Superscript reverse transcription-buffer, 6 µL 0.1 *M* DTT, 6 µL 10 m*M* dNTPs, 1 µL 40 U/µL RNasin, 2 µL 200 U/µL Superscript, and 1 µL H_2O. Add the premix to the RNA sample, mix and put 10 min at RT. Incubate 60 min at 42°C. Put on ice. When necessary, stop here, and store at –20°C.
5. OPTIONAL: After reverse transcription, the authors usually perform an RNaseA treatment, which significantly increased yields.

3.2.2 First-round PCR

1. Prepare a premix containing: 5 µL PCR buffer, 5 µL DMSO, 2.6 µL dNTPs (25 m*M*), 1 µL bovine serum albumin (10 mg/mL, Boehringer), 0.4 µL Amplitaq (5 U/µL, Perkin-Elmer), 0.04 µL DeepVent (2U/µL, Biolabs) and 22 µL H_2O. Add the mix to the cDNA sample.

2. Add 2 μL forward primer (20 pmol/μL), 2 μL reverse primer (20 pmol/μL), 10 μL RT product, two drops of mineral oil (Sigma Light Oil), and spin briefly (for primer sequences, *see* **Table 1**).
3. Perform the PCR reaction, cycling conditions; once 3 min 93°C, then 30× 1 min 93°C/1 min 58°C/4 min 72°C, and finally once for 7 min 72°C. Store at 4°C (*see* **Note 7**).

3.2.3 Second-round PCR

1. Prepare a premix containing: 5 μL Supertaq PCR buffer (HT Biotechnology), 5 μL 2 m*M* dNTPs, 2 μL tailed forward primer (20 pmol/μL), 2 μL reverse primer (20 pmol/μL), 0.05 μL Supertaq, and 33 μL H_2O (for primer sequences, *see* **Table 2**; *see* **Note 8**).
2. Add 3 μL first-round PCR product and a drop of mineral oil (Sigma Light Oil), and perform the PCR protocol as in **Subheading 3.2.2., step 8**. After PCR, store at 4°C (*see* **Note 9**).

3.3. In vitro Transcription/Translation

Protein synthesis from the amplified RT-PCR products can be performed in several ways. First, there is the option to perform the analysis using a radioactive or a nonradioactive labeling/detection system. Second, one can perform the in vitro transcription/translation in a coupled (one-tube) or an uncoupled reaction. Two protocols will be provided to show both alternatives; a coupled radioactive transcription/translation, based on the TnT T7 Quick Coupled Transcription/Translation System from Promega, and an uncoupled nonradioactive transcription/translation based on the Protein Truncation Test Kit from Boehringer Mannheim. The author prefers the more flexible format of the uncoupled system.

3.3.1. Uncoupled Nonradioactive Transcription/Translation

Transcription and translation, using the nonradioactive Protein Truncation Test Kit (Boehringer Mannheim), is essentially performed as recommended by the supplier. Signal in this system is generated by chemiluminescent detection of the synthesized proteins, after incorporation of biotin-labeled lysine.

1. Transfer 200 ng PCR product to a fresh Eppendorf tube containing 2.5 μL 4*T7 transcription mix from the kit. Add H_2O to a final reaction volume of 10 μL. Incubate for 15 min at 30°C.
2. Optional: Analyze 2.5 μL transcription reaction on a 1% agarose gel, to check the transcription product, its size, and its yield.
3. Transfer 20 μL translation mix from the kit to a fresh Eppendorf tube. Add 5 μL transcription reaction, mix carefully, and incubate for 1 h at 30°C (*see* **Note 10**).
4. Stop the reaction by adding 125 μL SDS sample buffer. Denature the sample for 2 min at 100°C. Store the reaction at –70°C (or –20°C).

5. Optional: Centrifuge the sample for 1 min in an Eppendorf centrifuge.
6. Load the gel with the samples (10–15 µL), controls, and protein markers.
7. After electrophoresis, the gel is washed and blotted on a PVDF Western Blotting Membrane (Millpore, Bedford, MA), according to standard Western blotting procedures.
8. Biotin-labeled proteins are detected with the BM Chemiluminescence Blotting Substrate POD (Boehringer Mannheim), using the supplier's recommendations. After blocking for 40 min at RT, the membrane is incubated with streptavidin-horseradish peroxidase conjugate (1:5000 dilution) for 30 min at RT.
9. Perform four 10-min, washing steps with TBS-Tween.
10. Add 1–5 mL detection solution (luminol/iodphenol); incubate for 1 min.
11. Expose to X-ray film (Kodak X-Omat R), depending on the signal, for a few seconds up to a few minutes.

3.3.2. Coupled Radioactive Transcription/Translation

Transcription and translation, using the TnT T7 Quick Coupled Transcription/Translation System (Promega), is essentially performed as recommended by the supplier. Signal in this protocol is generated by radioactive detection of the synthesized proteins after incorporation of ^{3}H-labeled leucine (*see* **Note 11**).

1. Remove the TnT Quick reagents from the –70°C. Put the TnT T7 RNA polymerase directly on ice (not too long) and, after thawing, store all components on ice. Rapidly thaw the rabbit reticulocyte lysate by hand warming.
2. Pipet into a 1.5-mL microcentrifuge tube: 10 µL TnT T7 Quick mix, 1 µL ^{3}H-leucine (5 mCi/mL, 160 Ci/mmol, Amersham), 0.7 µL tRNA^{nscend}tRNA, and up to 4 µL PCR product (50–500 ng) (*see* **Note 12**).
3. Mix and incubate the reaction for 60 min at 30°C.
4. Stop the reaction by adding 30 µL SDS sample buffer. Denature the sample for 2 min at 100°C. Store the reaction at –70°C (or –20°C) (*see* **Note 13**).

   For SDS-PAGE analysis of the translation products, the author uses the MiniProtean II gel system (Bio-Rad, Hercules, CA), which requires only a short electrophoresis time (1–1.5 h), and uses small amounts of reagents to prepare and stain a gel. Most frequently, the author uses a 12% PAA-gel, with a 3.75% stacking gel. This gel can be used to analyze peptides from 15 to 70 kDa (requiring 12–15% overlaps for genes analyzed in segments).
5. Optional: Centrifuge the sample for 1 min in an Eppendorf centrifuge.
6. Load the gel with the samples (10–15 µL), controls, and protein markers (*see* **Note 14**).
7. Electrophoresis is performed at a constant current of 30 mA (60 V) in the stacking gel and 40 mA (200 V) in the separating gel. Stop the run when the bromophenol blue dye reaches the bottom of the gel.
8. Remove the gel, place it in a plastic box, cover with staining solution, and incubate 15–30 min under gentle agitation (*see* **Note 15**).
9. Discard the staining solution, rinse briefly with destaining solution, remove it, and repeat until the protein markers are clearly visible.

Table 1A
Primer Sequences for PTT of Dystrophin Gene: Leiden Set

Set	Exons	PCR	Name	Localization	Length	Sequence
1		1st	1h	257–280	1345	CAAAAGAAAACATTCACAAAATGG
			1a	1601–1578		TTAGCCAGTCATTCAACTCTTTCA
	2–11	2nd	1d	295–314	1258	gc-[T7]-TCTAAGTTTGGAAGCAGCA
			1c	1511–1493		TGAGGCATTCCCATCTTGA
		1st	1b	1091–1111	1350	CGATTCAAGAGCTATGCCTAC
			1g	2440–2419		ACTCTGCAACACAGCTTCTGAG
	10–18	2nd	1f	1292–1312	1,174	[T7]-TTGCAAGCACAAGGAGAGATT
			1e	2426–2405		CTTCTGAGCGAGTAATCCAGCT
2		1st	2h	2276–2297	1327	cggatccACAAGGGAACAGATCCTGGTAA
			2a	3594–3617		GTCTCAAGTCTCGAAGCAAACTCT
	17–25	2nd	2d	2342–2364	1,244	gc-[T7]-AGGCAGATTACTGTGGATTCTGA
			2c	3544–3524		CCCACCTTCATTGACACTGTT
	1st		2b	3281–3299	1538	ATTGAGGGACGCTGGAAGA
			2g	4810–4787		cgggatcCTGCTTTTTCTGTACAATCTGACG
	23–32	2nd	2f	3320–3342	1411	gc-[T7]-GAGCATTGTCAAAAGCTAGAGGA
			2e	4689–4667		TCCACACTCTTTGTTTCCAATG
3		1st	3h	4365–4388	1533	TCACAGGCAGGTACAAGCAGTTGG
			3a	5897–5876		CAATGTCATCCAAGCATTTCAG
	31–38	2nd	3d	4517–4537	1093	gc-[T7]-GCCCAAAGAGTCCTGTCTCA
			3c	5568–5545		TTAAACTGCTCCAATTCCTTCAA
	1st		3b	5281–5301	1473	CACAAAGTGGATCATTCAGGC
			3g	6745–6723		gcgaattcACTGGCATCTGTTTTTGAGGAT
	36–45	2nd	3f	5300–5318	1450	[T7]-GCTGACACACTTTTGGATG

			3e	6710–6691		CTTCCCCAGTTGCATTCAAT
4		1st	4h	6404–6424	1463	GCAACGCCTGTGGAAAGGGTG
			4a	7866–7844		CGATCCGTAATGATTGTTCTAGC
	44–52	2nd	4c	6575–6601	1308	[T7]-GCTGAACAGTTTCTCAGAAAGACACAA
			4c	7843–7820		CTCTTGATTGCTGGTCTTGTTTT
	1st		4b	7489–7510	1543	AGCTCCTGGACTGACCACTATT
			4g	9031–9008		CTCTTGAAGTTCCTGGAGTCTTTC
	51–59	2nd	4f	7643–7663	1351	[T7]-TGGACAGAACTTACCGACTGG
			4e	8954–8933		CCCACTCAGTATTGACCTCCTC
5		1st	5h	8580–8603	1986	AAAAGTCTCTCAAATTAGGTCCC
			5a	10565–10544		ATCCATTGCTGTTTTCCATTTC
	58–68	2nd	5d	8827–8846	1383	gc-[T7]-ACAGAGCAGCCTTTGGAAG
			5c	10168–10146		TGGACACTCTTTGCAGATGTTAC
	1st		5b	9435–9456	1926	ACGAGACTCAAACAACTTGCTG
			5g	11352–11328		gcgaattcTATTCTGCTCCTTCTTCATCTGTC
	67–79	2nd	5f	9953–9972	1381	gc-[T7]-GGTGAAGTTGCATCCTTTGG
			5e	11292–11272		ATCATCTGCCATGTGGAAAAG

Set, number amplified segment of the dystrophin-coding sequence; Exons, exons amplified; PCR, primers to be used in the 1st or 2nd round PCR; Name, primer name; Localization, primer in relation to the dystrophin cDNA sequence (GenBank M18533); Length, size of amplified fragment (in bp); PTT, length of translation product (in kDa); Sequence, primer sequence, lower case letters indicating added tail sequences, [T7], 5'-ggatcctaatacgactcactataggaacagaccaccATG-3'. Sequences are used with permission from refs. *19* and *20* and Hogervorst et al. (unpublished).

Table 1B
Primer Sequences for PTT of Dystrophin Gene: London Set

Set	Exons	PCR	Name	Localization	Length	Sequence
1		1st	DMD1a	13–33	1206	CTTTCCCCCTACAGGACTCAG
			DMD1b	1218–1199		CTCTCCATCAATAGAACTGCC
	2–10	2nd	DMD1c	212–232	1003	[T7]-CTTTGGTGGGAAGAAGTAGAG
			DMD1d	1175–1154		CCAAATGCTGTGAAGGAAATGG
2		1st	DMD2a	1091–1111	1329	CGATTCAAGAGCTATGCCTAC
			DMD2b	2419–2399		GCGAGTAATCCAGCTGTGAAG
	9–18	2nd	DMD2c	1133–1153	1303	[T7]-ACCTCTGACCCTACACGGAGC
			DMD2d	2396–2377		CAGTTATATCAACATCCAAC
3		1st	DMD3a	2300–2319	1320	CATGCTCAAGAGGAACTTCC
			DMD3b	3619–3599		CTGAGTGTTAAGTTCTTTGAG
	17–25	2nd	DMD3c	2342–2362	1292	[T7]-AGGCAGATTACTGTGGATTCTG
			DMD3d	3594–3574		GTCTCAAGTCTCGAAGCAAAC
4		1st	DMD4a	3507–3526	1,346	CAATTCAGCCCAGTCTAAAC
			DMD4b	4852–4832		CAAAGCTGTTACTCTTTCATC
	25–33	2nd	DMD4c	3527–3547	1,323	[T7]-AGTGTCAATGAAGGTGGGCAG
			DMD4d	4810–4790		CTGCTTTTTCTGTACAATCTG
5		1st	DMD5a	4740–4760	1,199	GTCTGAGTGAAGTGAAGTCTG
			DMD5b	5938–5919		CCTTTCATCTCTGGGCTCAG
	33–38	2nd	DMD5c	4763–4785	924	[T7]-GTGGAAATGGTGATAAAGACTGG
			DMD5d	5647–5627		ATTGAAGTCTTCCTCTTTCAG
6		1st	DMD6a	5823–5842	802	CTCTAGAAATTTCTCATCAG
			DMD6b	6624–6605		GCATGTTCCCAATTCTCAGG
	37–44	2nd	DMD6c	5528–5548	1095	[T7]-GGAAAGGCCTCCATTCCTTTG
			DMD6d	6583–6564		CTGTTCAGCTTCTGTTAGCC

7		1st	DMD7a	6404–6424	1311	GCAACGCCTGTGGAAAGGGTG
			DMD7b	7714–7694		GTCACCCACCATCACCCTCTG
	43–51	2nd	DMD7c	6428–6449	1289	[T7]-CTACAGGAAGCTCTCTCCCAGC
			DMD7d	7677–7568		TCAAGCAGAGAAAGCCAGTC
8		1st	DMD8a	7583–7603	1308	CTAGAAATGCCATCTTCCTTG
			DMD8b	8890–8871		CTCAGGAGGCAGCTCTCTGG
	51–58	2nd	DMD8c	7616–7636	1296	[T7]-CCTGCTCTGGCAGATTTCAAC
			DMD8d	8872–8852		GGGCTCCTGGTAGAGTTTCTC
9		1st	DMD9a	8754–8773	1,317	GGGCCTTCAAGAGGGAATTG
			DMD9b	10070–10051		CCAGTCTCATCCAGTCTAGG
	58–68	2nd	DMD9c	8786–8807	1300	[T7]-CCTGTAATCATGAGTACTCTTG
			DMD9d	10046–10027		GGGCCGCTTCGATCTCTGGC
10		1st	DMD10a	9953–9972	1376	GGTGAAGTTGCATCCTTTGG
			DMD10b	11328–11308		CATGACTGATACTAAGGACTC
	67–79	2nd	DMD10c	9971–9993	1332	[T7]-GGGGGCAGTAACATTGAGCCAAG
			DMD10d	11263–11243		CATTGTGTCCTCTCTCATTGG
11		1st	DMD11a	11185–11206	2102	GATGGAGCAACTCAACAACTCC
			DMD11b	13286–13267		GTCAGAGGTAACAGATTTGC
	77–79	2nd	DMD11c	11214–11234	1,646	[T7]-GTTCAAGAGGAAGAAATACCC
			DMD11d	12859–12838		GTAACATTTGAATCAATTTGCC

Set, number amplified segment of the dystrophin coding sequence; Exons, exons amplified; PCR, primers to be used in the 1st or 2nd round PCR; Name, primer name; Localization, primer in relation to the dystrophin cDNA sequence (GenBank M18533); Length, size of amplified fragment (in bp); PTT, length of translation product (in kDa); Sequence, primer sequence, lower case letters indicating added tail sequences; [T7], 5'-ggatcctaatacgactcactataggaacagaccaccATG-3'. Adapted with permission from refs. *10* and *12*.

10. Wash the gel for 15 min with water.
11. Cover the gel with DMSO, and wash for 10 min under gentle agitation. Repeat once (*see* **Note 15**).
12. Treat the gel twice for 10 min with DMSO/PPO (*see* **Note 17**).
13. Wash the gel for 10 min with water (this step removes the DMSO/PPO; the gel becomes white).
14. Put the gel on 3MM paper. Dry at 60–70°C for at least 1 h (depending on the thickness of the gel and the percentage of acrylamide used).
15. Expose with X-ray film (e.g., Kodak X-Omat AR) (*see* **Note 18**).

4. Notes

1. Alternatively, RNA can be isolated from, e.g., cultured cells. Take a tissue culture flask (75 cm^2) with cells grown to 80–90% confluency. Discard culture medium, wash carefully with sterile and cold PBS, add 5 mL PBS, put the flask on ice, and collect the cells by scraping with a sterile wiper. Transfer the cells to a fresh tube, add 5 mL PBS to the original flask, and repeat the scraping. Collect all cells, centrifuge at 1500 rpm for 10 min, and carefully remove all supernatant by inverting the tube. Proceed with **Subheading 3.1.2., step 1**. Incubation of the cells with cycloheximide (100 µg/mL for 4–8 h), prior to harvesting of the cells, can be used to specifically increase the yield of the RNA transcribed from the mutated allele, frequently producing a less-stabile RNA molecule ***(13)***.
2. Always use sterile pipets, tubes, and solutions, keep the RNA samples cold, wear gloves, and work with DEPC-treated RNase-free solutions.
3. For cells isolated from 5 mL blood or cultured cells from one 75-cm^2 flask, the author uses 1–1.3 mL RNAzolB. RNAzolB contains chloroform and guanidinium chloride, it promotes the formation of complexes of RNA with guanidinium and water molecules, and abolishes hydrophilic interactions of DNA and proteins, which are thus removed from the aqueous phase.
4. To check the quality and amount of RNA, it can be analyzed on gel. Genomic DNA contaminations in the RNA samples often interfere with the RT-PCR, and should be prevented as much as possible.
5. Comparison with the standard is used to determine the RNA concentration. The RNA quality is sufficient when the 18S and 23S rRNA bands are clearly visible, and when no contaminating DNA band can be seen.
6. Alternatively, gene-specific primers can be used to prime the cDNA synthesis. In this case, scale down the amount of RNA to 200–500 ng, add 0.5 µL gene-specific primer (20 pmol/µL, **Table 1**), and anneal in 9.5 µL TE by incubation for 10 min at 65°C. Add, for a final volume of 20 µL: 4 µL RT buffer (Gibco-BRL), 2 µL 0.1 *M* DTT, 2.5 µL 10 m*M* dNTPs, 0.5 µL RNasin (40 U/µL, Promega), and 200 U Superscript.
7. The total volume of the PCR can be scaled down to 25 µL, using half of all the ingredients. For difficult PCRs, results can be improved by adding 0.1–0.2 U Deepvent (2 U/µL, Biolabs).
8. The tailed forward primer contains a T7 RNA polymerase promoter and a eukaryotic translation initiation (Kozak) sequence (5'-...<u>TAATACGACTCACTATAGG</u>

AACAG ACCACCATGg...-3', where the ATG should be in-frame with the dystrophin coding sequence.

9. Analysis of an aliquot of the RT-PCR sample (5–10 µL), using agarose gel electrophoresis (1% gel in TBE buffer), is used to determine the yield and size of the amplification products. An accurate estimate of the yield is required to determine the amount necessary for in vitro transcription/translation. Furthermore, at this step, the detection of abnormal product sizes points to the presence of genetic rearrangements (genomic deletions, duplications, and so on) or mutations affecting RNA processing (mostly splicing).
10. As a control for the in vitro transcription/translation reaction, the kit contains a luciferase-encoding control plasmid. When this template DNA is subjected to the in vitro transcription/translation, a 62-kDa protein should be synthesized. The translation reaction may be optimized by varying the Mg^{2+}-concentration. Since labeling of the translation products is achieved by incorporation of biotinylated lysine, it should always be checked whether the translated segment contains lysines.
11. Other ^{3}H-labeled amino acids or ^{35}S-labeled amino acids can also be used, although it should be checked that they are encoded by the translated region.
12. Unused lysate should be refrozen as quickly as possible. As a control for the in vitro transcription/translation reaction, the TnT Lysate System contains a luciferase-encoding control plasmid. When this template DNA is subjected to the in vitro transcription/translation, a 62-kDa protein should be synthesized. Good results are also obtained when the transcription/translation is reduced to a 12-µL reaction, with a ratio of PCR:TnT mix of up to 1:2.
13. When translation products do not appear to enter the gel (i.e., strong signal in the slot), adding 5% β-mercaptoethanol and omitting the boiling step may solve the problem.
14. As mol-wt markers, the author uses ^{14}C-labeled protein marker (Amersham) or prestained protein markers (Bio-Rad).
15. When ^{14}C-labeled or prestained protein markers are used, the Coomassie blue staining (**steps 9** and **10**) can be omitted.
16. **CAUTION:** DMSO is a hazardous organic chemical, therefore, these steps should be performed in a fume hood. DMSO is used to dehydrate the gel, enabling the subsequent infusion of PPO.
17. PPO, an organic scintillant, is used to convert the energy emitted by the isotope to visible light, enabling detection by exposure to X-ray film. The DMSO/PPO solution can be reused 2–3×. There are reagents that can be used to enhance the results for autoradiography, e.g., Amplify (Amersham) and Enhance (New England Nuclear).
18. Usually, translation products of 50 ng of a 1.5 kb PCR product in a 12-µL reaction can be easily detected after overnight exposure.

5. Problems And Pitfalls

Because a nested PCR protocol is required to amplify the target sequences, the procedure is sensitive to contaminations in the sample and ingredients of the

RT-PCR reaction. Any previous PCR analysis is a major source of contamination. A pre-PCR laboratory is thus essential to keep the RNA sample and primers physically separated from the RT-PCR and subsequent steps of the procedure. A control reaction (no RNA and/or no enzyme added) should always be part of the PTT, to exclude contaminations.

The most prominent failure of the PTT is the inability to amplify the target sequences from the RNA sample. In this respect, the reverse transcription reaction is technically the most critical step. Fresh constituents and fresh batches of enzyme are the best safeguards against any problems. Failure is often caused by bad-quality isolated RNA (low yields, degraded RNA, contamination with interfering chemicals and/or DNA). Control RT-PCR reactions, using a batch of good RNA and a 1:1 mixture of this RNA with the target RNA, are highly recommended to trace these problems. Amplification failure may also be caused by a failure of primer binding, either because the primer binding site is deleted or mutated. Similarly, amplification across (and beyond) translocation and inversion breakpoints will yield no product. In exceptional cases, amplification failure from a male DMD sample may indicate the existence of mutations affecting transcription (promoter mutations) or RNA maturation and/or stability.

Alternative splicing in the 3' end of the dystrophin gene, mostly of exons 71 and 78, may complicate the analysis of this region. First, each splice form produces a specific translation product, yielding a very complex overall picture. Second, one should realize that, when a specific exon is missing from all amplified transcripts, it is not scanned for mutations; the absence may in fact highlight the mutation, e.g., a mutation affecting splicing of the exon.

Occasionally, PCR products give poor yields in transcription/translation. This is often caused by poor-quality tailed forward primer. Because primers are synthesized 3' 5', the T7 RNA polymerase promoter sequence is synthesized last, and, when the coupling steps are inefficient, most primers will thus contain an incomplete T7-promoter sequence. Although such incomplete primers give normal yields in PCR, in vitro transcription will fail, as can be easily verified when the transcription products are analyzed on agarose gel. Reamplification of the tailed products with a specific T7-promoter primer is simple and effective, to both highlight and solve the problem.

Upon translation, some sets produce a range of undesired background translation products, usually derived from secondary sites of translation initiation. Although these products may disguise truncated products, in general, the translation pattern is constant and changes are easy to detect. Furthermore, truncated bands from such sets go together with a similar set of side products, thereby simplifying their detection. Tagging the translation products with a specific N-terminal protein sequence, e.g., a myc tag incorporated in the tailed forward primer sequence, has been reported as an effective procedure to reduce the background derived from secondary translation initiation *(14)*.

Detection of a unique truncated fragment should always be verified by a second assay, starting from an independent reverse transcription reaction. The author has experienced a few cases in which the truncated fragment could not be reproduced. The origin of these artifacts (false positives) is unclear, but it probably resides in the infidelity of the reverse transcriptase and/or polymerases used to copy and amplify the RNA. Other false positives, e.g., a truncated translation product without a detectable mutation at the DNA level, have never been reported.

False negatives in PTT, i.e., the failure to find mutations that are present, potentially have several origins, most frequently the intrinsic property of PCR to favor amplification of shorter products. For example, duplications will be detected only when they are small (below 1-kb exonic sequences), and when the primers used for amplification span the duplicated region. Similarly, insertions will be missed when the incorporated sequences go beyond a given size. Reduced separation of nearly full translation products, and the danger that small products run off the gel, make the end and beginning of each scanned segment critical regions. In segmented sets, these problems can be mostly bypassed by selection of large overlaps. Finally, mutations altering the splicing pattern are not detected when the mutated product increases beyond amplifyable size, e.g., when excision of an intron is abolished. In such cases, even minute levels of normally spliced transcripts yield the normal product, and thus obscure the detection of the altered major transcript and the disease-causing mutation.

Analysis of carrier-derived RNA samples, using PTT, is complicated by the presence of an mRNA molecule from the healthy allele. Consequently, unless it is specifically checked, e.g., using polymorphisms that are present in the coding region, one cannot be sure that transcripts from both alleles were amplified. Furthermore, expression of both alleles may be highly variable, e.g., as a result of nonrandom X-inactivation, positive selection of the healthy allele in somatic tissues, or when the mutated RNA is unstable as a consequence of the mutation itself.

Using RNA templates not derived from a disease-affected tissue, one should realize that the structure, i.e., the exon content, of the RNA may be different between tissues. Consequently, mutations influencing tissue-specific expression, including the use of tissue-specific promoters and tissue-specific splicing, will not be detected. In the case of the dystrophin gene, it should be recognized that blood-derived RNA frequently contains an additional exon X, spliced between exons 1 and 2, which is not present in muscle RNA *(15,16)*. Furthermore, dystrophin mutations have been detected in patients with X-linked dilated cardiomyopathy, which affect transcription in heart and skeletal muscle differently *(17)*, and which may easily remain undetected.

The PTT protocol provided does not detect mutations that affect absolute mRNA levels. The dystrophin gene contains an extensive 2.5-kb 3' untranslated region, which probably contains information regarding the stability of the dystrophin RNA, its turnover time, and its cellular localization. Potentially, mutations affecting these sequences, as well as those that affect poly(A)-addition and transcription termination, are disease-causing. Since they probably yield reduced levels of functional transcripts, they can be expected to have milder phenotypic consequences, and thus may present as BMD.

Finally, RT-PCR and PTT only detect mutations that alter the length of the transcript and/or cause premature translation termination. Amino acid substitutions thus go undetected. For DMD, nearly all mutations identified to date are truncating (*see* http://www.dmd.nl). Few mutations resulting in amino acid substitutions have been reported, and, for most of these, it is debatable if they are really disease-causing. Sequence comparisons between dystrophin, utrophin, and dystrophin-related proteins from a range of organisms have highlighted several regions of (absolute) amino acid sequence conservation ***(18)***. Potentially, these sites are candidates for disease-causing substitution mutations, as above, presumably with milder phenotypic consequences (BMD cases), because they interfere with protein–protein interactions and the proper localization of dystrophin in the muscle cell wall.

6. Discussion

The fact that PTT analysis is the best technique to scan the dystrophin gene for point mutations is examplified best by the report of Gardner et al. ***(12)***, which detected 17 mutations from 22 samples analyzed. PTT analysis of the dystrophin gene was recently simplified significantly by Whittock et al. ***(16)***, reporting a five-fragment PTT multiplex protocol covering the entire coding region (**Fig. 3**). The primers (**Table 2**) were selected so that the RT-PCR and translation products could be clearly recognized as independent fragments. PCR fragments vary between 1.6 and 3.7 kb, and translation products between 66 and 151 kDa (**Fig. 3**). Furthermore, to enable all PCR reactions to be performed under one set of conditions, primers were designed to have a melting temperature of at least 70°C (**Table 2**).

Roberts et al. ***(10)*** have published an alternative RNA-based protocol using chemical mismatch cleavage to detect the mutations. Although the protocol was successful, mutations were found in seven of seven samples analyzed; the high frequency of nondisease-causing sequence variations (polymorphisms) gave many false-positive results. Later, the authors switched to the PTT assay ***(12)***, mostly because it has the intrinsic advantage of revealing truncating, i.e., DMD disease-causing, mutations only.

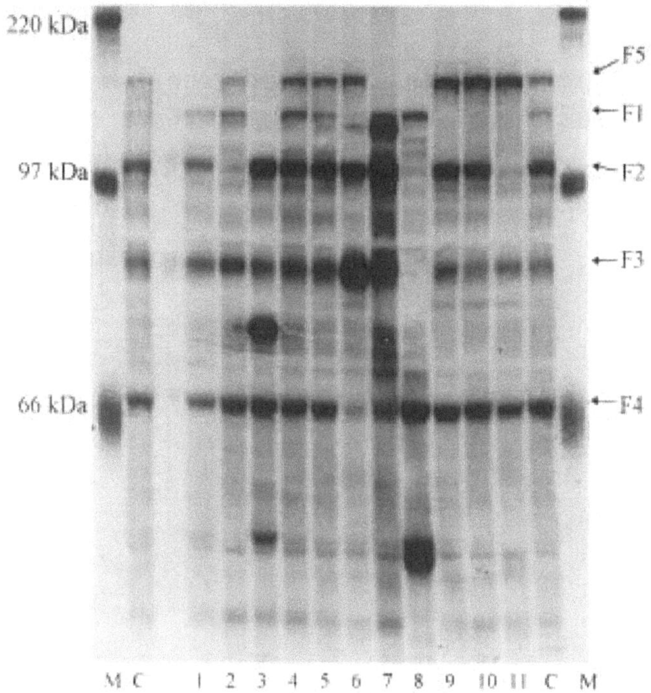

Fig. 3. Multiplex dystrophin PTT according to **ref. *16***. Dystrophin sequences were amplified using the primers given in **Table 2**. C, control sample; F1–F5, dystrophin translation products 1–5; M, protein marker. Lanes 1–11 contain patient samples showing several truncating mutations. PCR conditions can be found at http://www.dmd.nl/ptt.html.

6.1. Dystrophin Point Mutation Detection Using Other Techniques

Several techniques have been applied to detect point mutations, based on the amplification of individual exons of the dystrophin gene, but all had a low success rate, i.e., too few mutations were identified based on the percentage of the dystrophin-coding sequence scanned. The low efficiency in detecting mutations in these studies probably is because a large fraction of those affecting RNA processing are missed, partly because the intron–exon boundaries were not exhaustively analyzed. Several groups have reported mutation analysis of the 18 exons amplified with the two multiplex PCR reactions designed for the deletion detection, using techniques like SSCA, HA, DSCA, CMC, and direct sequencing (for overview, see http://www.dmd.nl/database.html).

Primer design, to cover all exons of the dystrophin gene effectively for mutation screening, was hampered by the fact that about one-half of the exon

Table 2
Primer Sequences for Multiplex Dystrophin PTT

Set	Exons	PCR	Name	Localization	Length	PTT	Sequence
F2		1st	NW1a	7–33	3511		CCCTCACTTTCCCCCTACAGGACTCAG
			NW1b2	3517–349			GGGCTGAATTGTCTGAATATCACTGAC
	1–23	2nd	NW1c	212–238	3272	132	[T7]-CTTTGGTGGGAAGAAGTAGAGGACTGT
	2–23		ExX-T7	242–268	3242	132	[T7]-GAAAGAGAAGATGTTCAAAAGAAAACA
			NW1d2	3483–3457			CTGCACTGTTTCAGCTGCTTTTTTAGA
F3		1st	NW2a	2293–2319	2871		GGTAAAGCATGCTCAAGAGGAACTTCC
			NW2b	5163–5137			TTATCTTCCACCAACGTCTCCTTCTTG
	17–35	2nd	NW2c	2342–2368	2772	112	[T7]-AGGCACATTACTGTGGATTCTGAAATT
			NW2d	5113–5086			CCTACCTCTGTGATACTCTTCAGGTGC
F4		1st	NW3a	4734–4760	2178		ATAAAAGTCTGAGTGAAGTGAAGTCTG
			NW3b	6911–6885			TAGCAATGTTATCTGCTTCCTCCAACC
	33–45	2nd	NW3c	4763–4789	2051	83	[T7]-GTGGAAATGGTGATAAAGACTGGACGT
			NW3d	6813–6787			CTGTCTGACAGCTGTTTGCAGACCTCC
F5		1st	NW4a	6398–6424	1712		CAAAGTGCAACGCCTGTGGAAAGGGTG
			NW4b2	8109–8083			TGCCACTGGCGGAGGTCTTTGGCCAAC
	43–53	2nd	NW4c	6428–6454	1635	66	[T7]-CTACAGGAAGCTCTCTCCCAGCTTGAT
			NW4d2	8062–8036			CTTTTGGATTGCATCTACTGTATAGGG
F1		1st	NW5a2	7487–7513	3842		CTAGCTCCTGGACTGACCACTATTGGA
			NW5b	11,328–11,302			CATGACTGATACTAAGGACTCCATCGC
	51–79	2nd	NW5c2	7520–7546	3744	151	[T7]-CCTACTCAGACTGTTACTCTGGTGACA
			NW5d	11,263–11,237			CATTGTGTCCTCTCTCATTGGCTTTCC

Set, number amplified segment of the dystrophin coding sequence; Exons, exons amplified; PCR, primers to be used in the 1st or 2nd round PCR; Name, primer name, ExX-T7 was designed to avoid amplification of exon X (and a premature stop codon); Localization, primer in relation to the dystrophin cDNA sequence (GenBank M18533); Length, size of amplified fragment (in bp); PTT, length of translation product (in kDa); Sequence, primer sequence, lower case letters indicating added tail sequences; [T7], 5'-ggatcctaatacgactcactataggaacagaccaccATG-3'. Adapted with permisison from **ref. *16*.**

Table 3
Primer Sequences for Amplification of Dystrophin Exons

Exon	Length	Forward primer	Reverse primer	Name
1	535	<u>gaagatc</u>tagacagtggatacataacaaatgcatg	TTCTCCGAAGGTAATTGCCTCCCAGATCTG AGTCC	PmF/R
2	233	cactaacacatcataatgg	gatacacaggtacatagtc	ex2-F/R
3	410	tcatccatcatcttcggcagattaa	caggcggtagagtatgccaaatgaaaatca	ex3-F/R
4	196	ttgtcggtctctctgctggtcagtg	caaagccctcactcaaacatgaagc	ex4-F/R
5	225	caactaggcatttggtctc	ttgtttcacacgtcaaggg	ex5-F/R
6	442	gaatagactcctagccttg	aacggatctggaaccatac	ex6-F2/R2
7	279	gcatggaagtaaatctcatggaac	gtgtagaaatgacaagtctcagatg	ex7-F/R
8	307	tcgtcttcctttaactttg	tcttgaatagtagctgtcc	ex8-F2/R2
9	278	tctatccactcccccaaacc	aacaaaccagctcttcac	ex9-F/R
10	290	gacattaattgtgtaacacc	ggatgacttgccattataac	ex10-F2/R2
11	303	caaaataaaactcaaaaaccacacc	cttccaaaacttgttagtcttc	ex11-F2/R
12	331	gatagtgggctttacttacatccttc	gaaagcacgcaacataagatacacct	ex12-F/R
13	351	gcaaatcatttcaacacac	tctttaaatcacagcacttc	ex13-F2/R2
14 + 15	431	tttgctgatgcttgattgtc	caatagcataggagagactaa	ex14+15-F/R
16	313	gcaaatgagcaaatacacg	ctctgagatagtctgtagcatgat	ex16-F2/R2
17	328	gtgctattttgatctgaagg	aagcttgagatgctctca	ex17-F2/R2
18	255	ggagtctcagattgagaaaagaatg	caagcagcacaaaatgagtacag	ex18-F/R
19	459	gatggcaaaagtgttgagaaaaagtc	ttctaccacatcccattttcttcca	ex19-F/R
20	357	tggctttcagatcatttctttc	aaatacctattgattatgctcc	ex20-F/R
21	319	gcaaaatgtaatgtatgcaaag	atgttagtaccttctggatttc	ex21-F/R
22	>191	caattaagtgattctcattc	gataagcgtgctttattgttttgac	ex22-F2/R
23	423	gtcataactgatagaagatcatc	tttacagtttacagtgtatcgttag	ex23-F/R
24	291	ttgggcctgtgtttagacata	aaatccaccccagctgtaaaa	ex24-F/R
25	258	tgtggcagtaatttttttcag	aggaaatcttagttaagtacg	ex25-F/R
26	299	atgtttcatcactgtcaataacg	ttcaagcattgttgcatttctttc	ex26-F/R

continued

Table 3 *(continued)*

Exon	Length	Forward primer	Reverse primer	Name
27	>260	tttcatgctattaagagagc	aactatgaccatgtattgac	ex27-F2/R2
28	275	gaagttttaataatgaaatggcaaaa	gtacctcttttaatactgcatat	ex28-F/R
29	242	ccaatgtatttagaaaaaaaaggag	gcaaattagattaaagagattttcac	ex29-F/R
30	261	tacagaaaagctatcaagag	caaacaaaaagaatggaagc	ex30-F/R
31	206	gttagttgttctttgtagag	gcccaacgaaaacacgttcc	ex31-F/R
32	265	ggcaaaattaaatcagtgcc	taatgaggaaagtcaagggg	ex30-F2/R2
33	401	tagatattgaccaccgctgc	ttgctaagactctaatcatac	ex33-F/R
34	338	cagaaatataaaagttccaaataagtg	catgttaatacttccttacaaaatc	ex34-F2/R2
35	271	ccgtttcataagcattaaatc	agcttctagccttttctc	ex35-F/R
36	215	tgtctaaccaataatgccatg	ctggtgtacaatttggaca	ex36-F/R
37	314	ctttctcactcttctcgctcac	ttcgcaagagaccatttagcac	ex37-F/R
38	238	ggtttatgtttcttataaaaagtaa	atttatttccactcctagtt	ex38-F/R
39	400	ggattaaagtgtgtgtttaa	accacctcaaaaatgttaaa	ex39-F/R
40	340	ctgcagccagaagtgcacta	ggaaatgcatccctcaaaga	ex40-F/R
41	274	gttagctaactgccctgggccctgtattg	tagagtagtagttgcaaacacatacgtgg	ex41-F/R
42	155	CACACTGTCCGTGAAGAAA CGATGATGG	CTTCAGAGACTCCTCTTGCTTAAAGAGAT	ex42-F/R
43	320	tgcaacaccatttgctacc	atcatttctgcaagtatcaag	ex43-F2/R2
44	268	cttgatccatatgcttttacctgca	tccatcacccttcagaacctgatct	ex44-F/R
45	547	aaacatggaacatccttgtggggac	cattcctattagatctgtcgccctac	ex45-F/R
46	373	ccagtttgcattaacaaatagtttgag	agggttaagaagaaataaagttgtgag	ex46-F2/R2
47	363	tgatagactaatcaatagaagcaaagac	aacaaaacaaaacaacaatccacatacc	ex47-F2/R2
48	506	ttgaatacattggttaaatcccaacatg	cctgaataaagtcttccttaccacac	ex48-F/R
49	439	gtgcccttatgtaccaggcagaaattg	gcaatgactcgttaatagccttaagatc	ex49-F/R
50	271	caccaaatggattaagatgttcatgaat	tctctctcacccagtcatcacttcatag	ex50-F/R
51	388	gaaattggctctttagcttgtgtttc	ggagagtaaagtgattggtggaaaatc	ex51-F/R
52	>160	gaagaaccctgatactaagg	catcttgctttgtgtgtccc	ex52-F2/R2

53	212	tcctccagactagcatttac	ttagcctgggtgacagtg	ex53-F2/R2
54	450	gtttgtcctgaaaggtgggttac	ttatcgtcttgaaccctcccaag	ex54-F/R
55	408	aatttagttcctccatctttctct	aaatacatcaggctgtataaaagc	ex55-F/R
56	337	tttctttrgtaattctgc	ctgaaattgggatgatttac	ex56-F2/R
57	258	gatattctgacatggatcgc	gtcactggattactatgtgc	ex57-F/R2
58	280	ttttgagaagaatgccacaagcc	aaaatatgagagctatccagacc	ex58-F2/R2
59	374	actctttctttcttccagtatgacc	gtaaagaagtagaccgtacCTTGAC	ex59-F2/R2
60	231	taaatattctcatcttccaatttgc	ttactgtaacaaaggacaacaatg	ex60-F2/R2
61	163	aatgagagaacataatttctctcc	aatcaagatgcaataaagttaagtg	ex61-F2/R2
62	185	taatgttgtctttcctgtttgcg	atacaggttagtcacaataaatgc	ex62-F/R
63	194	tactcatggtaaatgctaaagtc	tagcaaagtaactttcacactgc	ex63-F/R
64	180	ttctgatggaataacaaatgct	cattctaggcaaactctaggc	ex64-F/R3
65	347	tatgagagagtcctagctagg	taagcctcctgtgacagagc	ex65-F/R
66	211	gtctagtaattgttttctgctttg	ataagaacagtctgtcatttccc	ex66-F2/R2
67	286	aattgctactggaattgagttgg	aagaataaatatgttacctagaagg	ex67-F/R
68	352	taatcgaactgatatacacctcc	actaacagcaactggcacagg	ex68-F/R
69	231	gaacgtggtagaaggtttattaaa	ctaactctcacgtcaggctg	ex69-F/R
70	237	tggtcattagttttgaaatcatc	catcaaacaagagtgtgttctg	ex70-F/R
71	125	aaagcgtgtgtctccttcacc	atgtgttggtggtagcagcac	ex71-F/R
72	144	gatggtatctgtgactaatcac	atttcaatcaatatttgcctggc	ex72-F/R
73	202	acgtcacataagttttaatgagc	atgctaattcctatatcctgtgc	ex73-F/R
74	248	accaaaacctttgattttattttcc	tttctatgtgtgcaagtgtatgc	ex74-F/R
75	344	tcttttttactttttgatgc	agtgctctctgaggtttag	ex75-F/R
76	198	gtaattctgtttcttttggatgac	ctacctttcttcagacaacaaaat	ex76-F/R
77	270	taatcatggccctttaatatctg	gatactgcgtgttggcttcc	ex77-F/R
78	220	ttctgatatctctgcctcttcc	aatgagctgcaagtggagagg	ex78-F/R
79	349	agagtgatgctatctatctgcac	TGCATAGACGTGTAAAACCTGCC	ex79-F/R

Primer sequences (listed from 5' to 3') and relevant references can be found at http://www.dmd.nl/exonprim.html. All primer sequences are intronic, except those in capitals, which are exonic, and those underlined, which are tails added at the 5' end.

sequences were not present in the GenBank database. The author has nearly completed the set of dystrophin exon sequences by collecting unpublished sequences, by extending the shortest intronic segments, and by sequencing of the missing intron–exon boundaries *(4)*. **Table 3** shows a list of primer sequences to amplify all dystrophin exons. Using this list, amplified products can be generated to scan the entire dystrophin gene for point mutations, using the detection techniques mentioned. In collaboration with another Dutch group (Hofstra and Buys, Department of Medical Genetics, Groningen University), we are currently designing a denaturing gradient gel electrophoresis-based mutation scan of the entire dystrophin gene (for details see http://www.dmd.nl).

7. Acknowledgments

The author thanks S. Abbs for providing the details, primer sequences, and photograph (**Fig. 3**) of the dystrophin multiplex PTT. Unpublished dystrophin sequences used for primer design were provided by A. Beggs, J. Chamberlain, C. Oudet, and R. Worton (see http://www.dmd.nl/seqlist.html). The research performed to develop the protein truncation test was facilitated by grants from the Praeventiefonds (the Netherlands), Prinses Beatrix Fonds (the Netherlands), and the Muscular Dystrophy Group of Great Britain and Northern Ireland.

References

1. Monaco, A. P., Neve, R. L., Colletti-Feener, C., Bertelson, C. J., Kurnit, D. M., and Kunkel, L. M. (1986) Isolation of candidate cDNAs for portions of the Duchenne muscular dystrophy gene. *Nature* **323,** 646–650.
2. Koenig, M., Hoffman, E. P., Bertelson, C. J., Monaco, A. P., Feener, C. A., and Kunkel, L. M. (1987) Complete cloning of the Duchenne muscular dystrophy (DMD) cDNA and preliminary genomic organization of the DMD gene in normal and affected individuals. *Cell* **50,** 509–517.
3. Den Dunnen, J. T., Grootscholten, P. M., Bakker, E., Blonden, L. A. J., Ginjaar, H. B., Wapenaar, M. C., Van Paassen, H. M. B., et al. (1989) Topography of the DMD gene: FIGE and cDNA analysis of 194 cases reveals 115 deletions and 13 duplications. *Am. J. Hum. Genet.* **45,** 835–847.
4. Den Dunnen, J. T. and Bakker, E. (1997) The Leiden Muscular Dystrophy data pages. *http://www.dmd.nl/.*
5. Chamberlain, J. S., Gibbs, R. A., Ranier, J. E., Nga Nguyen, P. N., and Caskey, C. T. (1988) Deletion screening of the Duchenne muscular dystrophy locus via multiplex DNA amplification. *Nucl. Acids Res.* **23,** 11,141–11,156.
6. Beggs, A. H., Koenig, M., Boyce, F. M., and Kunkel, L. M. (1990) Detection of 98-percent DMD/BMD gene deletions by polymerase chain reaction. *Hum. Genet.* **86,** 45–48.
7. Hu, X., Ray, P. N., Murphy, E., Thompson, M. W., and Worton, R. G. (1990) Duplicational mutation at the Duchenne muscular dystrophy locus: its frequency, distribution, origin and phenotype/genotype correlation. *Am. J. Hum. Genet.* **46,** 682–695.

8. Abbs, S. J., Roberts, R. G., Mathew, C. G., Bentley, D. R., and Bobrow, M. (1990) Accurate assessment of intragenic recombination frequency within the Duchenne muscular dystrophy gene. *Genomics* **7,** 602–606.
9. Nigro, V., Nigro, G., Esposito, M. G., Comi, L. I., Molinari, A. M., Puca, G. A., and Politano, L. (1994) Novel small mutations along the DMD/BMD gene associated with different phenotypes. *Hum. Mol. Genet.* **3,** 1907–1908.
10. Roberts, R. G., Bobrow, M., and Bentley, D. R. (1992) Point mutations in the dystrophin gene. *Proc. Natl. Acad. Sci. USA* **89,** 2331–2335.
11. Roest, P. A. M., Roberts, R. G., Sugino, S., Van Ommen, G. J. B., and Den Dunnen, J. T. (1993) Protein truncation test (PTT) for rapid detection of translation-terminating mutations. *Hum. Mol. Genet.* **2,** 1719–1721.
12. Gardner, R. J., Bobrow, M., and Roberts, R. G. (1995) The identification of point mutations in Duchenne muscular dystrophy patients using reverse transcript PCR and the protein truncation test. *Am. J. Hum. Genet.* **57,** 311–320.
13. Carter, M. S., Doskow, J., Morris, P., Li, S., Nhim, R. P., Sandstedt, S., and Wilkinson, M. F. (1995) A regulatory mechanism that detects premature nonsense codons in T-cell receptor transcripts in vivo is reversed by protein synthesis inhibitors in vitro. *J. Biol. Chem.* **270,** 28,995–29,003.
14. Rowan, A. J. and Bodmer, W. F. (1997) Introduction of a myc reporter tag to improve the quality of mutation detection using the protein truncation test. *Hum. Mutat.* **9,** 172–176.
15. Roberts, R. G., Bentley, D. R., and Bobrow, M. (1993) Infidelity in the structure of ectopic transcripts: a novel exon in lymphocyte dystrophin transcripts. *Hum. Mutat.* **2,** 293–299.
16. Whittock, N. V., Roberts, R. G., Mathew, C. G., and Abbs, S. J. (1997) Dystrophin point mutation screening using a multiplexed Protein Truncation Test. *Genet. Testing* **1,** 115–123.
17. Milasin, J., Muntoni, F., Severini, G. M., Bartoloni, L., Vatta, M., Krajinovic, M., et al. (1996) A point mutation in the 5' splice site of the dystrophin gene first intron responsible for x linked dilated cardiomyopathy. *Hum. Mol. Genet.* **5,** 73–79.
18. Roberts, R. G. and Bobrow, M. (1998) Dystrophins in vertebrates and invertebrates. *Hum. Mol. Genet.* **7,** 589–595.
19. Roest, P. A. M., Roberts, R. G., Van Der Tuijn, A. C., Heikoop, J. C., Van Ommen, G. J. B., and Den Dunnen, J. T. (1993) Protein truncation test (PTT) to rapidly screen the DMD-gene for translation-terminating mutations. *Neuromusc. Disord.* **3,** 391–394.
20. Roest, P. A. M., Bout, M., Van Der Tuijn, A. C., Ginjaar, H. B., Bakker, E., Hogervorst, F. B. L., Van Ommen, G. J. B., and Den Dunnen, J. T. (1996) Splicing mutations in DMD/BMD detected by RT-PCR/PTT: detection of a 19AA insertion in the cysteine-rich domain of dystrophin compatible with BMD. *J. Med. Genet.* **33,** 935–939.

7

DNA-Based Techniques for Detection of Carriers of Duchenne and Becker Muscular Dystrophy

Egbert Bakker

1. Introduction

Duchenne muscular dystrophy (DMD) is the most frequent muscle disease in children. The incidence of DMD is 1/4000 live-born males; one-third of the patients are the result of new mutation. DMD, a progressive, lethal, X-linked neuromuscular disorder, and its milder, less-frequently occurring allelic variant, Becker muscular dystrophy (BMD), are caused by defects in the dystrophin gene, located on the X chromosome (Xp21), which is, with 2.4 Mb of the genomic sequence, the largest human gene known to date. It harbors 79 exons, which together produce a 14-kb transcript (mRNA) and code for a 427-kDa protein called dystrophin, a muscle-specific protein, which is located underneath the sarcolemma membrane. In DMD, patients' dystrophin is absent, except for an occasional revertant, dystrophin-positive fiber (< 3%). In BMD patients' muscle cells, the dystrophin protein is reduced and less functional than in normal muscle cells (*see also* Chapter 3).

In both DMD and BMD, partial deletions of the dystrophin gene occur in approx 60% of cases; duplications are detected in 5% of cases. Both deletions and duplications cluster in two recombination hot spots, one proximal and one central in the dystrophin gene (*1*; *see* Chapter 5). Site and size of these mutations are very heterogeneous. DNA analysis by Southern blot and cDNA probe hybridizations enable detection of both partial deletions and duplications in DMD/BMD *(1–3)*. Frameshifting mutations generally cause DMD; in BMD, the reading frame of the gene is usually intact. This frame-shift model complies with the phenotype in 92% of cases *(4)*. In the 35% of cases, in which no deletion or duplication is detected, microlesions, such as point mutations, are likely to be found. However, microlesions are more difficult to find in the large dystrophin

From: *Methods in Molecular Medicine, vol. 43: Muscular Dystrophy: Methods and Protocols*
Edited by: K. M. D. Bushby and L. V. B. Anderson

gene, because they do not seem to cluster in certain regions of the gene. Because this type of analysis is far from routine in most diagnostic laboratories (*5*; Chapter 6), microsatellite markers are used to reconstruct the affected, or at risk, haplotype.

1.1. Carrier Detection

Female relatives of DMD and BMD patients are at risk of carrying the gene defect and transmitting the disorder to half their sons. Mothers, sisters, nieces, aunts, and cousins of DMD patients often request genetic counseling and genetic testing, because this disease is incurable, severely disabling, and a cause of early death. The first question to answer, in such cases, is how reliable is the diagnosis of the index case? To verify if the diagnosis DMD or BMD has been established correctly, one could check if it meets the diagnostic criteria for DMD/BMD *(6)*. Strongly elevated creatine kinases, and absence of dystrophin on a muscle section, are powerful tools to establish the clinical diagnosis of DMD. Often, molecular genetic analysis, such as multiplex polymerase chain reaction (PCR) (*see also* Chapter 5), has been performed in parallel, to identify a deletion in the dystrophin gene. In 35% of cases, in which no gross rearrangement is detected, linkage analysis using microsatellite markers is applied to identify the at-risk or affected X-haplotype. Deletion/duplication mutation detection by quantitative Southern blotting and hybridization with cDNA probes or linkage (haplotype) analysis, by use of the many polymorphic markers in the dystrophin gene, facilitate carrier detection and prenatal diagnosis *(7)*. The techniques of quantitative Southern blot and haplotype analysis are described more extensively below.

2. Materials

2.1. Southern Blotting Reagents

2.1.1. General

1. Filter paper.
2. GB002 Filter paper (Schleicher and Schuell).
3. GB003 Filter paper (Schleicher and Schuell, no. 10426892).
4. Hybond N^+ membrane (Amersham).
5. Paper towels.
6. Plastic trays (20 × 16 cm).

Note: Equivalent consumables may be used.

2.1.2. Chemicals

1. 5 g Bromophenol blue (sodium salt) (Sigma, no. B7021).
2. 10 mL (10 mg/mL) Ethidium bromide (EtBr) (Amersham Pharmacia Biotech, no. 17-1328-01).

3. 500 g Multipurpose agarose (Boehringer, no. 1388991).
4. Sodium dodecyl sulfate (SDS) (USB).
5. Sodium hydroxide (NaOH) Baker).
6. Sodium chloride (NaCl) (Baker).
7. 1 g Spermidine (Sigma, no. S 0266).
8. Sucrose (BDH, London).

Note: Equivalent chemicals may be used.

2.1.3. Solutions

1. 0.5 *M* Ethylenediamine tetra aacetic acid (EDTA), pH 8.0 (Life Technologies, no. 15575-012).
2. 10X Tris-acetate EDTA (TAE) buffer (Life Technologies, no. 15558-034).
3. 10X Tris-borate EDTA (TBE) buffer (Life Technologies, no. 15581-028).
4. 1 *M* Tris-HCl, pH 7.5 (Life Technologies, no. 15567-019).
5. 1X TBE buffer/0.2 mg/L EtBr for 5 L: Dilute 0.5 L 10X TBE to 5 L with MilliQ water (Bedford, MA). Add 100 μL EtBr (10 mg/mL), and mix on a magnetic stirrer. Store at room temperature (RT).
6. 1X TAE for 2 L: Dilute 200 mL 10X TAE to 2 L with MilliQ water. Store at RT.
7. 1X TAE/0.2 mg/L EtBr for 5 L: Dilute 0.5 L 10X TAE to 5 L with MilliQ water. Add 100 μL EtBr (10 mg/mL), and mix on a magnetic stirrer. Store at RT.
8. 1X TBE for 2 L: Dilute 200 mL to 2 L with MilliQ water. Store at RT.
9. 10X Sucrose loading mix (SLM) for 100 mL: Dissolve 40 g sucrose in 20 mL MilliQ water, add 10 mL 10% SDS, 20 mL 0.5 *M* EDTA, and 10 mL 1 *M* Tris-HCl, pH 7.5, add MilliQ water to 100 mL and add 250 mg bromophenol blue.
10. 10% SDS (Life Technologies, no. 15553-019). 2X SLM for 100 mL: Dilute 20 mL 10X SLM to 100 mL with MilliQ water. Store at RT.
11. 2X standard sodium citrate (SSC)/0.2 *M* Tris, pH 7.5, for 2 L: Add to 1400 mL MilliQ water 200 mL 20X SSC and 400 mL 1 *M* Tris, pH 7.5. The solution can be stored for 1 mo at RT.
12. 20X SSC (Life Technologies, no. 15557-028).
13. Alkali solution 1 (0.4 *N* NaOH) for 5 L: Add MilliQ water to 80 g NaOH, to a total volume of 5 L. Dissolve on a magnetic stirrer for at least 15 min. Prepare fresh before use. For one gel, prepare half the amount.
14. Alkali solution 2 (0.4 *N* NaOH/0.6 *M* NaCl) for 5 L: Add MilliQ water to 80 g NaOH and 175.3 g NaCl, to a total vol of 5 L. Dissolve on a magnetic stirrer for at least 15 min. Prepare fresh before use. For one gel, prepare half the amount.
15. One Phor All Buffer Plus (OPA+), Amersham Pharmacia Biotech.

2.2. Short Tandem Repeat Protocol Reagents

2.2.1. General

1. Cassette 35 × 43 cm, Auto G (Konica, no. 1190 1090).
2. 14 cm Vinyl Sharktooth comb (Life Technologies, no. 21045-018).

3. 0.4 mm comb STS45,64 wells (Micronic, no. IB 80110).
4. Electrophoresis Constant Power Supply (Amersham Pharmacia Biotech, no. ECPS 3000/150).
5. Heatblock, Unitek HB-130 (Biozym, Hermeln, Germany).
6. Hooked spacer (Promega,).
7. 35 × 43 cm intensifying screen, Blue Regular (Konica, no. 1180 2190).
8. Vacuubrand pump (Dijkstra Vereenigde, no. MZ 2C).
9. Vacuubrand, pump carrier (Dijkstra Vereenigde, no. MZ 2).
10. Slab gel dryer (Pharmacia Biotech, model SE 1160).
11. Sequencing Gel Electrophoresis Apparatus (Life Technologies, model S2, 21105-036).
12. Spacer foam blocks (Life Technologies, no. 21965-017).
13. 0.4 mm Spacerset STC (Micronic, no. IB 80440).
14. 0.4 mm spacer set (Life Technologies, no. 21108-014).

2.2.2. Chemicals

1. Ammonium persulfate (APS).
2. 99–100% Acetic acid, p.a.
3. Bromophenol blue (Sigma, no. B5525).
4. Dimethyldichlorosilane in 1,1,1-trichloroethane (Repel silane) (Promega, no. H5101).
5. Formamide p.a.
6. Methanol c/z.
7. *N,N,N',N'*-Tetramethylethylenediamine (TEMED), 1 × 25 mL (Promega, no. V3161).
8. Sodium acetate (NaAc) p.a.
9. Xylene cyanol (Sigma, no. X4126).

2.2.3. Solutions

1. Size markers, M13 sequence ladder.
2. 3 *M* NaAc, for 2 L: Dissolve 816.4 g NaAc in 1 L MilliQ water in a glass beaker. Adjust the volume to 2 L with Elga water. Store at RT.
3. Acrylamide/*bis*-acryl sequencing solution (Life Technologies, no. 10324-010).
4. 10% APS, for 10 mL: Dissolve 1 g APS in 10 mL MilliQ water in a black-capped tube. Store this solution for a maximum of 1 mo at 4°C.
5. EDTA, 0.5 *M*, pH 8.0 (Life Technologies, no. 15575-012).
6. 10X TBE buffer (Life Technologies, no. 15581-028).
7. 0.5X TBE, for 5 L: Dilute 250 mL 10X TBE buffer to 5 L with MilliQ water in the plastic container. Store at RT.
8. 0.83X TBE, 0.5 *M* NaAc for 5 L: Add 417 mL 10X TBE and 833 mL 3 *M* NaAc to 2 L of MilliQ water. Adjust the volume to 5 L. Store at RT.
9. 5% Methanol, 5% acetic acid for 5 L: Add, in the fume cupboard, 250 mL methanol and 250 mL acetic acid to 4.5 L of MilliQ water. Store at RT.
10. 10% Methanol, 10% acetic acid for 2 L: Add 200 mL methanol and 200 mL acetic acid to 1600 mL MilliQ water (work in the fume cupboard). Store at RT.

3. Methods

3.1. Quantitative Southern Blot

If no deletion is detected by the multiplex PCRs, or if no DNA of the male patient is available, a set of three pairs of screening blots is prepared using *Hin*dIII and *Bgl*II, to speed up the screening procedure to a total of three rounds of simultaneous hybridization with three of 10 cDNA probes. Furthermore the cDNA probes 63-1/1 and 63-1/2 can be hybridized together: This also holds for the cDNA probes 63-1/3 and 63-1/4. In addition to patient DNA samples (if no male patient is available, DNA of one obligate or possible carrier per family is used) to be tested, DNA of a control person is added on each blot to act as a normal reference for the cDNA bands.

If DNA is available from the male patient and a deletion is detected by use of the multiplex PCR technique, or a duplication had been previously detected, quantitative Southern blotting will enable both determination of the full extend of the deletion and carrier detection for female relatives. For these tests, two so-called family blots are prepared. A family blot ideally contains DNA of the following individuals: one healthy female, the female counselee(s), a proven carrier for the deletion/duplication, and/or the patient. Total genomic DNA is digested by use of the restriction enzymes *Hin*dIII and *Bgl*II.

Together, the 10 cDNA probes detect all 79 exons of the dystrophin gene *(8)*. Some of these probes detect overlap. For *Hin*dIII, the normal restriction pattern of all 79 exons is known, for *Bgl*II, the majority of the bands are known: This facilitates the correct interpretation of the autorads (**Table 1**; **Fig. 1**).

If a deletion or duplication starts or ends within a *Bgl*II or *Hin*dIII exon fragment, an altered-size fragment (a so-called "junction fragment") will be detected. A new band will show up, or, if the altered band co-migrates with an existing band, an intensity difference will be detected (*see also* **Subheading 3.1.10.**).

The restriction enzyme digestion of genomic DNA is followed by agarose gel electrophoresis and Southern blotting. The genomic DNA used in this protocol is isolated from total blood, according to Miller et al. *(9; see also* Chapter 18). The concentration of the DNA is measured at OD260. Five μg of each DNA sample is digested by one or more restriction enzymes. After incubation, all samples are tested for complete digestion, if needed, an additional incubation step is performed.

The DNA fragments are separated according to size on an agarose gel, by use of an electric field applied across the gel. At neutral pH, the DNA fragments have a negative charge, and will therefore migrate toward the anode. The DNA fragments are separated according to their size: The smaller fragments will migrate faster through the gel than the larger fragments.

Table 1
Dystrophin cDNA Probes

CDNA probe	Exon	Insert releasing enzyme sites	Insert fragment (kb)	Band no.
XJ10	1–16	*Eco*RI	2.1	2
30–2	11–20	*Eco*RI	1.15	2
30–1	21–31	*Eco*RI	1.95	2
47–4	31–47	*Eco*RI/*Xba*I	1.35 + 1.15	2 + 3
7b8	44–52	*Bgl*I/Pst I/*Hae*III	1.5	1
63.1/1	53–58	*Eco*RI/*Bam*HI/*Bgl* II	1.2	2
63.1/2	59–65	*Eco*RI/*Bam*HI/*Bgl* II	0.75	4
63.1/3	66–74	*Eco*RI/*Bam*HI/*Bgl* II	0.9	3
63.1/4	75–78	*Eco*RI/*Bam*HI/*Bgl* II	0.35	5
63.1/c	79	*Xba*I	2.0	3

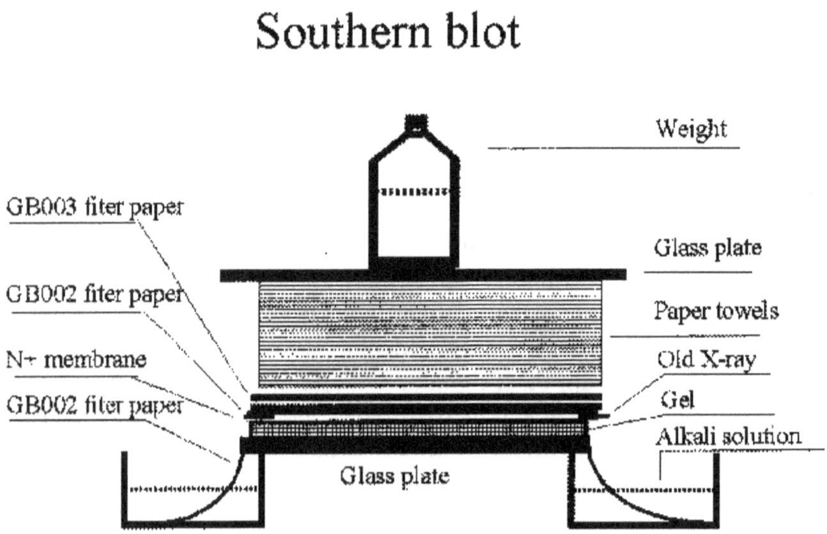

Fig. 1. Diagram of a Southern Blot, complete with those materials needed for preparation and process.

DNA fragments are denatured and transferred from the gel onto a nylon membrane (Southern blotting), using an alkali solution. After alkali blotting, the DNA fragments are bound to the membrane, and hybridization with a ^{32}P radiolabeled probe is used to detect specific fragments.

Based on a digestion of 5 µg genomic DNA, which is enough for one lane on the blot gel, the complete procedure takes 3 d.

3.1.1. Restriction Enzyme Digestion of Genomic DNA (d 1)

1. Determine the concentration (OD260) of each DNA sample to be tested, and calculate the volume in µL 5 µg.
2. First, pipet the amount of water into each tube (in µL) that you must add to get a volume (DNA + water) of 23 µL (or a multiple amount).
3. Add 1 µL spermidine and 3 µL 10X OPA + buffer (Pharmacia), or the buffer specific to the restriction enzyme, to each tube.
4. Add the calculated volume of each DNA sample. Use a new tip for every DNA sample. The total volume is 27 µL, or a multiple thereof.
5. Incubate 30 min in the 65°C incubator. Cool down to RT, and add 15 U (3 U for each µg of DNA) of restriction enzyme. Never add more enzyme than 10% of the total volume; glycerol inhibits enzyme activity.
6. Mix carefully, and spin down 5–10 s in the Eppendorf centrifuge.
7. Incubate overnight in the 37°C incubator.

Note: For some enzymes, different incubation temperatures are used.

3.1.2. Preparation of a Test Gel

For this gel, the Owl electrophoresis system is used, and a gel is casted in the casting tray.

1. Prepare a 0.8% agarose (MP from Boehringer Mannheim) test gel in 1X TBE buffer: Add 2.8 g agarose to 350 mL 1X TBE buffer in an Erlenmeyer, and mix.
2. Heat the mixture until the agarose is dissolved and the solution is boiling. Shake the mixture gently during the heating process to homogenize.
3. Add water to a final volume of 350 mL, and add 15 µL EtBr (10 mg/mL), and mix by gentle shaking.
4. Pour the melted agarose into the tray. The agarose should be allowed to cool to approx 60°C before pouring into the tray, by keeping the Erlenmeyer under running tap water.
5. Once the agarose has been poured, insert three combs (28 wells) in the grooves, at equal distances in the gel.
6. When the gel has solidified (30–45 min), lift the end gates from the chamber.
7. Place the gel tray in the buffer chamber filled with electrophoresis buffer (1X TBE–EtBr). Carefully remove the combs; to avoid damaging the wells, lift the comb straight up.

3.1.3. Preparation and Electrophoresis of Samples

1. Add 1.5 µL digested DNA# to 10 µL 2X SLM in a microtiter dish.
2. Load the samples on the gel, and run for 1–2 h at 100–150 V.
3. Make a photo of the gel, using a Polaroid camera or other gel-photo system.
4. Mark the slots on the photo, and write down the DNA numbers. Look critically to see whether all digestions are complete (*see* **Notes 1–3**). Record all additional steps performed.

3.1.4. Preparation of 20 × 25-cm Blot Gel

For this gel, the Owl electrophoresis system is used, and a gel is cast in the casting tray.

1. Pour a 0.7% agarose blot gel into 1X TAE buffer.
2. Preparation of a 0.7% agarose blot gel in 1X TAE-buffer: add 2.45 g agarose to 350 mL 1X TAE buffer in an Erlenmeyer, and mix.
3. Heat the mixture until the agarose is dissolved and the solution is boiling. Shake the mixture gently during the heating process to homogenize.
4. Add Elga water to 350 mL and 15 µL EtBr (10 mg/mL), and mix by gentle shaking.
5. The agarose should be allowed to cool to approx 60°C before pouring into the tray, by keeping the Erlenmeyer under cold running tap water. Pour the melted agarose into the tray.
6. Once the agarose has been poured, insert one comb (24 wells) in the groove, approx 2 cm from the top of the gel.
7. Once the gel has solidified (30–45 min), lift the end gates out of the chamber.
8. Place the gel tray in the buffer chamber filled with electrophoresis buffer (1X TAE–EtBr). Carefully remove the comb; to avoid damaging the wells, lift the comb straight up.
9. Heat the 10X SLM by keeping the tube under running hot tap water, to make it completely fluid. Add to the digested DNA samples (about 25 µL) 3 µL 10X SLM, and mix gently by pipeting up and down.
10. Load 25 µL of the sample into each slot. Write down the order in which the samples are loaded. Electrophorese overnight (12–16 h) at 40–50 V. A 2X overnight electrophoresis is performed in the case of specific enzymes.

3.1.5. Southern Blotting of the Gel (see also **Fig. 2**)

1. Prepare a fresh alkali solution for every blot. Alkali solution 1 is used to transfer the DNA, within 4–6 h, to the membrane. Alkali solution 2 is used in case of an overnight blotting procedure.
2. Clean all the glass plates and trays with water.
3. Put the gel on the UV transilluminator. Clean it with water before and after putting the gel on the transilluminator.
4. Cut the gel to the correct size (just above the slots, and just around the DNA).
5. Make a photo of the gel.
6. Turn the gel upside down between two glass plates.
7. Denature the gel 2× 15 min in the alkali solution, under gentle agitation.
8. Refresh the solution after 15 min. In the meantime, prepare everything needed for blotting.
9. Cut the following to size:
   a. Two GB002 papers 35 × 19 cm.
   b. One GB002 paper 19 × 20 cm.

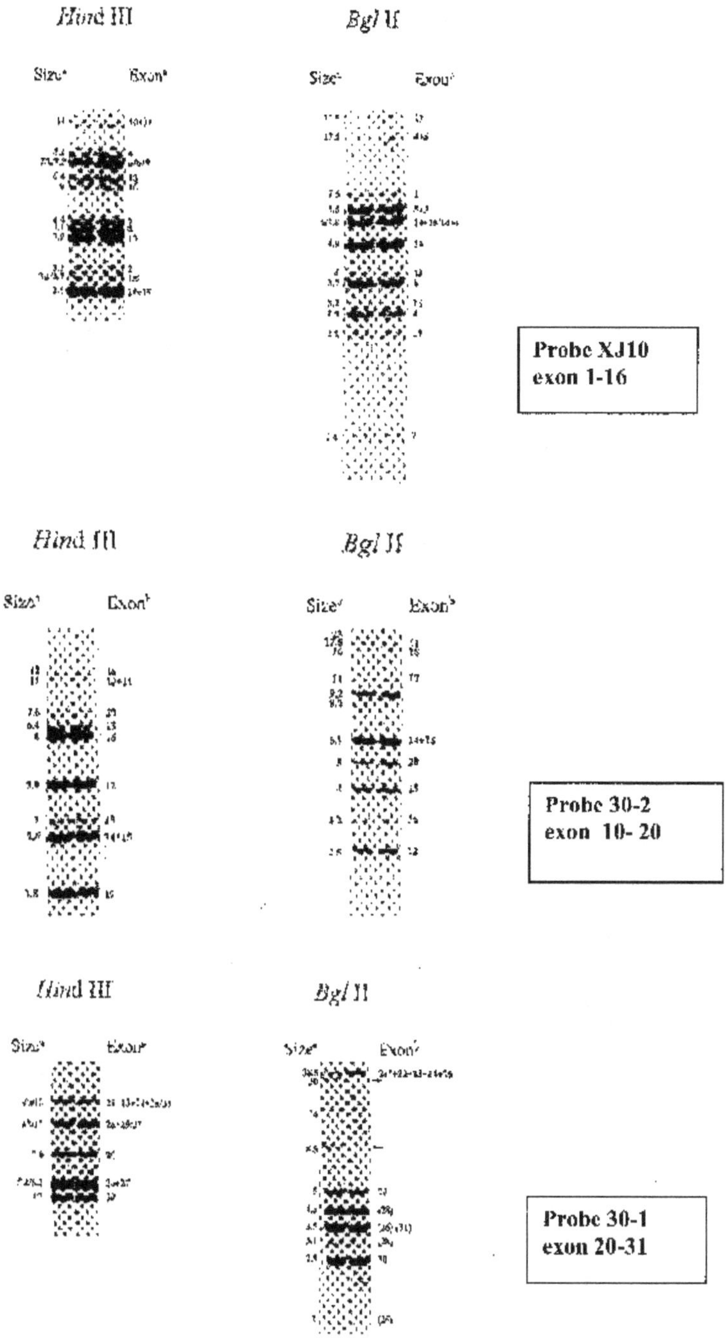

Fig. 2. *(this page and next two pages)* Example autoradiographs of cDNA blots after hybridization with the different cDNA probes. The bands are indicated according to their size (left, kb) and exon (right, exon number).

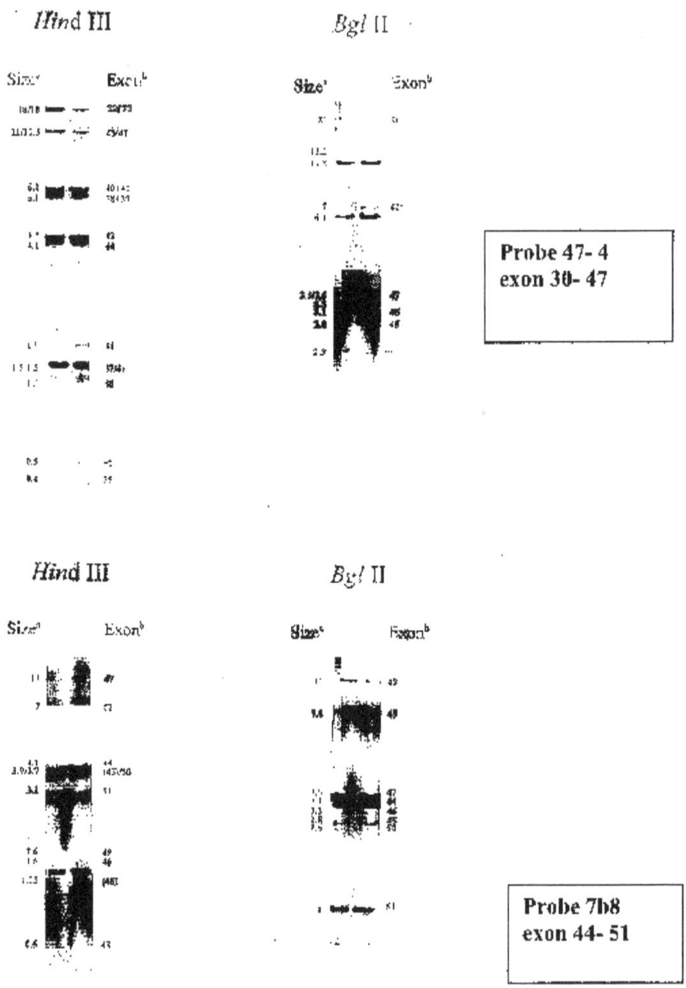

Fig. 2. (continued)

c. One Hybond N+ membrane (Amersham) 1 cm larger than the gel. With a black pen, mark the membrane with the date, and number of the gel (if more than one gel is blotted). Put water in a tray, and soak the membrane in it, then pour off the water, and leave the membrane in alkali solution for at least 5 min.
d. One GB002 paper, the same size as the gel.
e. One GB003 paper, the same size as the gel.

10. Start to build the blotting tower (*see also* **Fig. 1**): Put a glass plate on top of two plastic trays (20×16 cm), which contain the alkali solution.

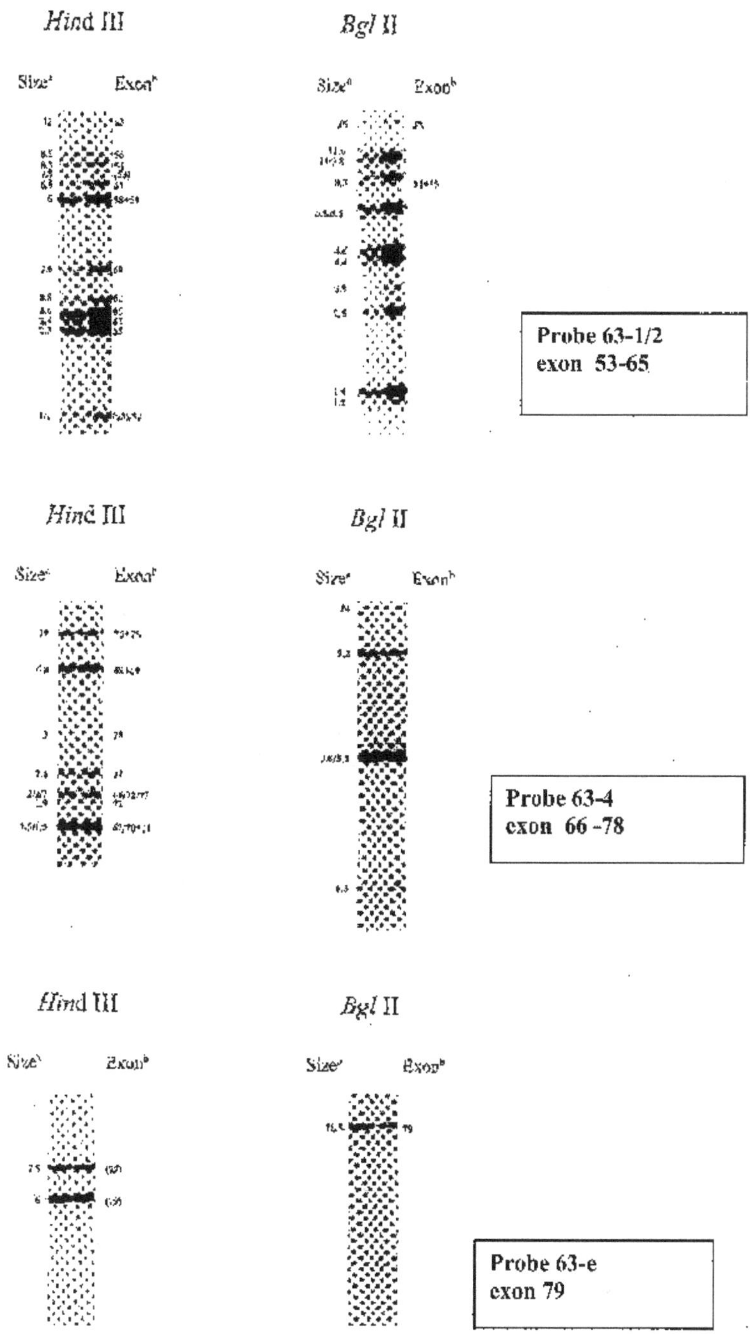

Fig. 2. (continued)

11. Soak the GB002 paper (20 × 19 cm) in the alkali solution, and put it on the other papers.
12. Add alkali solution to soak the paper bridge completely.
13. Put the denatured gel, still upside down, on a glass plate, and transfer it carefully to the GB002 paper bridge (be careful with a 0.5% gel).
14. Put slices of old X-ray film around and just under the edges of the gel, to ensure a capillary flow through the gel to the membrane.
15. Add alkali solution to soak the gel completely.
16. Put the membrane on the gel, with a marked corner to show the gel's orientation.
17. Soak the GB002 and the GB003 papers (with the same size as the gel) together in alkali solution, and put them on the membrane.
18. Fold paper towels or cellulose napkins (Uthermohlen) to about the same size as the gel. Make a pile about 10 cm high, and put this on the blotting tower.
19. Place a glass plate, together with a weight of about 250 g, on top. Do not use a weight when a 0.5% agarose gel is blotted.
20. Blotting takes place in 4–6 h (with alkali solution 1) or overnight (with alkali solution 2).
21. After blotting, remove the weight, glass plate, paper towels, and papers, and neutralize the membrane in 2X SSC/0.2 *M* Tris, pH 7.5, for 1–5 min, and dry it between filter paper.
22. Check the membrane for correct blotting and possible introduction of air bubbles, using an UV transilluminator. Cover it with Saran Wrap to protect the membrane. Mark all empty lanes and, if possible, the slots on the DNA side of the membrane. Check this with the Polaroid or print-out of the blot gel, before cutting the membrane.
23. Cut the membrane to the correct size for hybridization, and write on each piece the date, the enzyme, and the DNA numbers, with a black pen, on the DNA side.
24. Membranes (also called filters) are now ready for hybridization. Store the dried membranes at RT in envelopes ordered, e.g., by date.
25. Throw away remaining alkali solutions, the blotted gel, and all paper used in the procedure. Rinse the glass plates and trays with water, to remove all alkali solution. Clean the table with water.

3.1.6. Probe Preparation (d 3)

With a total of 10 dystrophin cDNA clones, all 79 exons of the dystrophin gene can be detected. The insert of the plasmid is released from the vector by use of restriction digestion (*see* **Table 1**). Alternatively, one could amplify the insert from the cDNA plasmid by use of primers specific for the plasmid used.

1. Label 1–10 ng insert cDNA with α [^{32}P-deoxycytidine triphosphate (dCTP), by use of the random priming hexanucleotide kit (Multi-prime Kit, Amersham).
2. The specific activity of the labeled probe should be >1 × 10^8 dps/s.

All hybridizations are carried out in plastic trays/containers, positioned in a gently shaking (GLF) water bath. Alternatively, glass bottles in rotating hybridization ovens may be used.

3.1.7. Prehybridization

1. Prehybridization of the dried membranes (filters) is carried out in a volume of 25 mL hybridization mix (125 m*M* $Na_2HPO_4 \cdot 2H_2O$, 7% SDS, 10% polyethylene glycol 8000, 1 mm EDTA) for one filter, and 40 mL for a maximum of six filters, in a small tray (15 × 8 cm) at 65°C. For a big tray (23 × 8 cm), 40 mL hybridization mix is used for one filter, and 60 mL is used for a maximum of six filters.
2. Pour the appropriate amount of preheated hybridization mix (65°C) into the cleaned trays. Optional: pipet 100 Fl of Herring sperm DNA solution (10 mg/mL, Life Technologies) for each 10 mL hybridization mix in the tray, to block the nonspecific attachment of the probe to the surface of the filter.
3. Mix gently, and place the filters, DNA-side-up, in the hybridization mix. After adding the filters, mix gently to completely cover the filters with hybridization mix. Place the cover on top of the tray, and incubate in the shaking water bath at 65° for 10–60 min.

3.1.8. Hybridization of the filters (d 3)

1. Remove (all) the filter(s) from the tray, and add all of the probe (approx 500 Fl) to the hybridization mix, and shake gently to get a homogeneous solution.
2. Place the filters back into the hybridization mix, one by one, DNA-side-up. After addition of a filter, mix gently to cover the filter with hybridization mix. Prevent trapping of air bubbles between/under the filters. Remove air-bubbles by replacing the filter in the solution.
3. Incubate overnight (12–16 h) at 65°C in the water bath under gentle shaking (to prevent the filters from adhering to one another).

3.1.9. Washing and Autoradiography of Filters (d 4)

1. Washing is done at 65°C in two shifts of 20 min each, in 0.1% SDS and a decreasing concentration of SSC: 2X, 1X, 0.3X (an optional wash in 0.1X can be done if more than 10 cpm per filter is measured on a Geiger counter). 20X SSC is 3.0 *M* NaCl, 0.3 *M* sodium citrate, pH 7.0.
2. Do not allow filters to dry at any stage during the washing procedure, because it may interfere with removing the bound probe after exposure.
3. Expose the filters (still damp), in Saran Wrap at –70°C, to sensitive Kodak X-OMAT. AR films are used for weak signals (approx 1–3 cpm per filter), and the Kodak Biomax MR or Konica AX films for strong signals (approx 3–10 cpm per filter).

3.1.10. Interpretation

After proper identification of the X-ray films, by date of the blot and the cDNA- probe hybridized, the DNA lanes on the X-ray film (DNA-nrs), the exposure time, and date of hybridization on the film, the bands can be interpreted by comparing the bands to the reference fragments in **Fig. 2**. A deletion or duplication should be detectable on blots *of* both *Hin*dIII and *Bgl*II.

For the interpretation of a screening blot, compare the pattern with the normal control sample (a healthy man or woman) on the same gel, and with the reference pattern in **Fig. 2**. Pay special attention to possible restriction fragment length polymorphisms (RFLPs) and their mode of inheritance; absence of bands, e.g., deletions (in a male DNA) or changed intensity, which could hint at less intense bands, a deletion (in female DNA) or more intense bands, which could hint to a duplication (in male and female DNA); possible junction fragments.

For the interpretation of a family blot, compare the pattern of the normal control sample (a healthy man or woman) with that of a patient or a proven carrier (if available), on the same gel. Pay special attention to possible RFLPs and their mode of inheritance, and possible junction fragments.

3.2. Dystrophin Gene Haplotype Analysis by Use of STRs

By use of multiple STR markers, a haplotype of the dystrophin gene can be formed and used to track its transmission in a family at risk. Haplotype analysis is a useful and reliable technique to estimate the carrier risk of women at risk in families in which no deletion or duplication is detected *(7,10)*. Sometimes, haplotype analysis is performed to confirm the segregation of a deletion, by detection of a null allele, also called hemizygosity. Many highly informative STRs are located in and around the dystrophin gene.

By use of these markers, the paternal and maternal X chromosomes can be differentiated. To assign a valid dystrophin haplotype, at least three informative markers are needed: one located in the coding region, and two flanking markers, one 5' and one 3' of the gene. Results of haplotype analysis are always displayed with the family data in a pedigree.

For standard haplotype analysis, an initial set of eight STRs, distributed over the dystrophin gene, could be used in duo sets of (STRs): 5' DYS1 and DXS1214, 5' DYS7 and DXS989, IVS44A and STR49, and 5' DYS2 and DXS1202. With these four sets of STRs, a highly informative haplotype can be created. Haplotypes are built from 3' to 5', are positioned on the chromosome Xpter → centromere. Preferably, allele lengths should be given in actual allele size (bp) for this allelic ladder, or rather the CEPH sample 134702 should be used as external standard for sizing the samples (**Table 2**). If necessary, additional markers can be chosen from **Table 3**. In families in which haplotype analysis has been performed previously, or in which a known deletion segregates, preselected markers are used.

Table 2
Combination of STR Markers and Internal Standards to be Used by Haplotype Analysis in New DMD/BMD Families

Combination of STRs	External marker CEPH 134702 alleles	Internal markers
5' DYS 1	175–181	164/194/232
DXS 1214	216–216	
5' DYS 7	133–133	104/164/232
DXS 989	181–183	
IVS44A	165–175	129/194/274
STR 49	227–251	
5' DYS 2	218–222	194/249/299
DXS 1202	281–283	

3.2.1. Amplification

Depending on which detection technique will be used, the PCR is set up. In case automatic sequencing equipment is used, specifically labeled fluorescent primers are used for detection on either the ALF (Pharmacia) or the ABI (Perkin-Elmer). For radioactive detection, unlabeled primers are used, and one of the bases (dCTP) is added, labeled with ^{32}P in the PCR mix.

Usually, 200 ng genomic DNA is used as a template for the amplification, in a total volume of 25 µL. See **Table 3** for the different annealing temperatures, buffers, and dilution of the products per marker. **Table 4** gives a pipet scheme to be used for one reaction in either of the PCRs. Normally, sufficient reaction mix is made to compensate for minor pipeting errors.

1. Prepare a dilution of the DNA samples 50 ng/µL in autoclaved water (MilliQ).
2. Pipet 4 µL DNA in the PCR tube, except in the blank 4 µL gautoclaved MilliQ water, place the tubes in the PCR tray. Fix the positions of the tubes in the tray by placing the retainer.
3. Prepare the reaction mix in a 1.5-mL tube, i.e., all ingredients except the template DNA (*see* **Table 4**). Note: Keep all ingredients on ice.
4. Start a PCR program in a PCR machine (**Table 5**) with a hot start of 95°C: Wait until 95°C is reached, and press pause.
5. Add 21 µL reaction mix to each of the tubes (pipet against the wall of the tube). Close the tubes with strips.
6. Put the PCR tray in the PCR machine, and press Run (9600) or Resume (9700/2400).

Table 3
Available STR's

Lab ID	Literature ID	Location	Allele length (bp)	Allele no.	Heterozygosity (%)
DXS 1068	AFM238yc11	Xp 11.4	245–259	11	67
5' DYS 8	DXS 8025	Xp11.4	181–201	10	76
DXS 8090	AFM338xa5	Xp 21	154–172	8	77
5' DYS 1	DMD.PCR10	3,5 kb 5' e1 b.	177–185	5	60
5' DYS 2	DMD.PCR11	1,2 kb 5' e1 b.	214–228	8	77
5' DYS 3	DMD.PCR12	3,5 kb 3' e1 b.	219–225	4	58
5' DYS 6	5'-5n3	Intron 1 m.	96–116	9	70
5' DYS 7	5'-5n4	Intron 4–5	133–155	8	64
STR07A	DXS 206	22 kb 3' e7	218–235	12	68
STR07B	DXS 206	23 kb 3' e7	227–241	8	44
5' DYS 5	5'-7n4	Intron 25–28	163–169	4	52
STR 44A	DXS 1238	13,8 kb 3' e 44	174–204	12	85
IVS44A	IVS44SK21	50 kb 3' e 44	158–181	10	84
IVS44B	IVS44SK12	50 kb 3' e 44	177–185	5	38
DXS1219	AFM297yd1	Intron 44	230–246	7	54
STR 44B	DXS 269	40 kb 5' e45	216–241	7	59
STR 45	DXS 1237	1,2 kb 3' e 45	156–184	15	87
DXS997	AFM217xa5	Intron 48	109–117	4	65
STR 49	DXS 1236	Intron 49	227–257	19	91
STR 50	DXS 1235	Intron 50	233–251	10	70
DXS 1067	AFM234vg7	5,5 kb 5' e 51	214–230	5	64
DXS 1036	AFM072zh3	Intron 51	145–151	4	62
DXS 1241	DMD.PCR7	Intron 55–57	245–255	5	51
DXS 1214	AFM283wg9	Intron 62–63	210–220	6	79
3' DYS 3	3' -19n8	3' e 63	140–150	5	58
DXS 992	AFM184xg5	> 20 kb 3' e79	201–211	11	87
DXS 1202	AFM260ye5	Xp22.12	265–283	8	80
DXS 989	AFM135xe7	Xp22	173–203	14	80

http://www.dmd.nl/rflpca.html

3.2.2. Electrophoresis

3.2.2.1. Protocol for the Separation of PCR Products on a Polyacrylamide Gel

This protocol describes the use of denaturing polyacrylamide gels (PAGs) for the separation of single-strand fragments of DNA. In the presence of free radicals, provided by ammonium persulfate and stabilized by TEMED, acrylamide and *bis*-acrylamide will form a crosslinked structure called poly-

Table 4
Pipet Scheme PCR-Reaction Mix (μL)

	PCR buffer		
Stock	ST	AT	STR
Geautoclaved MilliQ water	15	13.8	12.8
Buffer (10 * ST, 10 * AT, 5 * STR)	2.5	2.5	5
10 * dNTP mix[a]	2.5	2.5	2.5
25 m*M* $MgCl_2$	–	1.5	–
Primer F & R (25 pmol/μL)	0.5	0.5	0.5
Ampli Taq (5 U/μL)	0.2	0.2	0.2
End volume	21	21	21

[a]For a radioactive PCR, additional (^{32}PdCTP) is added.

Table 5
PCR Programs for STR PCR

	Time	Temperature (°C)	No. of cycles
Hot start	Max 99 min	95	1
Denaturation	5 min	95	1
Denaturation	30 s	94	
Annealing	30 s	55/60/65[a]	30
Elongation	30 s	72	
Elongation	5 min	72	1
Storage	4	4	1

[a]One of these, depending on the sequence.

Table shows the PCR programs for amplification of STRs. The PCR program ends in a 4°C cooling step.

acrylamide. Denaturing PAGs are polymerized in the presence of an agent (urea) that suppresses base pairing in nucleic acids. Denatured DNA fragments migrate through the gels at a rate that is almost completely independent of its base composition and sequence.

The PAGs are used for the separation of PCR products generated for the DNA analysis of multiple genetic diseases. After amplification of the various PCR products using the disease specific protocols, electrophoresis of the PCR products and autoradiography are performed according to this protocol. Furthermore, with minor adaptations, these gels can also be used for sequence analysis of generated PCR products.

The protocol first describes the preparation of a denaturing PAG, and continues with the electrophoresis, fixation, and drying of the gel, and finally ends with the detection of the DNA in the PAGs, using autoradiography.

3.2.3. Preparation of the Polyacrylamide Gel

1. Thoroughly clean the gel side of both a short and a long glass plate with warm water, soap, and a cleaning brush. Rinse afterwards with demiwater and 70% ethanol, respectively, and dry the plate with paper towels. Be careful not to touch the gel side of the glass plate after cleaning.
2. In the fume cupboard and wearing gloves, pour a small volume (5–10 mL) of Repel silane on the cleaned side of the glass plates. Spread the solution immediately with a paper towel over the whole plate, and allow the plate to dry for 2–5 min.
3. Rinse the treated side of the glass plates with 70% ethanol, and dry with paper towels.
4. Clean two identical spacers, and check the foam blocks. Replace them if they look too old. Put the spacers in correct position on the long glass plate (at the long sides with the foam blocks facing upward).
5. Place the small glass plate (with the gel side in downward position) on top of the long glass plate. Be sure to position the foam blocks against the top of the small glass plate, so that leakage of buffer during electrophoresis will not occur.
6. Keep the glass plates together by placing two clamps at the long sides of the glass plates.
7. Place the glass plates horizontally on a polystyrene tray, on a workbench covered with underlayment, to absorb excess acrylamide solution.
8. Clean the combs (64 wells or sharktooth) with water, and dry afterwards with paper towels. Also clean a 50-mL syringe.
9. Add 210 Fl 10% APS to 60 mL sequencing gel mix in a glass beaker, and mix the solution for a few seconds on a stirrer.
10. Add 43 Fl TEMED in the fume cupboard, and mix again on a stirrer for a few seconds.
11. Immediately start to pour the gel after addition of the TEMED, since polymerization is initiated. Take up the gel mix in the syringe. Introduce the nozzle of the syringe into the space between the two glass plates, and apply gel mix over the whole width of the glass plates, so that the flow of solution will be evenly across the plates. Keep the plates at an angle of about 10 degrees to enhance the flow.
12. When the space between the glass plates is completely filled, return the plates to the horizontal position. Accidentally trapped air bubbles can be removed using a hooked spacer. Insert the appropriate comb (64 wells, or sharktooth in downward position); avoid air bubbles trapped under the comb (*see* **Note 7**).
13. Place 4–5 100-mL bottles on top of the glass plates (or use two clamps) at the position of the comb, and allow the gel to polymerize for 45 min to 1 h. Leave the remainder of gel mix to check for polymerization. If the gel is left overnight, cover the ends of the gel with Saran Wrap, to prevent drying.

3.2.4. Electrophoresis

1. After polymerization, remove the bottles and clamps from the glass plates. Clean the upper side of the small glass plate with a moist tissue to prevent leakage during electrophoresis. One can use agarose, near the foam blocks of the spacer, to seal the upper side of the glass plate. Transport the gel cassette to the C-lab, and place the gel in position, small glass plate facing the electrophoresis apparatus. Tighten the screw knobs firmly.
2. Verify that the buffer chamber drain valve (at the right side of the apparatus) is closed, and fill the upper buffer chamber with approx 500 mL of 0.5X TBE buffer (or 1X TBE for sequencing gels).
3. Carefully remove the comb from between the glass plates, and immediately rinse the top of the gel with 0.5X TBE buffer, using a syringe and needle to remove any unpolymerized acrylamide.
4. If you are using a sharktooth comb (for sequencing gels), reinsert the comb between the glass plates with the teeth toward the gel. Insert the comb until the teeth just make contact with the surface of the gel. Do not allow the teeth to pierce the gel. A very slight indentation of the gel should be visible when the comb is properly inserted. Keep the comb in position with small clamps. Check correct position of the sharktooth comb by pipeting 5 µL loading buffer in every slot (*see* trouble shooting).
5. Fill the lower buffer compartment with approx 400 mL 0.83X TBE and 0.5 *M* NaAc buffer (or 1X TBE buffer for sequencing gels). Prevent airbubbles from obstructing buffer contact with the lower edge of the gel: Remove them with a syringe and a needle.
6. Close the upper and lower safety lids, and connect the power cords to the electrophoresis apparatus and the power supply. Set the power supply at 65 W, 50 mA, and 1800 V. If two apparatuses are connected to the power supply, the settings are 130 W, 100 mA, and 1800 V.
7. Prerun the gel for 15–30 min.
8. Meanwhile, prepare the samples for loading. Add 15 Fl loading mix to every STR–PCR sample (Sequence reactions of the size marker [M13, e.g., T-track] are already with sequence loading mix).
9. Denature the samples by running the denaturing program on the PCR apparatus (5 min 95°C; cool down to 4°C). Do not forget to denature the size markers before the first use of the day. Keep all denatured samples on ice.
10. Mark all lanes in which the size marker will be loaded (at least after every 16 lanes). Write down the order in which samples are loaded.
11. Stop the prerun, and again rinse the slots with electrophoresis buffer.
12. Load 2–4 Fl sample, using Multiflex Flat tips. The same tip can be used to apply all samples, if the tip is rinsed in electrophoresis buffer between loading two samples. Write down any abnormalities (sample swaps, overloading).
13. Start the electrophoresis, using the same settings as for the prerunning. Electrophoresis time depends on the size of the PCR product loaded. See disease-specific protocols for correct electrophoresis times.

14. Store PCR samples in the freezer in the C-lab, according to the general C-lab safety rules.

3.2.5. Fixation and Drying of the Gel

1. Turn off the power supply, take out the power cords, and open the safety lids. Open the buffer chamber drain valve (at the right side of the apparatus) to allow drainage of the buffer.
2. Turn on the heater of the gel dryer, and put it at 80°C (set the timer at > 2 h). The gel dryer is connected to a condensation trap. Empty the trap when the trap is half full.
3. Put paper towels in front of the apparatus, take out the glass plates, and dry the contaminated lower edge of the glass plates on the towels. Discard the contaminated towels in the appropriate waste.
4. Place the glass plates horizontally on a workbench, and remove the spacers from between the glass plates. Insert a pair of tweezers between the glass plates to remove the small glass plate. The gel will stick to one of the two glass plates. Write down to which one.
5. Fixate the gel, using one of two methods:

3.2.5.1. Method 1

1. Pour 5 L of 5% methanol, 5% acetic acid into the fixing tray.
2. Immerse the gel, together with its attached glass plate, gently in the fixative. Be careful that the gel stays on the glass plate, and does not start to float.
3. Allow the gel to fixate for 15 min.
4. Remove the gel from the fixative by carefully lifting the glass plate from the fluid, leaving excess of fixative in the tray.
5. Store the fixative in the tank. This solution can be used to fixate six gels. Note the number of times the solution is used on the tank.

3.2.5.1. Method 2

1. Place the glass plate with the gel in a fixing tray. Gently pour 10% methanol and 10% acetic acid on the gel, until coverage is complete.
2. Allow the gel to fixate for 15–30 min.
3. Take out the glass plate with the gel, leaving excess of fixative in the tray.
6. Discard the contaminated fixative in the appropriate liquid radioactive waste. Rinse the tray with water afterwards.
7. Cut a piece of GB002 paper and a piece of filter paper to size (approx 34 × 42 cm).
8. Place the GB002 paper neatly on the gel, trying to avoid air bubbles. The gel will stick to the paper.
9. Remove the paper, with the gel attached to it, and place it, gel-side-up, on the glass plate.
10. Completely cover the gel with Saran Wrap.
11. Place the piece of filter paper in the gel dryer. Position the gel in the gel dryer on top of the filter paper. Align all layers within the borders of the drying bed. Cover the gel with the mylar sheet, and return the silicone rubber flap in position.

12. Turn on the vacuum pump, and check that a vacuum is formed. Set the timer at 2 h.
13. Dry the gel for 30–40 min.
14. Clean the glass plates and the spacers in the C-lab. Measure possible radioactive contamination with the Geiger counter. The plates and spacers are brought back to the lab after complete removal of radioactive contamination.
15. Release the vacuum by removing the silicone rubber flap, turn off the vacuum pump, and take out the dried gel. A gel is properly dried when the Saran Wrap can be easily removed. Be aware of possible contamination of the Saran Wrap and the filter paper. Place the gel in a cassette. Never try to tear off the Saran Wrap.
16. Expose the gel to X-ray film under safelight illumination in the darkroom. Exposure takes place at RT. Label the cassette with your name and the date. The exposure time should be determined empirically, but can vary from 2 h to more than one night exposure. Depending on the isotope (^{35}S or ^{32}P) and the amount of radioactivity present in the gel, different films can be used: For sequencing gels, the Kodak Biomax MR can be used; for STR gels, the choice is between the sensitive Kodak X-OMAT AR films or the less sensitive Konica AX films. The exposure can also be performed using the PhosphorImager.
17. Development of exposed films is performed according to instructions of the supplier.
18. Mark the films as follows, writing directly on the film, not on (magic) tape (*see* Note 8): complete DNA numbers above the lanes or above/below the signal; date of electrophoresis; name of the STR above the lanes; marker lanes with G, A, T, or C code; exposure time; date of amplification.

3.2.6. Notes

1. Radioactive gels and PCR products are discarded in the appropriate radioactive waste container.
2. Decontamination of plastic ware used in the PCR procedure is according to the general rules for cleaning of PCR product contaminated materials.

4. Discussion

Southern blotting is more labor-intensive than PCR, usually takes several days to weeks, and requires high-mol-wt genomic DNA. With the above protocol, it is a quantitative and reliable technique, if the proper control samples are used. Quantitative Southern blot analysis, using dystrophin cDNA probes, has been used for more than 10 yr *(7)*. Deletions will be recognized in the patient's DNA as absent bands in the autoradiogram, and carriers show a reduced intensity of these bands. In families in which no male patient is available for DNA analysis, haplotype analysis often is used to give a better assessment of the carrier status for the females at risk. For example, **Fig. 3A** shows a pedigree of a Duchenne family, in which, initially, on creatine kinase (CK) and pedigree, the risk of being a carrier for individual 7 was estimated to be low (1–2%). However, DNA analysis on haplotype analysis showed an increase of the risk (50%): Individuals 1 and 7 shared a haplotype of six markers (data not shown), except for STR49. A hemizygous state indicates a deletion starting in intron

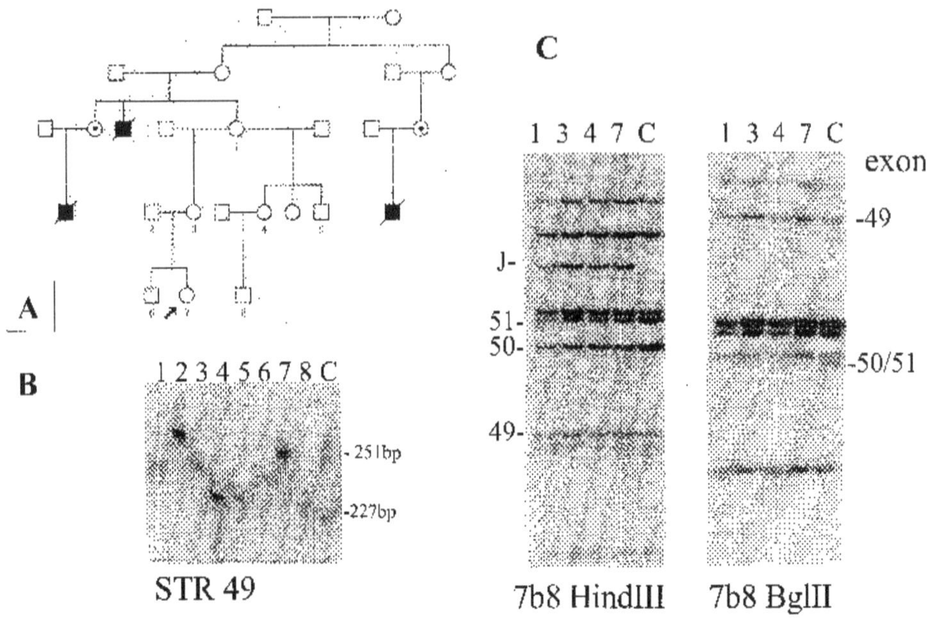

Fig. 3. **(A)** Pedigree of the family. **(B)** STR analysis in this family showed hemizygosity for STR49. Women 1, 3, 4, and 7 only show one (paternal) allele. Lane C is DNA of a female control sample CEPH 134702 shows two alleles. **(C)** The *Hin*dIII cDNA blot, hybridized with probe 7b8, shows a junction band (J) of a deletion for the exons 50–51 in the females at risk: 1, 3, 4, 7. All women also show on the *Bgl*II digest half intensity of the band (50/51). Lane C is DNA of a female control sample.

49. Southern blotting and hybridization with probe 7b8 confirmed this. Carrier females 1, 3, 4, and 7 show a junction band (J-band) that makes carrier detection relatively easy (**Fig. 3C**). Exon 49 is present, but exons 50 and 51 are deleted. The carrier risk for individual 7 now is 100%.

Because J-bands are found in less than 5% of the patients, carrier detection in normal Southern blotting is mostly based on band intensities, which require quantitative blotting conditions. J-bands are found in less than 3% of the deletions. Duplications appear in 5% of the patients' DNAs as a double-band intensity, compared to the normal situation. To increase the detection of junction fragments, large genomic probes (cosmids) were used, and were shown to be effective in 81% of precisely mapped deletions *(12)*. However, the competition hybridization needed for this technique appeared not robust enough to be used as a routine diagnostic test. The use of other restriction enzymes, such as *Bam*HI, *Kpn*I, or *Xba*I, however, was very successful in the hands of Yamagishi et al. *(13)*.

Alternatively, one could opt for the technically more demanding pulsed field gel electrophoresis or field-inversion gel electrophoresis techniques *(1)*, which are methods to separate long DNA fragments produced by rare cutting enzymes, and usually show J-bands for deletions larger than 20 kb.

If the protocol described here is followed consequently, and validation tests (successfully testing a set of known carriers) are performed, quantitative Southern blotting is a valuable diagnostic test.

Haplotype analysis in dystrophin gene is complicated by the very high intragenic recombination of 12% across the dystrophin gene ***(14,15)***: This demands combined use of flanking and intragenic markers. In the case of inconsistent results in linkage analysis, sampling errors and nonpaternity should also be borne in mind.

By use of informative polymorphisms STRs in the region corresponding to the deletion, STR analysis can confirm the presence of deletions, seen as quantitative differences in band intensity on a Southern blot. However, this means that DNA of the parents of the carrier woman should also be available. ST markers are very useful for this purpose ***(10)***. In **Fig. 3B**, an example of a segregating null allele is shown.

Risk calculations are performed by use of Baysian statistics ***(16)***. The high *de novo* mutation rate for DMD, however, often is a complicating factor in risk calculations, because of the presence of germline or somatic mosaicism. Approaches to risk calculation have been described in a report to which the reader is referred: the Proceedings of the (UK) Clinical Genetics Society Meeting on Germinal Mosaicism (1994) and risk calculations in DMD ***(17)***.

Although the possibilities for detecting microlesions (point mutations) in the dystrophin gene are increasing, for the near future, in about 30% of families, mutation detection will not be available. Fortunately, linkage analysis and CK determinations enable an accurate determination of carrier risks in these families. This may even be possible when no DNA from the patient is available.

5. Notes

1. Store the digested samples in the refrigerator or in the cold room.
2. When some of the samples are not completely digested, add more enzyme (10–20 U), and incubate again for 3–4 h at the appropriate temperature. The addition of spermidine (1 Fl) can also make a difference. If problems remain unsolved, perform **step 2**.
3. When digestions of a certain DNA sample are all incomplete or remain incomplete, it might be useful to perform a phenol extraction on the original DNA sample, to get rid of proteins, or other contaminants disturbing the digestion.
4. Preferably, preparation of the PCR should be executed in a pre-PCR-lab or in a downflow: Handling of PCR products should always be separated from this, to avoid contamination. Wear gloves.

5. **Caution:** Acrylamide is a potent neurotoxin, and is absorbed through the skin. The effects of acrylamide are cumulative. Wear gloves when handling acrylamide solutions. Although polyacrylamide is considered to be nontoxic, it should be handled with care, because of the possibility that it may contain small quantities of unpolymerized acrylamide.
6. Electrophoresis of the radioactive PCR samples takes place at the C-Lab. All steps carried out at the C-lab are performed according to the general C-Lab safety rules. **Caution:** Always wear a lab coat, gloves, and safety glasses, and protect yourself and others from radiation, using the radiation protection shields present at the C-Lab.
7. If the sharktooth comb is not in the correct position, try to carefully shift it or push it deeper into the gel.
8. Laboratories should be aware of the possibility of new mutation between alleles, especially with STR49. In the case of inconsistent results in linkage analysis, sampling errors and nonpaternity should be borne in mind.

References

1. Dunnen, J. T. den, Grootscholten, P. M., Bakker, E., Blonden, L. A. J., Ginjaar, H. B., Wapanaar, M. C., et al. (1989) Topography of the DMD gene: Fige- and cDNA analysis of 194 cases reveals 115 deletions and 13 duplications. *Am. J. Hum. Genet.* **45,** 835–847.
2. Koenig, M., Hoffman, E. P., Bertelson, C. J., Monaco, A. P., Feener, C., and Kunkel, L. M. (1987) Complete cloning of the Duchenne muscular dystrophy (DMD) cDNA and preliminary genomic organization of the DMD gene in normal and affected individuals. *Cell* **50,** 509–517.
3. Hu, X., Burghes, A. H., Bulman, D., Ray, P. N., and Worton, R. G. (1988) Partial gene duplications in Duchenne and Becker muscular dystrophies. *J. Med. Genet.* **25,** 369–376.
4. Koenig, M., Beggs, A. H., and Moyer, M. (1989) The molecular basis for Duchenne versus Becker muscular dystrophy: correlation of severity with type of deletion. *Am. J. Hum. Genet.* **45,** 498–506.
5. Roberts, R. G., Gardner, R. J., and Bentley, D. R. (1994) Searching for 1 in the 2,400,000, a review of dystrophin gene point mutations. *Hum. Mutat.* **4,** 1–11.
6. Bakker, E., Jennekens, F. G. I., de Visser, M., and Wintzen, A. R. (1997) Duchenne and Becker muscular dystrophies, in *Diagnostic Criteria for Neuromuscular Disorders,* (Emery, A. E. H., ed.), Royal Society of Medicine Press, London, pp.
7. Bakker, E., Veenema, H., den Dunnen, J. T., van Broeckhoven, C. H., Grootscholten, P. M., Bonten, E. J., van Ommen, G. J. B., and Pearson, P. L. (1989) Germinal mosaicism increases the recurrence risk for "new" Duchenne muscular dystrophy mutations. *J. Med. Genet.* **26,** 553–559.
8. den Dunnen, J. T. and Bakker, E. All detected microlesions in the dystrophin gene (http://www.DMD.nl).

9. Miller, S. A., Dykes, D. D., and Polesky, H. F. A simple salting out procedure for extracting DNA from human nucleated cells. (1988) *Nucl. Acids Res.* **16,**
10. Clemens, P. R., Fenwick, R. G., Chamberlain, J. S., Gibbs, R. A., de Andrade, M., Chakraboty, R., and Caskey, C. T. (1991) Carrier detection and prenatal diagnosis in Duchenne and Becker muscular dystrophy families using dinucleotide repeat polymorphisms. *Am. J. Hum. Genet.* **49,** 951–960.
11. Maniatis, Sambrook, and Fritsch (1993) *Molecular Cloning,* 2nd ed. 9.31.
12. Blonden, L. A. J., den Dunnen, J. T., van Paassen, H. M. B., Wapenaar, M. C., Grootscholten, P. M.. Ginjaar, H. B., et al. (1990) High resolution deletion breakpoint mapping in the DMD gene by whole cosmid hydridization. *Nucl. Acids Res.* **14,** 2111–2121
13. Yamagishi, H., Kato, S., Hiraishi, Y., Ishihara, T., Hata, J., Matsuro, N., and Takano, T. (1996) Identification of carriers of Duchenne/Becker muscular dystrophy by a novel method based on junction fragments in the dystrophin gene. *J. Med. Genet.* **33,** 1027–1031.
14. Abbs, S., Roberts, R. G., Mathew, C. G., Bentley, D. R., and Bobrow, M. (1990) Accurate assessment of intragenic recombination frequency within the Duchenne muscular dystrophy gene. *Genomics* **7,** 602–606.
15. Oudet, C., Hanauer, H., Clemens, P., Caskey, T., and Mandel, J. L. (1992) Two hot spots of recombination in the DMD gene correlate with the deletion prone regions. *Hum. Mol. Genet.* **1,** 599–603.
16. Bridge, P. J. (1994) *The Calculation of Genetic risks: Worked Examples in DNA Diagnostics.* The Johns Hopkins University Press, Baltimore.
17. Essen, A. J. van, Kneppers, A. L. J., Ginjaar, H. B., Kate, L. P. ten, Ommen, G. J. B., Buys, C. H. C. M., and Bakker, E., (1997) The clinical and molecular genetic approach to Duchenne and Becker muscular dystrophy. An updated protocol. *J. Med. Genet.* **34,** 805–812.

8

Fluorescence *In Situ* Hybridization Analysis for Carrier Detection in Duchenne/Becker Muscular Dystrophy

Jonathan K. Dore and Helen M. Kingston

1. Introduction

A variety of molecular techniques can be employed to determine carrier status in Duchenne/Becker muscular dystrophy (DMD/BMD). Some of these are described in other chapters of this book, and include linkage analysis using restriction fragment length polymorphism or CA repeats, single-strand conformational polymorphism (heteroduplex analysis, quantitative polymerase chain reaction (PCR), and fluorescence-based detection and direct point mutation analysis (*see* Chapters 5, 6, and 7). This chapter describes a method for fluorescence *in situ* hybridization (FISH) analysis that provides a simple method for carrier detection in families known to have a dystrophin deletion.

FISH is a molecular cytogenetic technique that has numerous applications *(1)*. Commercially available probes for whole chromosomes (chrs), satellite DNA, and many individual loci are available. These can be employed to determine the origin of marker chr and *de novo* unbalanced chromosomal segments, and to detect intrachromosomal rearrangements, cryptic translocations, and microdeletions. Specific gene deletions can be detected with appropriate probes, including intragenic deletions in large genes, such as the dystrophin gene.

FISH analysis in DMD/BMD was first described by Reid et al. in 1990 *(2)*. This technology has also been used to identify Xp21 contiguous gene deletions in complex glycerol kinase deficiency, which involves deletion of the genes for glycerol kinase, DMD, and/or congenital adrenal hypoplasia *(3)*. Evidence for somatic mosaicism in *de novo* dystrophin gene deletions has also been reported, using FISH techniques *(4)*.

From: *Methods in Molecular Medicine, vol. 43: Muscular Dystrophy: Methods and Protocols*
Edited by: K. M. D. Bushby and L. V. B. Anderson © Humana Press Inc., Totowa, NJ

Approximately two-thirds of boys with DMD, and a similar proportion of males with BMD, have one or more exons deleted from within the dystrophin gene *(5,6)*. Cosmid clones for *in situ* hybridization analysis are available for several exons within the two major deletion hot spots that encompass exons 45–52 and 3–19, making FISH a valuable technique in many carrier-testing situations. The technique described in this chapter is for FISH analysis using cosmid clones for exons 1, 3, 7, 8, 10, 13, 17, 19, 45, 47, 51, and 52 of the dystrophin gene. Cosmid clones are not available for all potentially deleted exons, but this problem could be overcome by using the PCR-amplified products corresponding to the deleted region as a probe, as described by Calvano et al. *(7)*.

When using FISH analysis for carrier detection, the gene deletion needs to be initially characterized in the affected male relative by PCR-based DNA-deletion screen (*see* Chapter 5). Cosmid clones corresponding to the deleted region are then hybridized directly to a standard metaphase chr spread to determine the presence or absence of signal on the X chrs of potential carriers. Noncarriers will demonstrate a signal on both X chrs, and carriers will demonstrate the signal on only one X chr, thus providing a definitive result. A minimum of 10 cells are analyzed to exclude false-negative results caused by hybridization failure. Cosmid clones for DMD/BMD FISH may contain an intronic sequence, and can therefore result in a false-positive signal, even when the corresponding exon is deleted. It is therefore important to confirm the validity of the method in the affected male or an obligate carrier from the family prior to carrier testing whether the cosmid probe corresponds to an exon at either end of the deleted region, or if the precise deletion end points are not known.

A major advantage of FISH analysis, compared to carrier-detection methods that utilize markers closely linked to, or within, the deleted region, is that it is not necessary to test intervening relatives. Once a deletion is identified in an affected male, any female relative at risk can be tested directly. As with other methods of carrier detection, a normal result from FISH analysis in the mother of an affected boy does not exclude the possibility of gonadal mosaicism. The FISH technique does, however, provide an effective method of detecting somatic mosaicism at relatively low levels *(4)*. FISH analysis can be used for the primary identification of mutations caused by deletions in obligate or potential carriers, when samples are not available from affected males in the family, and the mutation is unknown. FISH analysis can also be used to test for deletions in females presenting with limb-girdle dystrophy who may be manifesting carriers of DMD, but in whom there is no prior family history of MD.

Table 1
Cosmids

ICRFc104C0348	NRM1	Exon 1
ICRFc104A1047	NRM3	Exon 3
ICRFc104E0790	NRM7	Exon 7
ICRFc104F02123	NRM8/9	Exons 8 and 9
ICRFc104E0446	NRM10/11	Exons 10 and 11
ICRFc104F0393	NRM13	Exon 13
ICRFc104D02129	NRM17	Exon 17
ICRFc104B0281	NRM19	Exon 19
	CPT1	Exon 45
ICRFc104E0143	NRM46/47	Exons 46 and 47
ICRFc104C0461	NRM51	Exon 51
ICRFc104A1287	NRM52	Exon 52

2. Materials

2.1. Cosmid Probes

The cosmid probes used were developed for FISH by Charlesworth and Mountford. Each contains single exons or pairs of exons from the two chief deletion hot spots in the dystrophin gene. CPT-1 *(1)* was provided by van Ommen of Leiden University. The 11 NRM probes were obtained from the ICRF Reference Library by screening with dystrophin cDNA probes.

The cosmids, whose sizes range from 25 to 48 kb, are listed in **Table 1**.

2.2. Nick Translation of Probes

1. Probe DNA, prepared using commercial mini- or maxipreps. Store at –20°C.
2. BioNick Kit (Life Technologies).
3. Nick Columns (Pharmacia Biotech).
4. TNE buffer: 10 m*M* Tris-Hle, pH 8.0, 0.2 *M* NaCl, 1 m*M* ethylenediamine tetraacetic acid (EDTA).
5. Human Cot-1 DNA (Life Technologies).
6. Sonicated herring sperm DNA (Sigma).
7. Sodium acetate, 3 molar, pH 5.5.
8. Ethanol.
9. 50% Hybridization buffer (for 10 mL): 5 mL formamide, 2 mL 50% dextran sulphate, 1 mL 20X standard sodium citrate (SSC), 2 mL 0.5 *M* EDTA, 5 mL 1 *M* Tris-Hle, pH 7.6, 200 mL 5 mg/mL herring sperm DNA, 2 mL ultrapure water.
10. 70% Hybridization buffer: as above, except 7 mL formamide, no water.

2.3. Fluorescence In Situ *Hybridization*

1. 2X SSC.
2. RNase 10 mg/mL, store at –20°C.

3. Phosphate-buffered saline (PBS, Oxoid, Dulbecco A formula, pH 7.3).
4. 100 mg/mL pepsin, store at –20°C.
5. 1% acid-free formaldehyde, 1X PBS, 50 m*M* $MgCl_2$.
6. 70% Formamide, 2X SSC, pH 7.0.
7. Ethanol.
8. Plastic cover slips.
9. 4T buffer: 4X SSC, 0.05% Tween-20.
10. 4TM blocking buffer: 10 mL 4T, 0.5 g nonfat dried milk.
11. Fluorescein isothiocyanate (FITC) avidin conjugate (Vector, Burlingame, CA). Store at –20°C. Working solution: 5 mg/mL in 4TM blocking buffer. Make as required, avoid exposure to light.
12. Goat serum (Vector), store at –20°C.
13. Biotinylated antiavivin (Vector). Store at –20°C. Working solution: 5 mg/mL in 4T buffer/5% goat serum. Make as required.
14. DAPI-antifade: Citifluor AF1, 0.5 mg/mL DAPI.
15. Nail polish.

3. Methods

3.1. Probe Labeling (see Notes 3–5)

The following is a modification of the protocol supplied with the labeling kit.

1. Pipet into an Eppendorf tube on ice: 5 µL 10X deoxyribonucleoside triphosphate mix; 1 µg probe DNA; Ultrapure water, to give final volume of 45 µL; 5 µL 10X enzyme mix (keep at –20°C until required).
2. Mix and spin in a microcentrifuge for 1–2 s.
3. Incubate at 16°C for 1 h.
4. After 45 min, prepare a Nick Column by passing 10 mL TNE buffer through the column.
5. After 60 min incubation, add 5 mL stop buffer to the labelling mixture.
6. Load the probe mixture onto the column, followed by 400 µL TNE. Do not collect this fraction.
7. Position a 1.5-mL Eppendorf tube below the column, add a further 400 µL TNE, and retain this fraction.
8. Precipitate the probe by adding the following to the retained fraction:
   2 µL (20 µg) sonicated herring sperm DNA.
   7 µL Cot-1 DNA (i.e., 7X probe quantity) (*see* **Note 3**)
   41 µL 3 *M* NaAc, pH 5.5.
   900 µL 100% ethanol at –20°C.
9. Mix well and store at –20°C overnight.
10. Spin in a microcentrifuge at 13000 rpm for 15 min.
11. The pellet should now be visible on the uppermost surface of the Eppendorf. Without disturbing the pellet, remove all the supernatant using a Gilsen pipet.
12. Dehydrate by placing in a vacuum desiccator for 20–30 min.

13. Resuspend the probes in the following: 5 μL X centromere probe (biotin-labeled); 10 μL 70% hybridization buffer; and 60 μL 50% hybridization buffer.
14. Store at –20°C. This amount of probe is suitable for five reactions, using a 25 × 25 mm hybridization area.

3.2. Fluorescence In Situ Hybridization

1. Metaphase preparations should be prepared using standard culturing and harvesting techniques, using 3:1 methanol:acetic acid.
2. Care should be taken to ensure that preparations are free from cytoplasm, because this will inhibit probe-target hybridization.
3. Slides can be used immediately, and can be stored at room temperature (RT) for up to 2 mo, or at –20°C for 12 mo.
4. Slide pretreatment: (*see* **Note 9**). Incubate the slides in each of the following solutions:
   a. 2X SSC, 37°C, 2 min.
   b. 2X SSC, 100 mg/mL RNase, 37°C, 1 h.
   c. 2X SSC, 37°C, 2 min.
   d. PBS, 37°C, 2 min.
   e. 10 μg/mL pepsin, 0.01 *M* HCl, 37°C, 10 min
   f. PBS, RT, 2 min.
   g. 1% acid-free formaldehyde, 1X PBS, 50 m*M* $MgCl_2$, at RT for 10 min.
   h. PBS at RT for 2 min.

3.3. Probe Preparation

1. Aliquot 15 μL probe, as prepared in **Subheading 3.1., step 13**, into an Eppendorf tube.
2. Denature the probe by floating it in a 75°C water bath for 5 min. If this is carried out while the slides are in RNase, the probe and slides will be ready to use at the same time.
3. Transfer the probe to a 37°C water bath for 20 min to 2 h, to allow the competing out of repetitive sequence DNA by the Cot-1.

3.4. Slide Denaturation

1. Incubate the slides for 5 min in 70% formamide, 2X SSC, pH 7.0, at 75°C.
2. Pass the slides through an ascending ethanol series (70, 80, 90, and 100%) at –20°C, for 2 min in each.
3. Remove the slides from 100% ethanol, stand upright, and allow to dry at RT.

3.5. Hybridization (see Notes 10–13)

1. Prepare one 25 × 25-mm plastic cover slip for each probe.
2. Apply 15 μL denatured probe to the cover slip.
3. Ensuring that the target material is facing the probe, gently lower the dry slide onto the probe. Capilliary action will lift the cover slip toward the slide without the need to press the slide down, which could lead to loss of probe at the edges.
4. Label the slide with the probe name.
5. Incubate overnight in a humidified chamber at 37°C.

3.6. Stringency Washes and Signal Fetection (see Notes 14–17)

1. Carefully remove the cover slip and wash slides for 10 min in 50% formamide, 1X SSC, pH 7.0, at 43°C.
2. Wash for 10 min in 2X SSC at 43°C.
3. Pipet 50 µL 4TM blocking buffer onto a 25 × 25-mm plastic cover slip. Lower the slide toward the cover slip until capilliary action draws it toward the slide, then incubate, cover slip-side-up, for 5 min at RT.
4. Remove the cover slip, and apply a fresh plastic cover slip with 50 µL avidin–FITC working solution.
5. Incubate in the humid chamber for 15–30 min at 37°C.
6. Remove the cover slip, and wash 3× for 2 min in 4T buffer at RT.
7. Apply a fresh plastic cover slip with 50 µL biotinylated antiavidin working solution.
8. Incubate in the humid chamber for 15–30 min at 37°C.
9. Remove the cover slip, and wash 3× for 2 min in 4T buffer at RT.
10. Apply a fresh plastic cover slip with 50 µL avidin–FITC working solution.
11. Incubate in the humid chamber for 15–30 min at 37°C.
12. Remove the cover slip, and wash 3× for 2 min in 4T buffer at RT.
13. Wash slides for 2 min in PBS at RT.
14. Air-dry slides, but do not allow to dry completely.
15. Mount, using a glass cover slip with 10 µL DAPI antifade.
16. Seal edges of the cover slip with nail polish.
17. Store the slides in the dark in the refrigerator, until they are to be screened.

3.7. Fluorescence Microscopy (see Note 18)

Samples may now be viewed using a flourescence-equipped microscope with a DAPI and FITC filter set.

3.8. Interpretation of Results

1. Before using FISH analysis for carrier detection, the presence and extent of the dystrophin gene deletion in a given family must be determined. This is usually achieved by using a multiplex PCR method or analysis with cDNA probes on a DNA sample from an affected male. When no sample is available from an affected male, a deletion can be looked for in an obligate carrier or female relative at risk from the family, by FISH analysis using all the available FISH probes. Once a deletion is detected, appropriate clones can be identified for carrier-testing other female relatives.
2. Prior to carrier testing, an affected male relative or an obligate female carrier from the family should be tested with the selected FISH probes, to ensure that the deletion will be correctly identified. False-positive hybridization signals will be detected if the cosmid clone incorporates DNA sequence that overlaps with, but extends beyond, the deletion region within the dystrophin gene. This may occur when the probe corresponds to an exon at either end of the deletion. In such cases, reduced signals may be detected, but this may not be sufficiently reliable to form the basis of a diagnostic test.

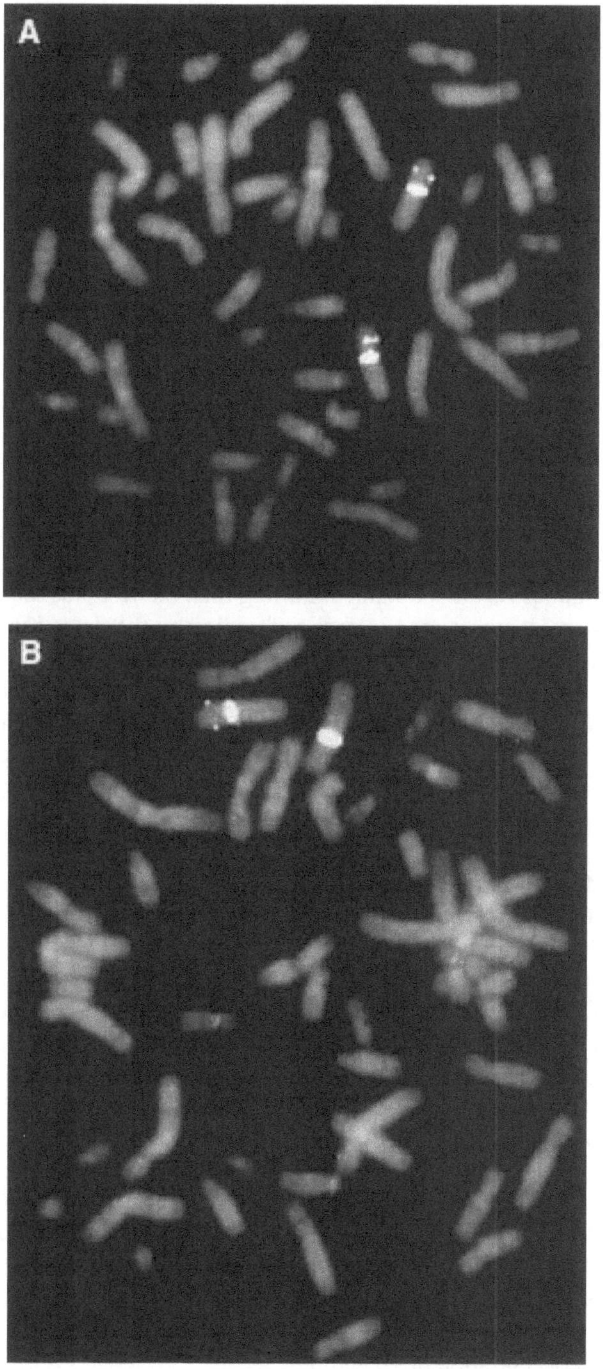

Fig. 1. FISH analysis in normal and carrier females.

3. If no sample is available from an affected male or obligate female carrier for *in situ* hybridization studies, then carrier test results in other female relatives may only be interpreted with certainty if the probe being used corresponds to an exon/exons contained within the deleted region that is/are flanked by other deleted exons.
4. For diagnostic use, a minimum of 10 cells are screened for each probe on each sample. It is necessary to analyze many more cells to determine the presence of somatic mosaicism, if this is suspected in a female relative from whom the deletion may have originated.
5. Only X chrs with a centromeric signal and one signal on each chromatid are scored as positive (**Fig. 1**). Chromosomes with a signal on only one chromatid are not scored. These are likely to be caused by the orientation of the chromatids or to reduced hybridization efficiency of the procedure, and could give a misleading result if scored.
6. In normal female cases, 8–10 of the cells screened will demonstrate signals on each X chr. A number of cells with one or no signals may also be seen, and, at this low level, this is considered to be a function of the hybridization efficiency of the procedure. If the results are unclear, more cells need to be screened until an unambiguous result is obtained. Failing this, the test must be repeated.
7. Deletions are demonstrated in carrier females by the detection of signals on one X chr only in all cells examined, and, in males affected, as no signal on the X chr. It is essential to run a control sample for each probe tested in a male. Testing a female relative's sample at the same time can provide an ideal control, since, if she is deleted, her normal X chr would act as a control for both samples.

4. Notes

1. Formamide is hazardous, and should be handled with caution at all times. Formamide should be handled in a safety cabinet: This may be mandatory under local safety regulations.
2. **CAUTION:** Gloves should be worn at all times. In addition to the health hazards posed by formamide and other chemicals used, contamination of the probes could lead to their possible degradation.
3. The method described here is for Biotin-labeling of probes, with signal detection and amplification using the biotin-avidin system. If probes are labeled with different reporter molecules, different detection systems will be required. If the probes are to be directly labeled with a fluorochrome (such as Spectrum Green), the use of Nick Columns is not recommended, because the directly labeled probe molecule is too large, and loss of probe will occur. More Cot-1 DNA may need to be added, if the Nick Column step is omitted.
4. When labeling the X centromere probe, the addition of Cot-1 DNA is not required. After the dehydration step, resuspend the probe in 70% hybridization buffer at a concentration of 10 ng/mL.
5. Probes can be precipitated at –70°C for 30 min as an alternative method to overnight at –20°C.

6. The use of slides coated to aid cell adhesion does not appear to be necessary for DMD screening, as long as care is taken with application of antifade (*see* **Note 17**).
7. If problems are encountered with chrs lifting off the slide, subsequent samples can be artificially aged by placing them on a hot plate at approx 40°C for 30 min prior to the pretreatment.
8. If the cell suspension is applied along the entire length of the slide, two different probes can be hybridized on the same slide. This is of particular use when a full 12-probe screen is required. Care should be taken to ensure that the quality of the metaphases is suitable for FISH on both parts of the slide (*see also* **Note 13**).
9. Although the method described is time-consuming, it is used to optimize the quality of the samples, and therefore to aid rapid screening. This is of particular use when numerous probes are used to test a patient, because time spent on pretreatment can be recouped during analysis. A number of alternative methods are available, however, and the following method has been found to work well on good-quality preparations.
   a. Incubate slides for 30 min in 2X SSC at 37°C.
   b. Pass through ascending ethanol series (70, 80, 90, 100%, 2 min in each).
   c. Denature and hybridize as described in **Subheading 3.2.6.**
10. A simple humid chamber for hybridization can be made by placing damp paper towels in a food container, such as a sandwich box, and placing this in a 37°C incubator.
11. In the humid chamber, sealing the edges of the plastic cover slips is not necessary. Slides have been left hybridizing for 55 h with no apparent ill effect.
12. Plastic cover slips are commercially available, or can be easily made by cutting up laboratory film, such as Parafilm, to the appropriate size. If using Parafilm, remove the backing paper, taking care not to touch the clean surface, and use clean-side-up.
13. If applying probes for two different exons to the same slide, use two separate 25 × 25-mm cover slips, and ensure that a space remains between the two cover slips when the slide is applied. Use a diamond-tipped pen to mark the border between the two probes. For the detection and amplification steps, a 25 × 50-mm plastic cover slip can be used.
14. It is important that the stingency wash solutions reach the correct temperature before use: Too low a temperature will result in excessive background; too high a temperature will reduce the signal intensity.
15. The 5-min 4TM step reduces nonspecific binding of the reagents to the slide. If nonspecific signals are seen on the slide itself, rather than on the chrs, it is likely to be a problem at this stage, and not with the stringency washes.
16. It is not necessary to carry out the signal detection and amplification stages in the dark, although exposing the slides to direct sunlight should be avoided.
17. Take care not to use too much antifade or to apply cover slips to slides that are too wet. This can cause the chrs to lift off the slide.
18. The use of a CCD camera PC-based image capture and storage system (such as SmartCapture) is useful, but not essential, for DMD screening. If the signal strength is poor, such a system can be used to enhance the image and obtain a

result, when previously the FISH reaction would need to be repeated. The system is of most use as an archive of representative cells from patients studied.

References

1. Trask, B. J. (1991) Fluorescence in situ hybridization: applications in cytogenetics and gene mapping. *Trends Genet.* **7,** 149–154.
2. Reid, T., Mahler, V., Vogt, P., Blonden, L., Van Ommen, G. J. B., Cremer, T., and Cremer, M. (1990) Direct carrier detection by in situ suppression hybridization with cosmid clones of the Duchenne/Becker muscular dystrophy locus. *Hum. Genet.* **85,** 581–586.
3. Worley, K. C., Lindsay, E. A., Bailey, W., Wise, J., McCabe, E. R. B., and Baldini, A. (1995) Rapid molecular cytogenetic analysis of X-chromosomal microdeletions: fluorescence in situ hybridisation (FISH) for comlex glycerol kinase deficiency. *Am. J. Med. Genet.* **57,** 615–619.
4. Bunyan, D. J., Crolla, J. A., Collins, A. L., and Robinson, D. O. (1995). Fluorescence in situ hybridisation studies provide evidence for somatic mosaicism in de novo dystrophin gene deletions. *Hum. Genet.* **95,** 43–45.
5. Den Dunnen, J. T., Grootscholten, P. M., Bakker, E., Blonden, L. A., Ginjaar, H. B., Wapenaar, M. C., et al. (1989) Topography of the DMD gene, FIGE and cDNA analysis of 194 cases reveals 115 deletions and 13 duplications. *Am. J. Hum. Genet.* **45,** 835–847
6. Forrest, S., Cross, G. S., Speer, A., Gardner-Medwin, D., Burns, J., and Davies, K. E. (1987) Preferential deletion of exons in Duchenne and Becker muscular dystrophies. *Nature* **329,** 638–640.
7. Calvano, S. Memeo, E., Piemontese, M. R., Melchionda, S., Bisceglia, L., Gasparini, P., Zelante, L. (1997) Detection of dystrophin deletion carriers using FISH analysis. *Clin. Genet.* **52,** 17–22.
8. Blonden, L. A. J., Grootscholten, P. M., den Dunnen, J. T., Bakker, E., Abbs, S., Bobrow, M., et al. (1991) 242 Breakpoints in the 200-kb deletion prone P20 region of the DMD gene are widely spread. *Genomics* **10,** 631–639.

9

DNA-Based Prenatal Diagnosis for Duchenne and Becker Muscular Dystrophy

Ann Curtis and Daisy Haggerty

1. Introduction

Progressive muscle wasting, which leads to severe disability and early death, make Duchenne and Becker muscular dystrophies (DMD/BMD) highly distressing disorders to both patient and family. Diagnosis in pregnancy, therefore, is frequently considered by couples in which the woman has a family history of either disorder. However, prenatal diagnosis is not always straightforward. It is frequently complicated by the high new mutation rate associated with the dystrophin gene, and, related to this, the high incidence of mosaicism in the germline. In addition, family structure is not always ideal, because samples from vital members may be unavailable.

1.1. Source of Fetal Tissue

Prenatal diagnosis for DMD and BMD, using molecular genetic methods, is routinely carried out on DNA extracted from tissue of embryonic origin obtained by chorionic villus sampling (CVS) or by amniocentesis. CVS, either transvaginal or transabdominal, is the procedure of choice, because sufficient DNA can be extracted from a small number of villi obtained relatively early in pregnancy, at about the tenth week. This allows a prediction on the status of the fetus to be obtained within the first trimester. Amniocentesis is not usually performed earlier than the fifteenth week of pregnancy, and, because small numbers of cells are obtained, it is often necessary to culture the cells in vitro prior to DNA extraction and analysis. This further step extends the time between sampling and test result, and may lead to late termination of the pregnancy in the event of an affected fetus. Both CVS and amniocentesis are relatively invasive procedures that present a small risk to the pregnancy.

From: *Methods in Molecular Medicine, vol. 43: Muscular Dystrophy: Methods and Protocols*
Edited by: K. M. D. Bushby and L. V. B. Anderson © Humana Press Inc., Totowa, NJ

Other approaches to prenatal diagnosis that may overcome these problems of safety and acceptability are under development, but not yet in routine practice. One potential noninvasive source of fetal material is to use cells that have crossed the placenta and entered the maternal circulation during pregnancy *(1,2)*. A second alternative approach, which avoids the need to terminate an affected pregnancy, often the outcome of conventional prenatal diagnosis, would be to perform preimplantation diagnosis (reviewed in ref. ***3***) on one or two single blastomeres taken from 8–10-cell embryos following in vitro fertilization. Unaffected embryos are selected and transferred for continuation of a normal pregnancy.

1.2. Fetal Sex

The initial step in the prenatal diagnosis of an X-linked disorder, such as DMD or BMD, is to determine the sex of the fetus, because it is only necessary to perform the subsequent DNA analysis on male pregnancies. Sex can be determined by inspection of the karyotype in fetal cells, or by the polymerase chain reaction (PCR) to detect sequences specific to the X and Y chromosomes (chrs) *(4)*. A result from either of these procedures is available within one day, and therefore does not significantly delay the dystrophin gene analysis.

1.3. Contamination of Chorionic Villus Biopsies

An important part of the laboratory procedure leading to a prenatal diagnosis is the confirmation that the fetal DNA sample is uncontaminated with maternal DNA. If fetal sexing had been performed by cytogenetic analysis, then all of the cells investigated may have been of male origin. However, the lack of detectable maternal DNA should still be demonstrated by typing the fetal DNA sample with a polymorphic marker for which the mother is heterozygous. This allows the presence of only a single maternal allele to be confirmed. Hentemann et al. *(5)* reported that a 2% level of maternal contamination in a chorionic villus biopsy (CVB) was undetectable using 25 cycles of PCR, but, with 30 cycles, 0.2% contamination was detected.

1.4. Importance of Family Testing Prior to Pregnancy

The dystrophin gene, which extends over 2.4 Mb of genomic DNA and is fragmented into 79 exons, is the largest human gene identified *(6,7)*. Both the location within the gene, and the molecular nature of the mutations that are pathogenic in DMD and BMD, are variable. However, 60–65% of the mutations that underlie DMD are large deletions, located in two deletion-prone regions, encompassing exons 2–20 at the proximal end and exons 45–53 in the midportion of the gene; a further 5–10% of mutations are duplications *(8,9)*. In BMD, the proportion of mutations that are large deletions and duplications is

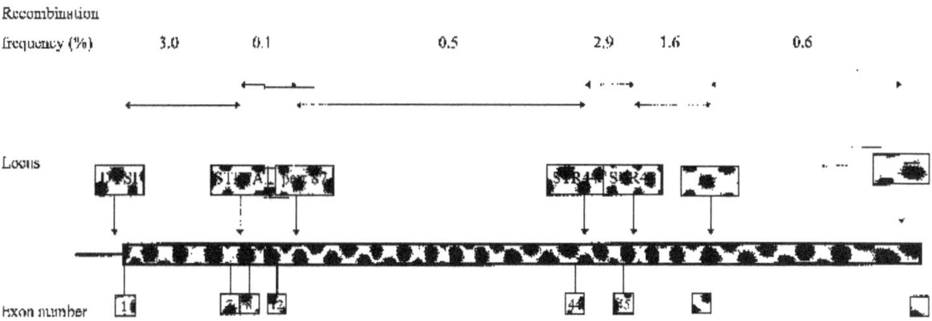

Fig. 1. Recombination frequencies within the dystrophin gene *(10,11)*. Particular 'hot spots' of recombination are observed at the 5' end of the gene and within intron 44.

higher, at 85% ***(10)***. The remainder are point mutations or small rearrangements that show no significant clustering. Therefore, before pregnancy, it is desirable that the specific familial pathogenic mutation has been identified. If this has not been possible, then polymorphic markers within the dystrophin gene must be informative, before prenatal testing can proceed with confidence. This prior knowledge allows the laboratory analysis to proceed efficiently when a woman does become pregnant, by focusing only on specific regions of the gene, thus generating a timely result.

A large number of polymorphic markers have been located within and at the 5' and 3' ends of the dystrophin gene and the relative positions of some of these are shown in **Fig. 1**. These represent both biallelic restriction fragment length polymorphisms (RFLPs) and simple tandem repeats (STR). STR markers are generally used, in preference to RFLPs, because they tend to be more informative. A list of useful STR markers is presented in **Table 1**.

1.5. Accuracy of Prenatal Diagnosis in DMD and BMD

The degree of accuracy of the prenatal test is dependent on whether a mutation has been identified in an affected male relative, and, if not, the location and number of polymorphic markers that are informative in the family. There is an unusually high level of recombination across the dystrophin gene, which is estimated at approx 10%, and, within this, hot spots occur, as illustrated in **Fig. 1** ***(11,12)***. Additional factors, which must also be considered, are the family structure and the carrier status of the mother of the fetus, including the high incidence of germline mosaicism ***(13,14)***. When the mother is a definite carrier of a dystrophin gene mutation, as determined by family history or previous DNA studies, then prenatal diagnosis can be discussed with confidence. However, the high rate of sporadic mutation in DMD and BMD means that the

Table 1
Microsatellite Markers Useful for Dystrophin Gene Analysis

Marker	Location	PIC/HET[a]	A/C[b]	Fragment size	% Midi Atto gel/ run time	Ref.
5' DYS I	5' Brain promoter	0.608	60°C/28	177–185 (5alleles)	10%/3 h	***15***
5' DYS II	5' Brain promoter	0.768	50°C/30	214–228 (8 alleles)	12%/3.5 h	***15***
5' DYS MSA	Muscle promoter	0.57[a]	50°C/30	56–88 (10 alleles)	7%/1.5 h	***16***
5'-5n3	Intron 1	0.70	61°C/28	96–116 (9 alleles)	8%/2 h	***17,18***
5'-5n4	Intron 4/5	0.64	58°Ca/28	133 (8 alleles)	8%/2 h	***18***
STR 7A	Intron 7	0.68[a]	55°C/30	218–235 (12 alleles)	12%/3.5 h	***25***
5'-7n4	Intron 25–28	0.52	60°C/28	165 (4 alleles)	10%/2 h	***18***
STR 44	Intron 44	0.87[a]	61°C/30	174–204 (12 alleles)	10%/3 h	***19***
IVS 44-SK21	Intron 44	0.84	56°C/30	158–181 (10 alleles)	10%/2.5 h	***20***
STR 45	Intron 45	0.887[a]	61°C/30	156–184 (13 alleles)	10%/2.5 h	***19***
STR 48	Intron 48	0.64	58°C/30	109–117	8%/2 h	***21,22***
STR 49	Intron 49	0.933[a]	61°C/30	227–257 (19 alleles)	12%/4 h	***19***
STR 50	Intron 50	0.716[a]	61°C/28	233–251 (6+ alleles)	12%/4 h	***19***
DMD I	Intron 57	0.50	55°C/28	245–255 (5 alleles)	12%/4 h	***23***
STR 62/63	Intron 62/63	0.38[a]	60°C/30	187–203 (3 alleles)	10%/3 h	Unpub.
3'-19n8	Intron >63	0.53	63°C/28	140–150 (5 alleles)	8%/2.5 h	***17,18***
3'-STRHI	Intron 64	0.68[a]	50°C/30	93–108 (5 alleles)	8%/2 h	Unpub.
3' DYS-CA	3' UTR (exon 79)	0.46	60°C/28	127–135	8%/2.5 h	***24***
MP1P	3' UTR (exon 79)	0.22	55°C/30	78/82 (2 alleles)	7%/1.5 h	***26***

[a]Useful STR markers.
[b]A/C indicates the primer-specific annealing temperature/number of cycles.

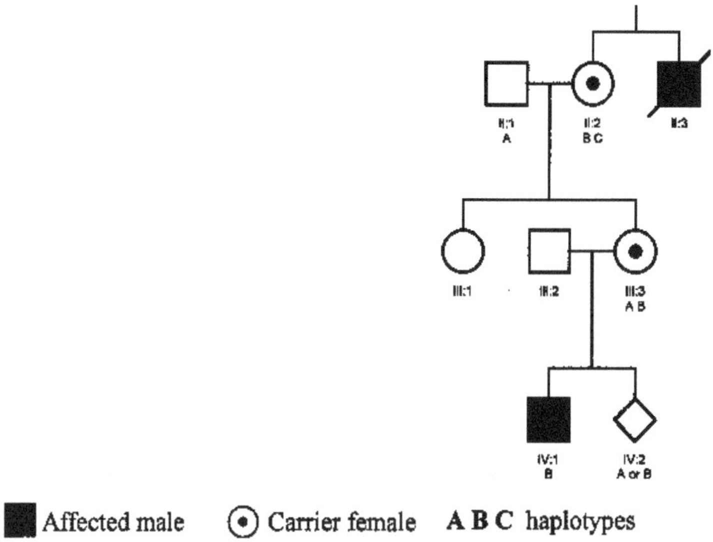

Fig. 2. Prenatal diagnosis where there is a strong family history of DMD or BMD. III:3 has an affected son and a deceased affected uncle. She, and her mother, II:2, are therefore, obligate carriers of a dystrophin gene mutation. Her sister, III:1, has a carrier risk of 50%. The identification of a mutation in IV:1 will allow accurate prenatal testing for III:3 and will allow the possibility of direct carrier testing as well as accurate prenatal diagnosis for III:1. If a mutation is not detected in IV:1, then haplotypes can be constructed using polymorphic markers across the gene to identify the haplotype which is tracking with the mutant dystrophin gene in II:2, III:3 and IV:1. In the example shown here, the presence of haplotype **A** in the male fetus, IV:2, indicates that it has low risk of being affected and haplotype **B** indicates a high risk. The precise risk will depend on the actual markers used to generate the haplotypes.

mother of an isolated case has only a 0.66 prior probability of carrying the causative mutation herself.

1.5.1. Causative Mutation in Affected Male is Known

When a dystrophin gene mutation is identified in an affected male, highly accurate prenatal diagnosis is available to female relatives (**Figs. 2** and **3**). If the defect is a deletion or a point mutation, it is generally a straightforward laboratory procedure to test for the presence of that particular mutation in a male fetus, giving a prediction that is 100% accurate. In the case of a duplication, which may be technically more difficult to identify, dosage analysis should be performed, when possible. Alternatively, the closest flanking markers to the duplication may be used to track the defective gene in the fetus. The

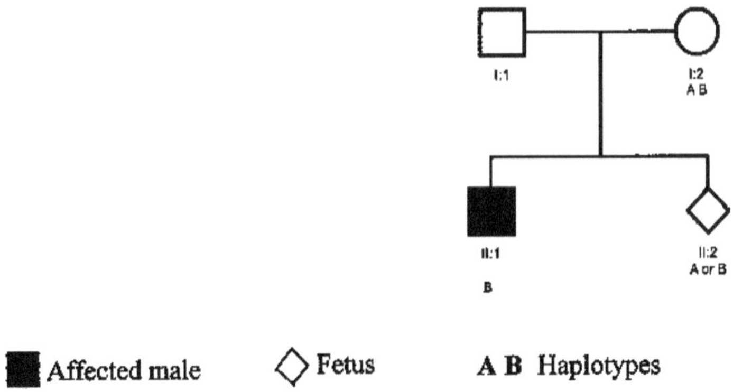

Fig. 3. Prenatal diagnosis where there is an apparent isolated case of DMD or BMD. The detection of a mutation in II:1 allows highly accurate prenatal testing for his mother I:2 in subsequent pregnancies. Failure to identify a mutation means that haplotypes using markers across the gene must be constructed to enable distinction of the high risk and low risk alleles in I:2. In this example, the presence of haplotype **B** in DNA from the male fetus II:2 would predict a high risk of DMD/BMD and of haplotype **A**, a low risk. Precise risk estimates will depend on the markers used to generate the haplotypes.

risk of error here would be equivalent to that of a double recombination event between the two markers.

1.5.2. Causative Mutation in Affected Male is not Known

If it has not been possible to locate the causative mutation in DNA from an affected male, then prenatal diagnosis can be performed by testing for the high risk X chr in the fetal DNA, based on haplotype data (**Figs. 2** and **3**). Informative haplotypes should be generated prior to CVB, using at least four polymorphic markers, evenly distributed between the 5' and 3' ends of the gene (**Fig. 1** and **Table 1**), to maximize the chance of detecting recombination events, which would otherwise lead to inaccurate predictions. The risk of error then is the sum of the chance of double recombination between the markers used.

1.5.3. Risks from Germline Mosaicism

If the causative mutation in an isolated case is not present in the somatic DNA of his mother, the most recent figures ***(14)*** suggest that she retains a 20% risk of being a germline carrier for that mutation. Therefore, the mother has a prior 5% risk of having another affected son, and may choose prenatal diagnosis, based on detection of the mutation in a future pregnancy.

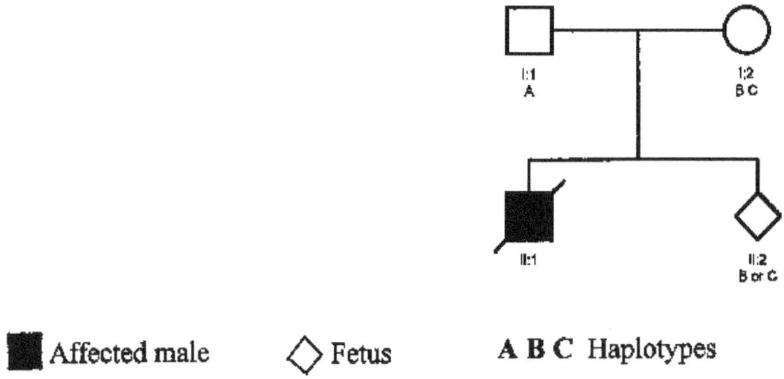

Fig. 4. Prenatal diagnosis where there is an apparent isolated case of DMD or BMD for whom DNA testing is not possible. If analysis of DNA from II:1 is not possible, then prenatal testing is usually not possible for female members of the family. In the example shown here it is impossible to associate either haplotype **B** or **C** with the disease.

1.5.4. Dystrophin Gene Analysis Results Are not Available from Affected Male

In the case of an isolated affected male for whom DNA analysis results are unavailable, e.g., because he died without storage of suitable tissue or DNA samples, then prenatal testing may not be possible for his female relatives, as illustrated in **Fig. 4**. An exception to this would be if a mutation could be identified in the affected child's mother. Testing for previously unidentified dystrophin gene mutations in the DNA from a male fetus could be performed, but it would be very difficult to give reassurance about the outcome, if a mutation were not detected.

When a woman is an obligate carrier, based on her family history, but dystrophin gene analysis results are not available for any affected male relatives (**Fig. 5**), then two approaches to prenatal diagnosis can be considered. First, if time permits prior to pregnancy, deletion and duplication analysis, based on dosage differences, and point mutation searching may be performed on DNA from the obligate carrier herself. Detection of a mutation would allow highly accurate prenatal testing to be performed. Second, if no mutation is found or this approach was not possible, then haplotypes can be generated (using at least four informative polymorphic markers spanning the gene), which allows the identification of the grandparental X chromosome in the fetal DNA. If this is of grandpaternal origin, then DMD/BMD can be excluded in the fetus, but, if it is of grandmaternal origin, then the fetus is predicted to be at high risk.

Figure 6 illustrates an example of a woman whose carrier status is unknown, but for whom prenatal exclusion can be offered, in the absence of DNA results

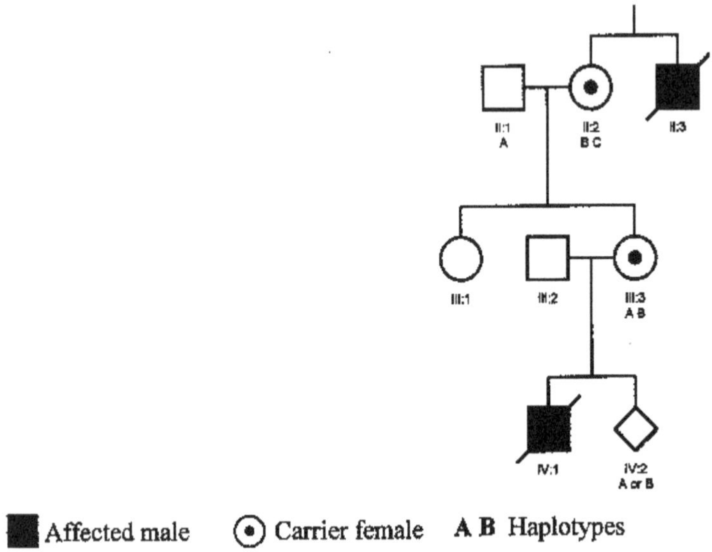

Fig. 5. Prenatal diagnosis where there is a strong family history of DMD or BMD but DNA analysis in affected members of the family is not possible. In the absence of DNA results from an affected male, prenatal diagnosis is possible by haplotype analysis. In the example shown here, the presence of the grandmaternal haplotype, **B**, predicts a high risk that the male fetus, IV:2, will be affected and the presence of the grandpaternal haplotype, **A**, predicts a low risk. Precise risks will depend on the markers used to generate the haplotypes.

from her affected brother. Detection of the grandpaternal haplotype will exclude the disease in the fetus, but the presence of the grandmaternal haplotype leaves the fetus with a 50% risk. If a couple chooses to terminate a pregnancy based on a 50% risk that the child will be affected, then analysis of the dystrophin protein in the fetal tissue may give an indication as to the disease status of the fetus. If appropriate, the fetal DNA could then be screened for dystrophin mutations, allowing accurate prenatal diagnosis in subsequent pregnancies. This form of exclusion testing is not possible for mothers of isolated cases, because a new mutation in the mother can be of paternal or maternal origin (**Fig. 7**).

2. Materials

2.1. DNA Extraction from Chorionic Villus Biopsies 1 (Suitable for Use in PCR; see Note 1)

1. CVB buffer: 150 m*M* sodium chloride (NaCl), 25 m*M* ethylenediamine tetra-acetic acid (EDTA). Adjust to pH 7.4. Autoclave, and store at 4°C in 0.5-mL aliquots.

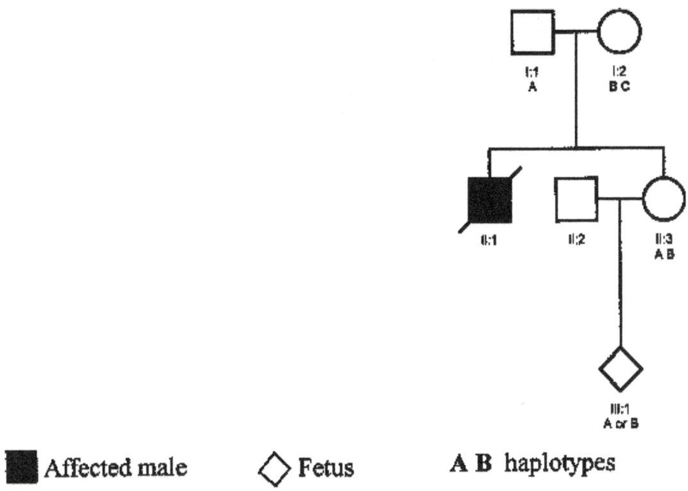

Fig. 6. Prenatal diagnosis where there is an apparent isolated case of DMD or BMD but DNA analysis in affected members of the family is not possible. In the absence of DNA results from the affected male, prenatal exclusion only is possible by haplotype analysis. In the example shown here, the presence of the grandpaternal haplotype, **A**, predicts that the fetus, III:1, has a low risk of being affected. However, the presence of the grandmaternal haplotype, **B**, leaves the fetus with a risk close to 50%.

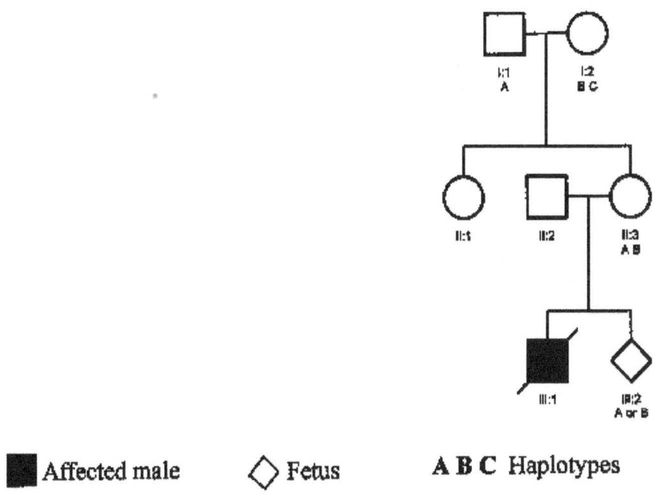

Fig. 7. Prenatal diagnosis for the mother of an apparent isolated case of DMD or BMD for whom DNA testing is not possible. Prediction of disease status in the male fetus III:2 is not possible in the absence of dystrophin gene analysis results from the affected male III:1. If II:3 represents a new mutation, then this could have arisen on either her maternally or paternally derived X chromosome.

2. Sodium dodecyl sulphate (SDS): Prepare a 10% solution and filter sterilize. Store in aliquots at room temperature (RT).
3. Proteinase K (Sigma): Prepare a solution at 1 mg/mL in sterile dH_2O. Aliquot, and store at –20°C.
4. Phenol, watersaturated (*see* **Note 2**). The authors purchase this from Rathburn Chemicals, .
5. Chloroform mix: Prepare a solution of chloroform and octan-2-ol at a ratio of 24:1.
6. NaCl: Prepare a 5 *M* solution in dH_2O. Autoclave, and store at 4°C.
7. Absolute ethanol: Store at 4°C.
8. 70% ethanol in dH_2O: Store at 4°C.
9. Ammonium acetate: Prepare a 7.5 *M* solution in sterile dH_2O. Store at 4°C.
10. Tris-EDTA (TE) buffer: 10 m*M* Tris-HCl pH 7.5, 1 m*M* EDTA, pH 8.0. Autoclave, and store at 4°C.
11. 1.5 mL microcentrifuge tubes with screw tops.
12. Disposable mini-Pasteur pipets with fine tips (Alpha Laboratories, Eastleigh, Hampshire, UK).

2.2. DNA Extraction from Chorionic Villus Biopsies 2 (Recommended for Use in Southern Blotting; see Note 1)

1. Urea buffer: 8 *M* urea, 0.3 *M* NaCl, 10 m*M* Tris-HCl, pH 7.5, 10 m*M* EDTA, 2% SDS. Filter-sterilize, and store as 300-μL aliquots at 4°C.
2. Sterile needles: 19G (buff), 21G (green), 23G (blue).
3. 2 mL syringe.
4. Items 2–5 and 10 detailed in subheading 2.1. above.
5. Absolute ethanol: Store at –20°C.
6. 70% ethanol in dH_2O: Store at –20°C.
7. Solution A: 5 m*M* Tris HCl, pH 7.5, 0.05 m*M* EDTA, pH 8.0, 1 m*M* NaCl. Autoclave, and store at 4°C.
8. Solution B: 0.5 m*M* Tris-HCl, pH 7.5, 5 m*M* EDTA, pH 8.0, 0.1 m*M* NaCl. Autoclave, and store at 4°C.
9. RNase A: Prepare a solution at 5 mg/mL in TE buffer, boil for 5 min (*see* Note 3), and store in aliquots at –20°C.
10. Sodium perchlorate ($NaClO_4$): Prepare a 6 *M* solution in sterile dH_2O. Store at 4°C.
11. NaAc: Prepare a 3 *M* solution in sterile dH_2O, and store at 4°C.

2.3. DNA Extraction from Cultured Amniocytes

This method is based on the Nucleon 1 DNA extraction kit supplied by Scotlab,

1. 2-mL microcentrifuge tubes with straight sides.
2. Solution B (*see* **Note 4**): 400 m*M* Tris-HCl, pH 8.0, 60 m*M* EDTA, 150 m*M* sodium chloride. Autoclave, and then add SDS to 1%.
3. $NaClO_4$: Prepare a 5 *M* solution in sterile distilled water (*see* **Note 4**). Store at RT.
4. Chloroform stored at –20°C.

5. Nucleon silica suspension (*see* **Note 4**).
6. Absolute ethanol, stored at –20°C.
7. 70% ethanol in dH_2O: Store at –20°C.
8. TE buffer: *See* subheading 2.1., item 10.

2.4. Determination of DNA Concentration

1. Standard DNA of known concentration, such as native λ DNA.
2. 10X sucrose loading buffer containing the following: 0.25% bromophenol blue, 0.25% xylene cyanole, 65% w/v sucrose dissolved in dH_2O.
3. Tris-acetate EDTA (TAE) electrophoresis buffer: Dilute to 1X concentration from a 10X stock solution containing 48.4 g Tris-base, 5.7 mL glacial acetic acid, 10 mL 0.5 *M* EDTA, pH 8.0, per L.
4. 0.8% agarose gel (SeaKem LE, supplied by Flowgen), approximate dimensions 12 × 13 cm, prepared in 1X TAE electrophoresis buffer (*see* **item 3**, above) and containing 5 µL solution of 10 mg/mL ethiduim bromide.
5. Horizontal electrophoresis tank appropriate for the prepared gel.
6. Test fetal DNA from CVB or amniocytes.

2.5. Fetal Sexing by PCR

1. *Taq* polymerase: The authors use *Taq* polymerase purchased from Promega, at a concentration of 5 U/µL, which is stored at –20°C.
2. 10X PCR amplification buffer containing 15 m*M* $MgCl_2$: This buffer is supplied by the manufacturer of the *Taq* polymerase, optimized for each batch of enzyme, and is stored at –20°C.
3. Deoxynucleoside triphosphates (dNTPs): Prepare a working stock containing a mixture of deoxyadenosine triphosphate, deoxycytidine triphosphate, deoxyguanosine triphosphate, and deoxythimidine triphosphate, each at 2 m*M*, in sterile dH_2O. These can be purchased individually as 100 m*M* stocks from Boehringer Mannheim Ltd. Both 100 m*M* and 2 m*M* stocks should be stored at –20°C.
4. Oligonucleotide primers (sequences shown in **Table 2**): Prepare each of the three oligonucleotides (X-Y primer, X-specific primer, and Y-specific primer) at a concentration of 10 µ*M* in sterile dH_2O.
5. Sterile dH_2O.
6. Control female (XX), control male (XY), and test fetal DNA samples.

Table 2
Primer Sequences for Determination of Fetal Sex by PCR

Primer	Sequence (5–3')
Common X-Y	GAA TTC TTA ACA GGA CCC ATT TAG GAT TAA
X-specific	CTG CAG AAA CAA GCT CAT CAG CGT GAC TAT
Y-specific	GTA CTA CCT TTA GAA AAC TAG TAT TTT CCC

Adapted with permisison from **ref. *4***.

7. 1.0% agarose gel (SeaKem LE, supplied by Flowgen), approximate dimensions 12 × 13 cm, prepared in 1X TAE electrophoresis buffer (*see* **Subheading 2.4., item 3**), and containing 5 µL solution of 10 mg/mL ethiduim bromide.
8. 10X sucrose loading buffer: *see* **Subheading 2.4., item 2**.
9. Mol-wt marker, such as pBR322 digested with *Bst*N1 (*see* **Note 5**), and prepared at 0.5 µg/10 µL in 1X sucrose loading buffer (*see* **Subheading 2.4., item 2**).

2.6. Direct Detection of Deletions and Duplications

The materials required for the detection of deletions and duplications using PCR based approaches are listed in Chapter 5, **Subheadings 2.1., 2.2.**, and **2.3.**, and those for Southern blotting are in Chapter 5, **Subheading 2.4.**

2.7. PCR of Microsatellite Markers

1. Items 1–3, and 5 detailed in subheading 2.5. above for PCR amplification.
2. Oligonucleotide primers as appropriate (*see* **Table 3**), prepared as 10 µ*M* solutions in sterile dH_2O.

2.8. Separation of Microsatellites on Denaturing Gels

2.8.1. Rapid Separation Using Midi Gels (see **Note 6**)

1. Midi Atto-type gel apparatus, (GRI), approximate dimensions 15 × 15 cm, gel thickness 0.75 mm. Glass plates should be cleaned with ethanol before assembling the cassette.
2. 40% w/v Acrylogel solution (19:1 ratio of acrylamide to *bis*-acrylamide) supplied by BDH (London).
3. 8 *M* urea solution: Prepare in dH_2O, and stored at RT.
4. 10% ammonium persulphate (APS): Prepare in dH_2O, and store at –20°C in 1 mL aliquots. Once thawed, use within 48 h.
5. *N,N,N′,N′*-tetramethylethylenediamine (TEMED [Sigma]).
6. Formamide loading buffer: 95% formamide, 10 m*M* EDTA, pH 8.0, 0.05% xylene cyanole, 0.05% bromophenol blue.
7. Tris-borae–EDTA (TBE) electrophoresis buffer: Dilute to 0.6X concentration from a 10X stock solution containing 108 g Tris-base, 55 g orthoboric acid, 40 mL 0.5 *M* EDTA, pH 8.0, per L.
8. Suitable mol-wt marker ladder, such as pBR322 digested with *Msp*1 (*see* **Note 7**).
9. Silver (Ag) staining solution 1 (fixer): 10% ethanol, 0.5% acetic acid, prepared in dH_2O.
10. Ag staining solution 2 (stain): 0.1% Ag nitrate dissolved in dH_2O.
11. Ag staining solution 3 (developer): 1.5% NaOH, 1.5% formaldehyde freshly prepared before use in dH_2O.
12. Ag staining solution 4 (neutralizer): 0.75% Na carbonate in dH_2O.
13. Hot air gel drier (Bio-Rad, Hercules, CA).
14. Cellophane membrane (Bio-Rad).

Table 3
Primer Sequences of Microsatellite Markers Used for Dystrophin Gene Analysis

Marker	Forward primer (5'–3')	Reverse primer (5'–3')	Ref.
5' DYS I	ACT GTA AAT GAA ATT GTT TTC TAA GTG CC	GTT AAC AAA ATG TCC TTC AGT TCT ATC C	*15*
5' DYS II	TCT TGA TAT ATA GGG ATT ATT TGT GTT TGT TAT AC	ATT ATG AAA CTA TAA GGA ATA ACT CAT TTA GC	*15*
5' DYS MSA	ATC CCA TCC TGT TCT ATT TT	ACT GGC ATG CAT TAT TTT GT	*16*
5'-5n3	TTC AGT TTC TCT CGG TGT TCC T	TAC ACC TGC ACA TGT GAT GAA A	*17,18*
5'-5n4	GTC AGA ACT TTG TCA CCT GTC	GAA GGG AAA ATG ATG AAT AAA ACT	*18*
STR 7A	TTC TGG TTT TCT GGT CTG	GAA TCA ATC TCT CTG TCA AG	*25*
5'-7n4	GTG AAG CTA CAA AAA TAT TAG AG	CAA CAA TAT CTC ACC ATA CTT G	*18*
STR 44	TCC AAC ATT GGA AAT CAC ATT TCA A	TCA TCA CAA ATA GAT GTT TCA CAG	*19*
IVS 44-SK21	GGT TTG CTG AAC AGC TCC AG	GCT CAG TGA ATG AAT AGC ACA C	*20*
STR 45	GAG GCT ATA ATT CTT TAA CTT TGG	CTC TTT CCC TCT TTA TTC ATG TTA	*19*
STR 48	TGG CTT TAT TTT AAG AGG AC	GTT TTC AGT TTC CTG GGT	*21,22*
STR 49	CGT TTA CCA GCT CAA AAT CTC AAC	CAT ATG ATA CGA TTC GTG TTT TGC	*19*
STR 50	AAG GTT CCT CCA GTA ACA GAT TTG G	TAT GCT ACA TAG TAT GTC CTC AGA C	*19*
DMD I	ATA ACT TAC CCA AGT CAT GT	TGT CTG TCT TCA GTT ATA TG	*23*
STR 62/63	TTC TTC GTC GAT ACC CCC ATT CCA	CTC TTT GAG TTT GAA GTT ACC TGA	Unpub.
3'-19n8	AGC CCC ATT CTG TAC ATC AAA T	AAC GAC TTC CCC CAC TCT GT	*16,17*
3' STR HI	ACG ACA AGA GTG AGA CTC TG	ATA TAT CAA ATA TAG TCA CTT AGG	Unpub.
3' DYS-CA	GAA AGA TTG TAA ACT AAA GTG TGC	GGA TGC AAA ACA ATG CGC TGC CTC	*24*
MP1P	ATC AGA GTG AGT AAT CGG TTG G	ATC TAG CAG CAG GAA GCT GAA TG	*26*

2.8.2. Separation on Sequencing Gels (see **Note 6**)

1. Bind solution: 3 µL methacryloxypropyltrimethoxysilane (Sigma), 1 mL 5% acetic acid/90% ethanol. Clean one of the gel plates with bind solution. It is important to ensure that the gel will adhere to one plate, when the cassette is dismantled following electrophoresis. This plate will act as a support while the gel is being stained.
2. 1X TBE electrophoresis buffer: Dilute from 10X stock (*see* **Subheading 2.8.1., item 7**).
3. 6% denaturing polyacrylamide sequencing gel: Prepare gel using sequencing-grade acrylamide such as Sequagel (National Diagnostics) in 5.2 *M* urea and 1X TBE buffer. Polymerize with TEMED (*see* **Subheading 2.8.1., item 5**) and APS (*see* **Subheading 2.8.1., item 4**).
4. Formamide loading buffer: 98% formamide, 10 m*M* EDTA, pH 8.0, 20 m*M* NaOH, 0.05% xylene cyanole, 0.05% bromophenol blue.
5. Ag staining fixer: 1.8 L dH_2O, 200 mL glacial acetic acid.
6. Ag staining solution: Dissolve 2 g Na nitrate in 2 L dH_2O, then add 3 mL formaldehyde, in a fume cupboard.
7. Ag staining developer: Prepare a solution of Na thiosulphate at 10 mg/mL. Dissolve 60 g sodium carbonate in 2 L dH_2O, then add 3 mL formaldehyde and 400 µL Na thiosulphate solution in a fume cupboard. Store at 4°C. Ensure that this solution is at 4°C before use.
8. Tray sufficiently large to hold a sequencing gel plate.
9. APC Na sequence film (Promega).
10. Light box.

3. Methods

3.1. DNA Extraction from CVBs 1 (Suitable for Use in PCR; see Note 1)

1. Place the CVB sample (usually 20–30 mg) into 500 µL CVB buffer in a 1.5-mL tube.
2. Mix well, and centrifuge at high speed (1300 rpm) in a microcentrifuge for 2 min.
3. Discard as much of the supernatant as possible.
4. Add 500 µL CVB buffer, 5 µL 10% SDS, and 50 µL proteinase K. Mix well.
5. Incubate at 37°C for 16 h, or overnight, on a circular rotating platform, or in a shaking water bath.
6. Freshly prepare a premix of 600 µL water saturated phenol and 600 µL chloroform mix.
7. Take 500 µL of the lower organic layer of this phenol–chloroform mix, and add to the digested CVB mixture. Shake well for 1 min and centrifuge at high speed for 1 min.
8. Transfer the upper, aqueous layer to a clean tube, using a mini-Pasteur pipet, leaving behind any opaque matter at the interface.
9. Repeat the extraction with a further 500 µL phenol–chloroform mix.

10. Transfer the upper, aqueous layer to a clean tube, and extract with 500 µL chloroform mix. Shake well for 1 min, and centrifuge at high speed for 1 min.
11. Transfer the upper aqueous layer to a clean tube, add 43 µL 5 *M* NaCl, and mix well.
12. Add 2 vol of ethanol at RT, and mix gently by tilting the tube back and forth till the strands of DNA become visible.
13. Pellet the DNA by centrifuging for 5 s. Drain away the ethanol mixture, and air-dry for a few minutes.
14. Dissolve the DNA pellet completely in 50 µL sterile dH_2O. Add 25 µL 7.5 *M* ammonium acetate, and mix well.
15. Add 300 µL ethanol at RT, and precipitate the DNA by gently mixing the contents back and forth.
16. Pellet the DNA, by centrifuging for 5 s at high speed, and drain off the ethanol mixture.
17. Wash the DNA in 1 mL 70% ethanol, centrifuge for 10 s, and completely drain off the ethanol.
18. Resuspend the DNA in 50 µL sterile TE buffer.

3.2. DNA Extraction from CVBs 2 (Recommended for Use in Southern Blotting; see Note 1)

1. Place biopsy sample into a 1.5-mL microcentrifuge tube containing 300 µL urea buffer (*see* **Note 8**). Allow to lyse for 16 h, or overnight, at RT on a rotating platform.
2. Pass the sample through a series of three needles with decreasing bore size.
3. Extract with an equal volume of chloroform mix. Shake for 1 min, and centifuge at high speed (1300 rpm) in a microcentrifuge for 1 min.
4. Transfer the upper aqueous layer to a clean tube, leaving the debris at the interface, and extract once more with an equal volume of chloroform mix, as above.
5. Transfer the upper aqueous layer to a clean tube, and add 2 vol of ice-cold absolute ethanol. Mix gently, but thoroughly. Centrifuge at high speed in a microcentrifuge for 1 min. Discard the supernatant.
6. Wash the pellet in ice-cold 70% ethanol. Centrifuge as above, and discard the supernatant, removing as much of the liquid as possible.
7. Dissolve the pellet in 250 µL solution A. When the pellet is thoroughly dispersed, add 25 µL solution B.
8. Add RNaseA to a final concentration of 50 µg/mL (3 µL). Incubate at 37°C for 1 h on a rotating platform.
9. Add 10% SDS to a final concentration of 0.5% (15 µL), and proteinase K to a final concentration of 50 µg/mL (15 µL). Mix by gentle inversion of the tube, and incubate at 37°C for 3–4 hr
10. Add one-tenth vol of 6 *M* $NaClO_4$, and incubate for 1 h at 37°C.
11. Extract with an equal volume of fresh water-saturated phenol–chloroform mix (1:1). Shake well, and centifuge at high speed in a microcentrifuge for 1 min.
12. Transfer the upper aqueous layer to a clean tube, leaving behind any proteinaceous debris at the interface. Extract with an equal volume of chloroform mix. Centrifuge as above.

13. Repeat **step 12**.
14. Transfer the aqueous phase to a clean tube, and add one-twentyfifth vol of 3 *M* NaAc, and mix well.
15. Precipitate the DNA with 2 vol of ice-cold absolute ethanol. Rock the tube gently to allow the DNA to precipitate.
16. Wash the pellet in 1 mL 70% ice cold ethanol to remove excess salt. Drain the pellet, and allow to air-dry.
17. Dissolve the DNA in 50–100 µL TE buffer.

3.3. DNA Extraction from Cultured Amniocytes

This method is based on the Nucleon 1 DNA extraction kit supplied by Scotlab.

1. Transfer 3×10^6 cultured amniocytes to a 2 mL microcentrifuge tube in culture medium. Centrifuge at low speed (600 rpm), and discard the supernatant.
2. Add 340 µL solution B, and vortex to resuspend.
3. Add 100 µL 5 *M* $NaClO_4$ solution, and mix on a rotary mixer for 20 min.
4. Incubate for a further 20 min at 65°C, gently mixing from time to time.
5. Add 580 µL ice-cold chloroform and rotary mix for 20 min.
6. Centrifuge at high speed (1300 rpm) for 1 min.
7. Without disturbing the separated phases, add 50 µL Nucleon silica suspension, and briefly allow to settle through the upper aqueous phase. Centrifuge at high speed for 4 min.
8. Remove the DNA-containing phase above the Nucleon silica plug to a 1.5-mL tube.
9. Centrifuge at high speed for 30 s, to pellet any residual Nucleon silica. Transfer supernatant to a clean 1.5-mL tube.
10. Add 880 µL ethanol, and invert occasionally to precipitate DNA.
11. Centrifuge at high speed for 5 min to pellet DNA, and discard supernatant.
12. Add 1 mL ice-cold 70% ethanol, and repeat **step 11**.
13. Dissolve pellet in 50 µL sterile TE buffer.

3.4. Determination of DNA Concentration

1. Dilute the standard DNA to provide the following range of concentrations, in µg/µL: 0.1, 0.25, 0.5, 0.75, and 1.0.
2. Mix 1 µL of each of the dilutions with 10 µL 1X sucrose loading buffer. Prepare the fetal DNA samples by adding 0.5, 1.0, and 2 µL to 10-µL aliquots of 1X sucrose loading buffer. Load all the samples into the wells of a 0.8% agarose gel.
3. Electrophorese at 10 V/cm for 1 h.
4. View the gel with UV illumination, and assess the concentration of the fetal DNA sample by comparison with the range of known standards (*see* **Note 9**).

3.5. Fetal Sexing by PCR (see Note 10)

1. In a 1.5-mL microcentrifuge tube, cooled on ice, prepare a master mix of the components of the amplification reaction (*see* **Note 11**). For each DNA sample to

be amplified (*see* **Note 12**), mix the following: 2.5 µL 10X *Taq* polymerase buffer, 2.5 µL 2 m*M* dNTPs, 1.25 µL X-Y primer at 10 µ*M*, 0.625 µL X-specific primer at 10 µ*M*, 3.125 µL Y-specific primer at 10 µ*M*, 1 U *Taq* polymerase, and water, to allow a total reaction volume of 24 µL per sample (*see* **Note 13**).

2. Aliquot 24 µL master reaction mix into thin-walled 0.5-mL PCR tubes. Add 200–500 ng DNA to each tube in a volume of 1 µL. Substitute with 1 µL sterile dH_2O in the no-DNA control tube. Mix well by flicking the base of the tube.
3. With some thermal cycling machines, it is necessary to overlay with one drop light mineral oil to prevent evaporation.
4. Perform the PCR under the following cycling conditions: one cycle of 94°C for 4 min; 30 cycles of 94°C for 1 min, 52°C for 1 min, 72°C for 1 min; one cycle of 72°C for 10 min.
5. Electrophorese the PCR products through a 1% agarose gel, together with a suitable mol-wt marker at 10 V/cm for 2 h. The X-specific fragment is 771 bp, and the Y-specific fragment is 947 bp.
6. View the bands under UV illumination, and photograph. An example is shown in **Fig. 8**.

3.6. Direct Detection of Deletions and Duplications

Procedures for the detection of deletions and duplications are discussed in detail in Chapter 5. For specific comments concerning the detection of deletions and duplications in prenatal samples, *see* **Notes 14, 15**, and **16**.

3.7. PCR of Microsatellite Markers

Polymorphic microsatellite markers are used to detect maternal contamination of CVBs, and as gene-tracking markers, when the disease-causative mutation has not been identified in an affected male relative.

1. In a 1.5-mL microcentrifuge tube, cooled on ice, prepare a master PCR mix (*see* **Note 11**). For each DNA sample to be amplified (*see* **Note 17**), mix the following: 2.5 µL 10X *Taq* polymerase buffer, 2.5 µL 2 m*M* dNTPs, 1.25 µL forward and reverse primer at 10 µ*M*, 0.5 U *Taq* polymerase, and water, to allow a total reaction volume of 24 µL per sample.
2. Aliquot 24 µL master reaction mix into thin-walled 0.5-mL PCR tubes. Add 100–150 ng DNA to each tube in a volume of 1 µL. Substitute with 1 µL sterile dH_2O in the no-DNA control tube. Mix well by flicking the base of the tube.
3. With some thermal cycling machines, it is necessary to overlay with one drop of light mineral oil to prevent evaporation.
4. Perform the PCR under the following cycling conditions: one cycle of 94°C for 4 min; 28 - 30 cycles of 94°C for 1 min, specific annealing temperature for 1 min, 72°C for 1 min; one cycle of 72°C for 10 min (*see* **Table 1** for annealing temperatures and cycle numbers specific to individual primer pairs).

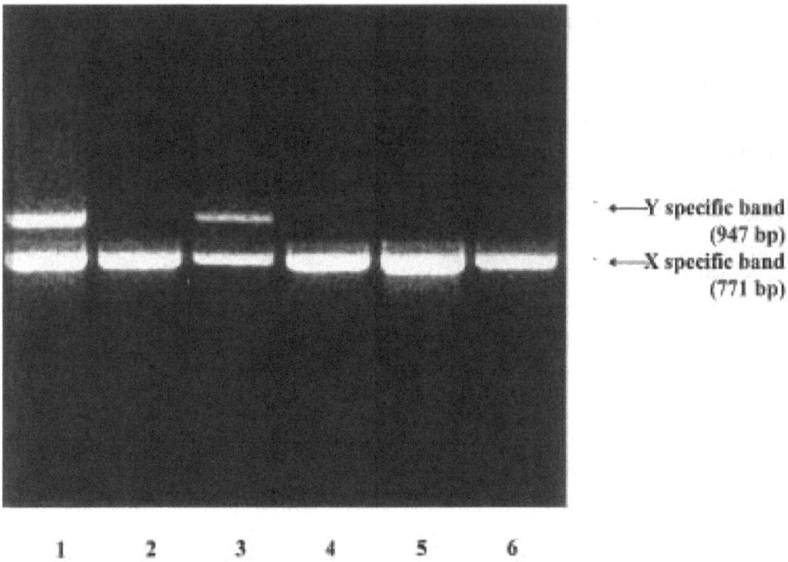

Fig. 8. Sex determination in CVB samples using the polymerase chain reaction. Photograph of a 1% agarose gel stained with ethidium bromide showing X chromosome specific (771 bp) and Y chromosome specific PCR fragments (947 bp). Lane 1, male control sample; lane 2, female control sample; lane 3, male CVB sample; lane 4, female CVB sample; lanes 5 and 6, test CVB sample with 1 µL and 0.5 µL DNA respectively, which was identified as female.

3.8. Separation of Microsatellites on Denaturing Gels

3.8.1. Rapid Separation Using Midi Gels (see **Note 6**)

1. For a gel of dimensions 15 × 15 × 0.75 cm, prepare 20 mL denaturing acrylamide gel solution, as follows: Mix 5 mL Acrylogel solution (this is sufficient for a 10% acrylamide gel, [*see* **Note 18**]), 1.2 mL 10X TBE, 12.5 mL 8 *M* urea, 0.3 mL 10% APS, 15 µL TEMED, dH_2O to a volume of 20 mL. Pour into the cassette, and allow to polymerize overnight, covered with clingfilm.
2. Rinse the wells several times with 0.6X TBE buffer.
3. Heat 1 L 0.6X TBE buffer to approx 60°C, and prerun the gel at 100 V for 10–20 min (*see* **Note 19**).
4. Mix 10 µL PCR product with 10 µL formamide loading buffer, and heat at 95°C for 4–5 min (*see* **Note 20**).
5. Load 6 µL denatured sample into each well (*see* **Note 21**). One lane should contain the mol-wt ladder.
6. Electrophorese the gel at a constant current of 1.7 mA/cm for 1.5–4 h (*see* **Table 4**). The xylene cyanole and bromophenol blue dye fronts will give an indication of how far the DNA fragments have migrated (*see* **Table 4**).

Table 4
Migration of DNA Fragments Relative to Tracking Dyes in Denaturing Polyacrylamide Gels

% gel	Recommended DNA fragment range (bp)	Relative position of bromophenol blue (bp)	Relative position of xylene cyanole (bp)
4.0	>250	30	155
6.0	60–250	25	110
8.0	40–120	20	75
10.0	20–60	10	55

7. Dismantle the apparatus, leaving the gel adhered to one of the plates (*see* **Note 22**), and stain as follows:
8. Pour 500 mL Ag stain solution 1 (fixer) onto gel, and agitate gently for 5 min (*see* Note 23). Pour away the fixing solution. Cover with 500 mL Ag stain solution 2, and agitate gently for 15 min. Pour off the solution 2 (*see* Note 24), and rinse the gels briefly in dH_2O. Cover with 500 mL Ag stain solution 3 (developer), agitate gently for 20–30 min, during which time the bands will appear. Bands representing single-stranded fragments appear reddish in color. Discard solution 3, and replace with 500 mL Ag stain solution 4. Shake gently for 10 min.
9. Discard and cover the gel with dH_2O. It can be photographed to obtain a permanent record, or, alternatively, it can be dried between cellophane sheets using a hot air gel drier and stored.
10. Interpret the results. Examples are shown in **Figs. 9**, **10**, and **11**.

*3.8.2. Separation on Sequencing Gels (*see **Note 6***)*

1. Pre-electrophorese the sequencing gel for 30 min at 60–100 W, allowing the gel to heat to about 50°C.
2. Take a 2.5-µL aliquot of the amplification reaction, and denature by adding 2.5 µL formamide loading buffer. Mix well, and heat at 95°C for 5 min.
3. Load the samples, and electrophorese for 3 h at 60–100 W.
4. Dismantle the cassette, leaving the gel adhered to one plate (*see* **Note 22**).
5. Stain the gel as follows: Cover the gel with fixer solution, and shake very gently for 20 min. Pour off the fixer and retain for reuse. Wash the gel 3× for 2 min each wash in dH_2O. Cover with the Ag stain solution, and leave for 30 min. Pour off, and wash quickly in dH_2O for about 20 s. Add developer solution, and rock gently until bands appear. This usually takes 5–10 min. Add the retained fixer to the developer in the tray to stop the reaction. Wash in dH_2O.
6. Drain all of the liquid from the surface of the gel, and allow to air-dry overnight.
7. Place the gel, supported by the glass plate, onto a light box situated in a darkroom. With the darkroom lights off, place the glossy side of a piece of APC Ag sequence film against the gel. Switch on the light box for 45 s, then develop the film (*see* **Note 25**).

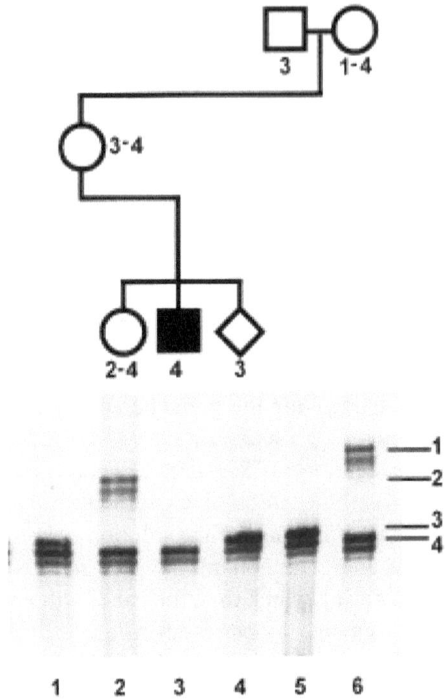

Fig. 9. Prenatal diagnosis using the marker 5'-5n4. PCR fragments were separated on a 8% denaturing polyacrylamide Midi Atto gel which was silver stained. The male fetus, shown in lane 4 has inherited allele 3 which is the opposite maternal allele to that inherited by his affected brother (lane 3). Allele 3 was inherited by the mother (lane 1) from her unaffected father (lane 2). The fetus, therefore, is predicted to be at low risk of developing DMD using this marker.

8. Number the alleles from the top of the gel, and interpret the result. An example is shown in **Fig. 10**.

4. Notes

1. Two methods are described for extraction of good-quality DNA from CVB. The first method is rapid, and is recommended for further analysis by PCR. The second method is more lengthy, but gives a greater yield than the first, and is therefore applicable when the subsequent analysis is by Southern blotting.
2. Fresh water-saturated phenol is a colorless liquid, but it will oxidize over a period of time, which causes the phenol to become discolored, and it should not be used in this state. 8-hydroxyquinoline can be added at a concentration of 0.1%, to reduce oxidation.
3. Most supplies of RNaseA are contaminated with DNase. This can be inactivated by boiling for 5 min without significant reduction in the activity of the RNase.

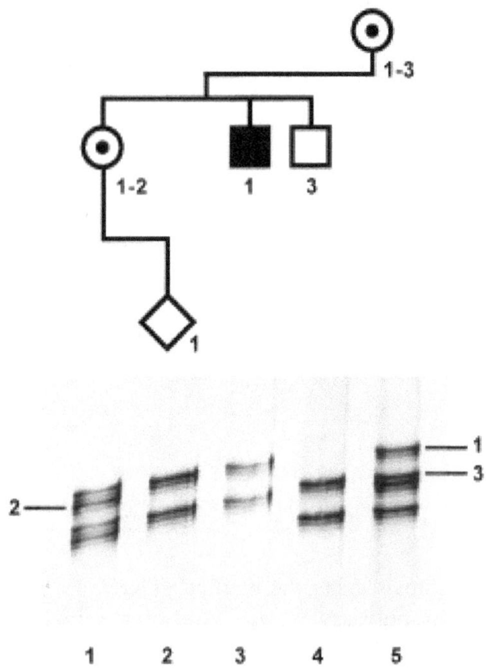

Fig. 10. Prenatal diagnosis using the marker STR 45. PCR fragments were separated on a 10% denaturing polyacrylamide Midi Atto gel which was silver stained. Each allele is detected as two distinct groups of bands as seen in lanes 2, 3 and 4 (male samples). Both the mother (lane 1) and grandmother (lane 5) of the fetus are obligate carriers (full pedigree not shown). The high risk allele is allele 1 as it is present in the affected male (lane 3) and in both obligate carriers. The male fetus, shown in lane 2 has inherited allele 1 from his carrier mother and therefore, is predicted to be at high risk of developing DMD using this marker.

4. This reagent is provided in the Nucleon DNA Extraction kit (Scotlab).
5. pBR322 DNA digested with *Bst*NI, gives fragments of 1857, 1058, 506, 929, 383, 121, and 13 bp. It can be purchased from New England Biolabs (Beverly, MA), and then diluted to the required concentration of 0.5 µg/10 µL with 1X sucrose loading buffer. Alternatively, a stock can be prepared as follows: Mix 10 µg native pBR322 DNA with 10 U *Bst*N1 and 5 µL 10X *Bst*NI digestion buffer. Make up to a total volume of 50 µL, and incubate at 37°C for 4 h. Remove 2 µL, and add 8 µL sucrose loading buffer. Check that digestion is complete, by electrophoresing this aliquot through a 1% agarose gel. Make the stock digest mix up to 200 µL (0.5 µg/10 µL) with 1X sucrose loading buffer.
6. Two methods are described for the separation of microsatellites on denaturing gels. The first, using a Midi Atto gel apparatus, is simple and inexpensive to perform, and the dried gel can be stored as a permanent record. However, resolu-

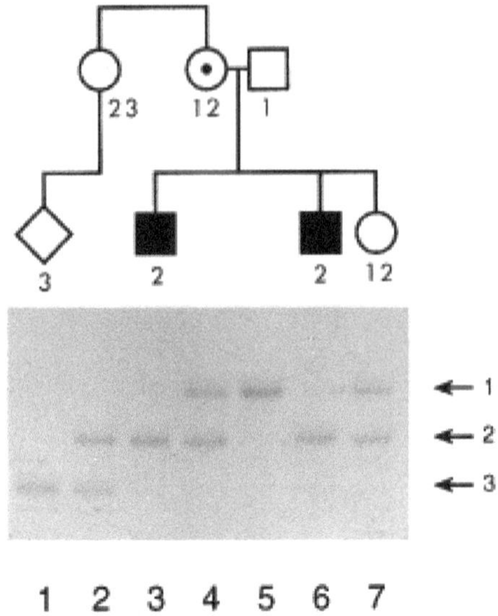

Fig. 11. Prenatal diagnosis using the marker STRH1. PCR fragments were separated on a 6% denaturing polyacrylamide sequencing gel which was silver stained. The aunt (lane 4) of the fetus is an obligate carriers as she has two affected sons. The high risk allele is allele 2 as it is present in both affected males (lanes 3 and 6). The male fetus, shown in lane 1 has inherited allele 3 from his mother and therefore, is predicted to be at low risk of developing DMD using this marker. It should be noted that, because the aunt and mother of the fetus are sisters, they should share a common paternal allele (allele 2). Assuming that their father was unaffected, the aunt either represents a new mutation or the father was a germ line mosaic.

tion of single repeat units can be difficult to achieve in large fragments. The second procedure recommended here is separation on sequencing-type gels, when excellent resolution of the alleles is obtained. However, the gels can be cumbersome to stain, and specialist film is required to obtain a permanent record.

7. pBR322, digested with *Msp*1, produces DNA fragments that are within an ideal size range for comparison with the microsatellite PCR products. The sizes are 622, 527, 404, 307, 242, 238, 217, 201, 190, 180, 160 (×2), 147 (×2), 123, 110, 90, 76, 67 bp. Digested DNA can be purchased from New England Biolabs and diluted to 0.5 µg/10 µL with 1X sucrose loading buffer, and used directly. Alternatively, native pBR322 can be digested with *Msp*1, according to the protocol detailed in **Note 5**.
8. 300 µL urea buffer is recommended for a sample weighing approx 20–30 mg. The volume should be adjusted for any significantly different amount of tissue.
9. This procedure also provides an indication of the quality of the DNA, because any degradation will be observed on the gel. Good quality, high mol-wt DNA will appear as a tight band migrating with, or slightly behind, the native λ DNA.

10. This PCR involves a set of three primers *(4)*. The forward, X-Y primer recognizes a sequence on both the X and Y chrs within the pseudoautosomal regions. The two reverse primers are specific for the X or the Y chr. In a male sample, both X and Y chrs produce amplification products of different sizes. In female samples, a single band is seen on the gel, representing the products from both X chrs.
11. In order to avoid contamination of a PCR mix with products of previous amplifications, it is recommended that two sets of pipets are available, one set for preparing reaction mixes, and a second set for analysis of the products.
12. Samples to be amplified should include the test fetal DNA, control male (XY) DNA, control female (XX) DNA, and a no-DNA control.
13. The final concentrations of the primers in the PCR mix are X-Y primer at 0.5 μ*M*, X-specific primer at 0.25 μ*M*, and Y-specific primer at 1.25 μ*M*. These concentrations give PCR products from the X and Y chrs in male samples of approximately equal intensity.
14. If analysis is by PCR, normally only one multiplex set of primers will be required, corresponding to that of the deletion or duplication previously identified in an affected male relative. However, care should be taken to ensure that one or two pairs of primers are included, which will amplify exons that are not within the deleted/duplicated region. These will produce a product, even in the presence of a deletion, thus controlling the integrity of the reaction components. In the case of a duplication, such control sets of primers are required as internal standards for dosage comparisons.
15. For duplication detection by dosage, it is very important that the fetal DNA is accurately quantified, and that 100–150 ng is used per PCR amplification.
16. If Southern blotting is to be performed, then it is recommended that DNA is extracted according to the protocol in **Subheading 3.2.**
17. Besides one tube for each DNA sample, set up a no-DNA control tube.
18. The acrylamide percentage of the gel will vary according to the size of the PCR fragments to be separated (*see* **Table 1**). The volume of Acrylogel solution should be adjusted accordingly, and compensated by the volume of water used.
19. When the gaskets are removed during assembly of the apparatus, the sides of the gel cassette can be sealed using fine silicone tubing of approx 0.9 mm diameter. This prevents leakage of current through the sides of the gel, which would cause distortion of the lanes as electrophoresis proceeds.
20. Disconnect the gel, and place it beside the heating block, so that the samples can be loaded directly into the wells of the gel.
21. The volume of sample loaded into the gel can be adjusted according to the efficiency of the PCR. This varies for different microsatellite markers.
22. Take care to avoid touching the gel, even when wearing gloves, because finger marks are easily detected by the Ag solution.
23. The gel will float off the plate when covered with fixer. The plate can be carefully removed at this stage without damaging the fragile gel.
24. The Ag stain solution can be reused 3–4× after which the amount of Ag becomes depleted for efficient staining.

25. When a permanent record has been made, the gel can be removed from the plate by soaking in water for 20 min, then scraped off, using a plastic instrument that will not scratch the glass. The plates should then be cleaned thoroughly with soap and water, and wiped with ethanol before reuse.

References

1. Lo, Y. M. D. (1994) Noninvasive prenatal diagnosis using fetal cells in maternal blood. *J. Clin. Pathol.* **47,** 1060–1065.
2. Simpson, J. L. and Elias, S. (1993) Isolating fetal cells from maternal blood: advances in prenatal dignosis through molecular technology. *JAMA* **270,** 2357–2361.
3. Handyside, A. H. (1993) Diagnosis of inherited disease before implantation *Reprod. Med. Rev.* 2, 51–61.
4. Ellis, N., Taylor, A., Bengtsson, B. O., Kidd, J., Rogers, J., and Goodfellow, P. (1990) Population structure of the pseudoautosomal boundary. *Nature* **344,** 663–665.
5. Hentemann, M., Reiss, J., Wagner, M., and Cooper, D. N. (1990) Rapid detection of deletions in the Duchenne muscular dystrophy gene by PCR amplification of deletion-prone exon sequences. *Hum. Genet.* **84,** 228–232.
6. Koenig, M., Monaco, A. P., and Kunkel, L. M. (1988) The complete sequence of dysrophin predicts a rod-shaped cytoskeletal protein. *Cell* **53,** 219–228.
7. Roberts, R. G., Coffey, A. J., Bobrow, M., and Bentley, D. R. (1993) Exon structure of the human dystrophin gene. *Genomics* **16,** 536–538.
8. Forest, S., Cross, G. S., Speer, A., Gargner-Medwin, D., Burn, J., and Davies, K. E. (1987) Preferential deletion of exons in Duchenne and Becker muscular dystrophies. *Nature* **329,** 638–640.
9. Den Dunnen, J. T., Grootscholten, P. M., Bakker, E., Blonden, L. A., Ginjaar, H. B., Wapenaar, M. C., et al. (1989) Topography of the DMD gene, FIGE and cDNA analysis of 194 cases reveals 115 deletions and 13 duplications. *Am J. Hum. Genet.* **45,** 835–847.
10. Bushby, K. M. D., Gardner-Medwin, D., Nicholson, L. V. B., Johnson, M. A., Haggerty, I. D., Cleghorn, N. J., Harris, J. B., and Bhattacharya, S. S. (1993) The clinical, genetic and dystrophin characteristics of Becker muscular dystrophy. II. Correlation of phenotype with genetic and protein abnormalities. *J. Neurol.* **240,** 105–112.
11. Abbs, S., Roberts, R. G., Mathew, C. G., Bentley, D. R., and Bobrow, M. (1990) Accurate assessment of the intragenic recombination frequency within the Duchenne muscular dystrophy gene. *Genomics* **7,** 602–606.
12. Oudet, C., Hanauer, H., Clemens, P., Caskey, T., and Mandel, J. L. (1992) Two hot spots of recombination in the DMD gene correlate with the deletion prone regions. *Hum. Mol. Genet.* **1,** 599–603.
13. Bakker, E., Veenema, H., Den Dunnen, J. T., van Broeckhoven, C. Grootscholten, P. M., Bonten, E. J., and van Ommen, G. J. B. (1989) Germinal mosaicism increases the recurrence risk for new DMD mutations. *J. Med. Genet.* **26,** 553–559.
14. van Essen, A. J., Abbs, S., Baiget, M., Bakker, E., Boileau, C., van Broeckhoven, C., et al. (1992) Parental origin and germline mosaicism of deletions and duplications of the dystrophin gene: a European Study. *Hum. Genet.* 88, 249–257.

15. Feener, C. A., Boyce, F. M., and Kunkel, L. M. (1991) Rapid determination of CA polymorphisms in cloned DNA: Application to 5' region of the dystrophin gene. *Am. J. Hum. Genet.* **48,** 621–627.
16. Oudet, C., Heilig, R., Hanauer, A., and Mandel, J. L. (1991) Nonradioactive assay for a new microsatellite polymorphism at the 5' end of the dystrophin gene and estimates of intragenic recombination. *Am. J. Hum. Genet.* **49,** 311–319.
17. King, S. C., Stapleton, P. M., and Love, D. R. (1994) Two new dinucleotide repeat polymorphisms at the DMD locus. *Hum. Mol. Genet.* **3,** 523.
18. King, S. C., Roche, A. L., Passos-Bueno, M. R., Takata, R., Zatz, M., Cockburn, D., Seller, A., Stapleton, P. M., and Love, D. R. (1995) Molecular characterisation of further dystrophin gene microsatellites. *Mol. Cell. Probes* **9,** 361–370.
19. Clemens, P. R., Fenwick, R. G., Chamberlain, J. S., Gibbs, R. A., et al. (1991) Carrier detection and prenatal diagnosis in Duchenne and Becker muscular dystrophy families using dinucleotide repeat polymorphisms. *Am. J. Hum. Genet.* **49,** 951–960.
20. Kochling, S., Den Dunnen, J. T., Dworniczak, B., and Horst, J. (1995) Two polymorphic dinucleotide repeats in intron 44 of the dystrophin gene. *Hum. Genet.* **95,** 475–477.
21. Saad, F. A., Busque, C., Vitiello, L., and Danieli, G. A. (1993) DXS997 localised to intron 48 of dystrophin. *Hum. Mol. Genet.* **2,** 2199.
22. Saad, F. A., Busque, C., Vitiello, L., and Danieli, G. A. (1994) DXS997 localised to intron 48 of dystrophin. *Hum. Mol. Genet.* **3,** 1034.
23. Powell, J. F., Fodor, F. H., Cockburn, D. J., Monaco, A. P., and Craig, I. W. (1991) A dinucleotide repeat polymorphism at the DMD locus. *Nucl. Acids. Res.* **19,** 1159.
24. Oudet, C., Heilig, R., and Mandel, J. L. (1990) An informative polymorphism detectable by the polymerase chain reaction at the 3' end of the dystrophin gene. *Hum. Genet.* **84,** 283–285.
25. Kneppers et al. DMD data pages, Leiden University,
26. Roberts, R. G., Montandon, A. J., Bobrow, M., and Bentley, D. R. (1989) Detection of novel genetic markers by mismatch analysis. *Nucl. Acids Res.* **17,** 5961–5971.

10

Molecular Diagnosis and Genetic Counseling of the Manifesting Carrier of Duchenne Muscular Dystrophy

Eric P. Hoffman and James Giron

1. Introduction

The large majority of female carriers (heterozygotes) of Duchenne or Becker muscular dystrophies (DMD/BMD) show no overt clinical symptoms. Although most carriers have been reported to have heart abnormalities by imaging technologies (echocardiography), the majority of female carriers do not show overt cardiac dysfunction *(1–3)*.

Rarely, some families segregating DMD in males can show female carriers who exhibit clinical symptoms. The symptoms of such manifesting carriers vary greatly in severity, and can mimic either DMD or BMD in males *(4–7)*. Of the 123 manifesting carriers that the authors have studied, common presentations were proximal weakness, asymptomatic hyperCKemia, and myalgias, with age of presentation ranging from the neonatal period to 49 yr of age; even older ages of presentation have been reported *(8)*. Some female manifesting carriers may present with a more severe and more complex phenotype than is typical for DMD in males: These patients generally have cytogenetic abnormalities involving the dystrophin gene (translocations, inversions, insertions). The authors have found an increasing number of isolated female cases of hyperCKemia referred for testing for carrier status, and a relatively high proportion of such asymptomatic hyperCKemi patients test positive as carriers of DMD (this is elaborated on below) *(4,8)*.

It is important to distinguish between manifesting carriers with a positive family history, and those who are isolated cases. Familial manifesting carriers have male relatives with typical DMD or BMD. Isolated cases of girls or women who are found to be carriers of DMD in the absence of a family history of DMD or BMD are termed isolated manifesting carriers.

From: *Methods in Molecular Medicine, vol. 43: Muscular Dystrophy: Methods and Protocols*
Edited by: K. M. D. Bushby and L. V. B. Anderson

The authors have seen about equal numbers of both familial and isolated manifesting carriers. However, this could represent ascertainment bias based on the referral population (familial manifesting carriers may be expected to be more common). The authors and others ***(4,6,7)*** have found excellent correlation among serum creatine kinase (SCK) levels, extent of dystrophin deficiency in muscle biopsy, and clinical severity in isolated carriers. However, familial manifesting carriers show considerable discrepancy among clinical, laboratory, and biochemical findings; this can be attributed to ascertainment bias on the part of the family, patient, and physicians, although this is a speculative explanation. There are many possible variables that can alter the amount of dystrophin in a patient's muscle (*see* below), and this may be the reason that X-inactivation/phenotype correlations have been more difficult to draw in other studies ***(5,9)***.

Girls and women who are manifesting carriers (both isolated and familial) represent one of the greatest challenges for diagnosis and genetic counseling ***(10)***. Much of the difficulty in detecting and counseling these patients results from the fact that they are mosaics of both mutant and normal dystrophin genes, and that the extent of mosaicism can change dramatically as a function of time (patient age). The many variables that contribute to the clinical phenotype, histopathological picture, biochemical findings, and genetic findings have been studied in some detail ***(11)***.

Before describing the pragmatic aspects of diagnosis and counseling of these patients, it is important to understand a number of the variables influencing phenotype (clinical and histological) in manifesting carriers. First and foremost, the patterns of X-inactivation are critical. All females show X-inactivation (also termed "lyonization"), in which either the maternal or paternal X chromosome (chr) is inactivated in each cell of the body. The X-inactivation event occurs early in embryogenesis (~100-cell stage), and is typically random; about 50% of cells opt to inactivate the maternal X chr, and the other 50% the paternal X. Because there is substantial mixing of cells during development, muscle tissue, and each myofiber, usually ends up with half the nuclei using the father's X chr, and half the mother's X chr. In the great majority of familial carriers of DMD who are asymptomatic, half the myonuclei have the normal X active (usually paternally derived X), and half have the maternal X with the mutant dystrophin gene active. This results in each myofiber making approx 50% of dystrophin, because half the myonuclei are producing dystrophin and half are not. In manifesting carriers, there is almost always skewed X-inactivation, in which a preponderance of cells use the abnormal X, and a minority of cells use the normal X ***(6,12)***.

One may anticipate that the amount of dystrophin produced in a carrier's muscle is correlated with the percentage of myofiber nuclei with the normal X (good dystrophin gene) active; e.g., a typical asymptomatic familial carrier, in whom myofibers have 50% of nuclei with the normal (paternal) X active, and 50% with the mutant (maternal), should show 50% of normal dystrophin levels in her muscle biopsies. This has been shown not to be true, because of additional important variables: nuclear domains, biochemical normalization, and genetic normalization. Nuclear domains are localized regions of a single myofiber, which are served by a single myonucleus; a dystrophin-positive nucleus with the normal X active will provide dystrophin protein to a region surrounding it, but not to distant reaches of the myofiber. Thus, individual myofibers typically appear mosaic regarding dystrophin expression, with some regions of the myofiber staining dystrophin-positive and some dystrophin-negative.

If nuclear domains were kept to a distinct and strict size, then each positive myonucleus would make dystrophin for it's specific nuclear domain, and each negative nucleus would show it's nuclear domain as dystrophin-negative. This should result in 50% of dystrophin in a typical, nonmanifesting carrier of DMD. However, this scenario also proves to be false, because of biochemical normalization, and genetic normalization (**Fig. 1**). Both of these are dynamic processes that alter the dystrophin content in a carrier muscle. Biochemical normalization refers to the diffusion of dystrophin within a syncytial myofiber, from regions that are positive into regions that are negative. Thus, the nuclear domain of a dystrophin-positive nucleus is probably much larger than the nuclear domain in a normal, noncarrier female, because dystrophin protein will diffuse into the nuclear domain of a dystrophin-negative nucleus. In this manner, biochemical normalization leads to the gradual diffusion of dystrophin in the myofiber, where negative regions are rescued, and the carrier muscle will gradually gain more dystrophin, with time, through this process (**Fig. 1**). Because dystrophin is a large, membrane-bound protein, it is probably capable of relatively limited diffusion; this hypothesis has been borne out by experimental and patient studies. Thus, biochemical normalization may result in a doubling of the dystrophin content, but probably not much more, e.g., a manifesting carrier with 10% of myonuclei, with the normal X active, shows 20% of normal dystrophin levels in her muscle because of biochemical normalization *(11)* (**Fig. 1**).

An even more dynamic process is genetic normalization (**Fig. 1**), which results in an everincreasing proportion of dystrophin-positive nuclei in carrier muscle, as a function of age, because dystrophin-negative regions of a myofiber

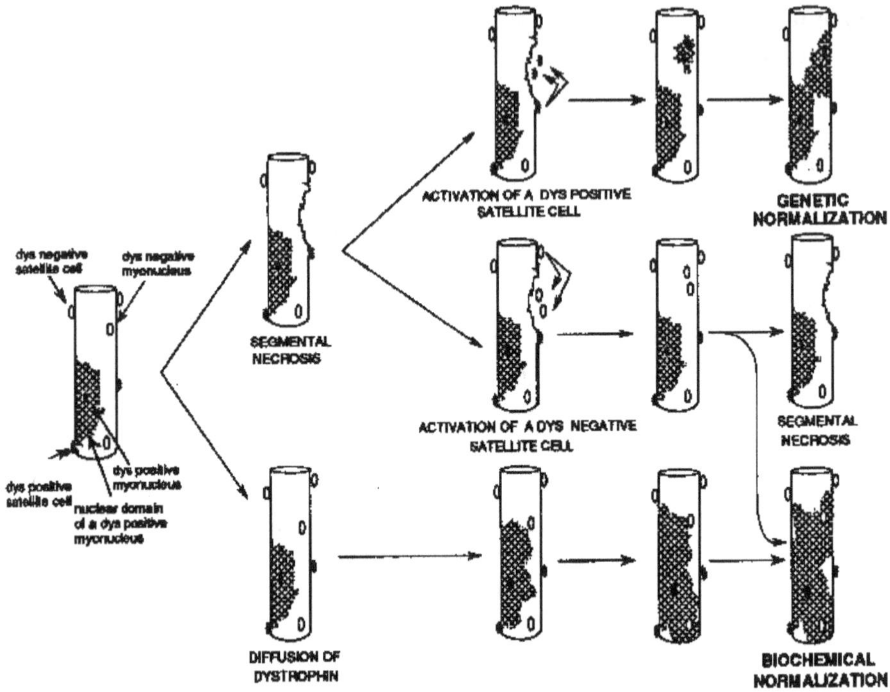

Fig. 1. Schematic diagram of the different cellular processes leading to changes in dystrophin-positive and dystrophin-negative nuclei, and to changes in distribution of dystrophin protein in female heterozygote muscle. Reproduced with permission from **ref.** ***11***.

are subject to segmental necrosis (death), but dystrophin-positive regions remain viable. If a dystrophin-negative region becomes necrotic, it may be regenerated by dystrophin-negative myoblasts; the proportion of nuclei with the normal X active will not change in that myofiber. However, the newly regenerated dystrophin-negative region of the myofiber is subject to further rounds of necrosis. On the other hand, it is possible that the necrotic region is regenerated by dystrophin-positive myoblasts, and this will change the X-inactivation pattern of the myofiber, in which it has more normal dystrophin genes than it started with. With advancing age, there is a constant selective pressure in muscle, where dystrophin-negative regions of myofibers will undergo multiple cycles of degeneration/regeneration, unless regenerated by dystrophin-positive myoblasts, at which point that region of the myofiber is no longer subject to segmental necrosis (**Fig. 1**). An additional fact that influences this genetic normalization of carrier muscle is the progressive histopathology of dystrophin-negative regions: If enough degeneration/regeneration occurs in a region of the muscle, then fibrosis and failed regeneration ensues, leading to replacement of the negative region with fibrofatty connective tissue. Thus, in older carriers, regions of muscle that were unable to regenerate as dystrophin-positive lose most or all dystrophin-negative myofibers to fibrofatty, endstage muscle, leaving only dystrophin-positive fibers remaining ***(13)***.

There are some pragmatic diagnostic and counseling consequences of the complex, dynamic processes occurring in carrier muscle. First, it is far more accurate to assay X-inactivation patterns in blood than it is in muscle. The patterns seen in blood almost certainly reflect the pattern that was present in the patient's muscle early in her life, before genetic normalization, biochemical normalization, and permanent death of myofibers took place. Second, it is always best to diagnose female carriers by muscle biopsy at young ages. The younger a patient is, the less chance that the complicating variables have had a dramatic effect on the biochemical and genetic patterns in the muscle tissue.

To illustrate this scenario, the authors have seen older, wheelchair-bound manifesting carriers who show only 5% of the normal X active in their peripheral blood, yet their muscle biopsy contains predominantly dystrophin-positive myofibers, with levels of 70–80% dystrophin by immunoblot. In this case, much of the dystrophin-negative muscle showed failed regeneration and had turned to fibrofatty connective tissue, leaving only the relatively small number of dystrophin-positive myofibers remaining in the atrophic muscle.

Regarding identification of female carriers, there are distinctly different methods employed for familial and isolated carriers. In the authors' opinion, muscle biopsy is rarely indicated for familial carriers: DNA testing (mutation detection, linkage analyses [*see* Chapters 7 and 8]) and laboratory testing (SCK measurements) are more appropriate methods. The difficulty in using muscle biopsy to identify familial carriers is best understood in terms of SCK: Elevations of SCK result from dystrophin-negative regions of myofibers, and about 70% of asymptomatic carriers have elevations of SCK because of these negative regions. It is may not be worthwhile to biopsy an asymptomatic carrier with high SCK, because the CK elevations indicate that she is almost certainly a carrier. Carriers can have normal CK levels, but these same carriers probably have very few dystrophin-negative regions in their muscle. If they have few dystrophin negative regions (because of biochemical and genetic normalization [*see* above]), then dystrophin testing of muscle biopsy may not be sensitive or accurate, because there are few if any dystrophin-negative fibers upon which to base a carrier diagnosis by muscle biopsy. Thus, the authors discourage the biopsy of potential familial carriers. If a potential carrier in a DMD pedigree is not satisfied with the risk assigned to her (ambiguous risks can be common in pedigrees with no deletion mutation present), then the authors suggest genetic linkage studies and consideration of a fetal muscle biopsy, in certain cases (*see* Chapter 23).

Muscle biopsy is strongly indicated for isolated female dystrophy patients, or isolated hyperCKemia patients, who are potential carriers of DMD or BMD. In our experience, about 10% of isolated female dystrophy and hyperCKemia patients will test positive for mosaicism of dystrophin by muscle biopsy immunofluorescence, and be diagnosed as isolated carriers (*4*; *see* Chapters 20 and 21). These patients are then referred for DNA studies and genetic counseling, as described below.

Establishing a prognosis in female carriers can be difficult. The authors have found that X-inactivation patterns in peripheral blood DNA is the most accurate indicator of prognosis: The greater the extent of skewing of X-inactivation, the more severe the phenotype that is expected ***(13)***. However, the authors' experience is that normalization processes that occur in these patients' muscles slow the progression of the disorder from that seen in males. Thus, in general, female manifesting carriers will have a slower progression, and many in fact improve with age. There is clearly a threshold at which the progression of the disease outraces the normalization processes: A girl with only 1% of nuclei producing dystrophin will not have much chance of rescuing the muscle by genetic and biochemical normalization before fibrosis and failed regeneration set in. Prognostic predictions based on X-inactivation patterns in peripheral blood DNA appear more accurate for isolated carriers than for familial carriers; the authors concluded that this was the result of ascertainment bias on the part of the patient, her family, and her physician ***(13)***.

The authors have diagnosed an increasing number of isolated carriers who were referred for dystrophin testing based solely upon the incidental finding of elevated CK. These asymptomatic hyperCKemia patients are often young girls, and many of them show a mosaic pattern of dystrophin expression in their biopsy diagnostic of the carrier state. Many or most of these girls will probably not show any symptoms, because the proportion of fibers producing dystrophin predominates over those that are dystrophin-negative. Consistent with this, the authors typically find random patterns of X-inactivation (50% maternal, 50% paternal) in their peripheral blood DNA.

DNA analysis and genetic counseling of female carriers is even more complex than is their diagnosis ***(10)***. Typically, deletion analysis is the first DNA testing offered to male patients with DMD or BMD; however, this testing is more difficult in female patients because of heterozygosity for deletions. In other words, males have only one X chromosome, and either all the exons of the dystrophin gene are there or some are missing. Female carriers have two X chrs, only one of which is mutated. Thus, deletion testing involves distinguishing between two copies of each exon and one copy (heterozygous state for a deletion mutation). This testing is typically done by Southern blot analyses, which are generally expensive and time-consuming. Despite these difficulties, deletion testing is indicated for all isolated females who have been diagnosed as carriers by biopsy testing.

X-inactivation assays are used in conjunction with linkage analyses to provide genetic counseling to the families of isolated manifesting female carriers *(10)*. This method is described in detail below. In brief, all isolated manifesting carriers show skewed X-inactivation. Because these girls and women show dystrophin deficiency in muscle that is much more dramatic than seen in asymptomatic carriers, it can be assumed that the more active X chr harbors the mutant dystrophin gene. X-inactivation patterns are determined using an androgen receptor methylation assay in peripheral blood DNA. The more active X chr is identified (that harboring the mutant dystrophin gene), and it is determined whether this at-risk X was derived from the mother or the father (*see* **Figs. 2–4**). If the more active X was derived from the father, then the dystrophin gene mutation must represent a new mutation in the father's germline (**Fig. 2**). The authors' empirical findings to date suggest that about 90% of isolated female manifesting carriers receive their mutant dystrophin gene from their father *(12)*. In such paternally derived dystrophin gene mutations, female siblings of the manifesting carrier have about a 20% risk of being a carrier (gonadal mosaicism risk). The mother and father have no risk of having male children with DMD, because the father cannot pass on his abnormal dystrophin gene to a son. The manifesting carrier is herself a carrier of DMD, thus, half of her male offspring would be expected to have DMD. The normal and abnormal dystrophin genes are followed through the family by linkage analysis, using CA repeat loci distributed throughout the dystrophin gene (*see* **Figs. 2** and **4**).

If the dystrophin gene mutation in an isolated manifesting carrier is derived from the mother (maternal X more active), then the mother may herself may be an asymptomatic carrier, or the mutation may have arisen as a new mutation in the mother's germline (**Fig. 3**). Bayesian risk estimates suggest that 66% of such mothers will be carriers, but 33% will not (new mutation). These risks can be modified by taking SCK measurements in both the mother, and in any female siblings. Any future male children of the mother are at relatively high risk for DMD, so genetic counseling and prenatal diagnosis (based on deletion or linkage testing) should be offered to the mother. Similarly, each of the female siblings of the patient has between a 15 and 50% risk of being a carrier of DMD, and should also be offered DNA linkage and/or deletion testing, and genetic counseling.

The remainder of this chapter focuses on isolated carriers of DMD (either manifesting, or asymptomatic incidental hyperCKemia). As mentioned above, familial carriers (both manifesting and asymptomatic) are best tested and counseled using standard DNA testing (dystrophin gene deletion, and/or dystrophin gene linkage analyses).

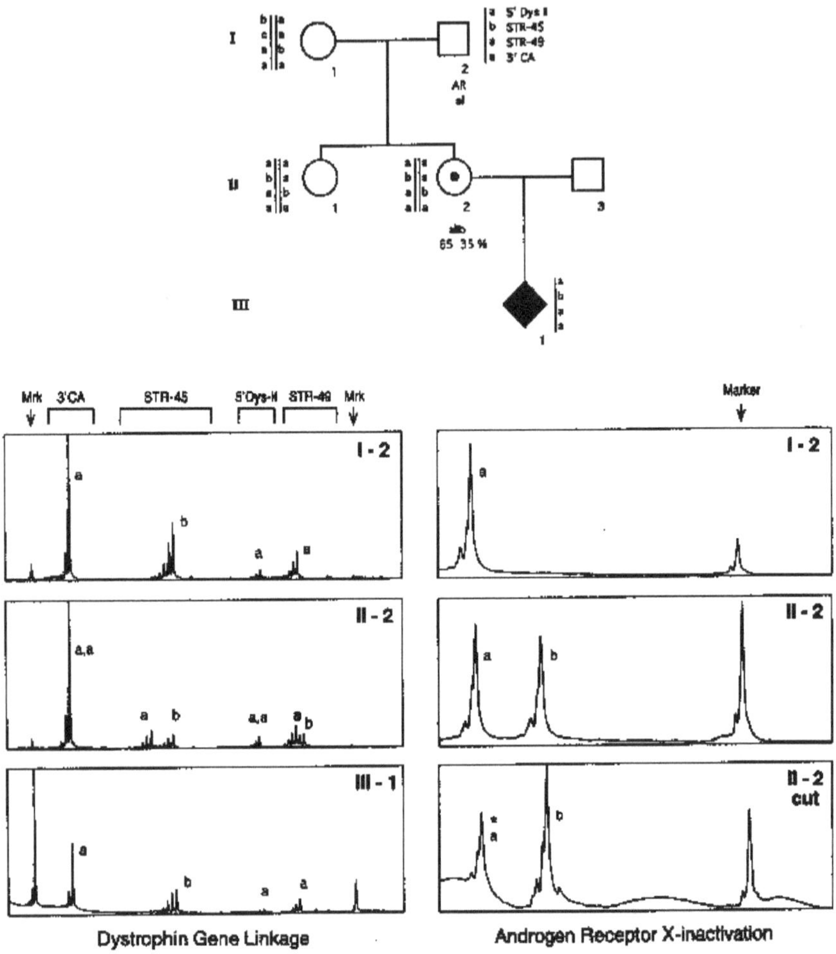

Fig. 2. Prenatal diagnosis in an isolated carrier detects an affected fetus with the grandpaternal dystrophin gene (family 1). Shown is the pedigree of the proband/consultand (II-2), with data on X-inactivation patterns and inheritance using the androgen receptor (right panels), and dystrophin gene linkage using multiplex fluorescent dinucleotide repeats (left panels). The code for haplotypes of the dystrophin gene and androgen receptor are shown near individual I-2. The quantitation of percentage of each X active is shown below the androgen receptor alleles in individual II-2. Individual II-2 showed the paternal androgen receptor gene to be active in 65% of nuclei, suggesting that her grossly elevated serum creatine phosphokinase (CPK) and easy fatigue were probably a consequence of a paternally derived *de novo* dystrophin gene mutation (right panels, "a" allele marked with an asterisk). The paternally derived dystrophin gene was defined in the proband, and it was determined that the male fetus of the proband inherited this at-risk dystrophin gene. The fetus was assigned a high relative risk *(85%)*, but was carried to term. The term baby was a male with persistent serum CPK in excess of 19,000 IU/L, and was diagnosed with DMD. Experimental data is shown for a subset of individuals, with all results summarized on the pedigree. Reprinted with permission from **ref. *10***.

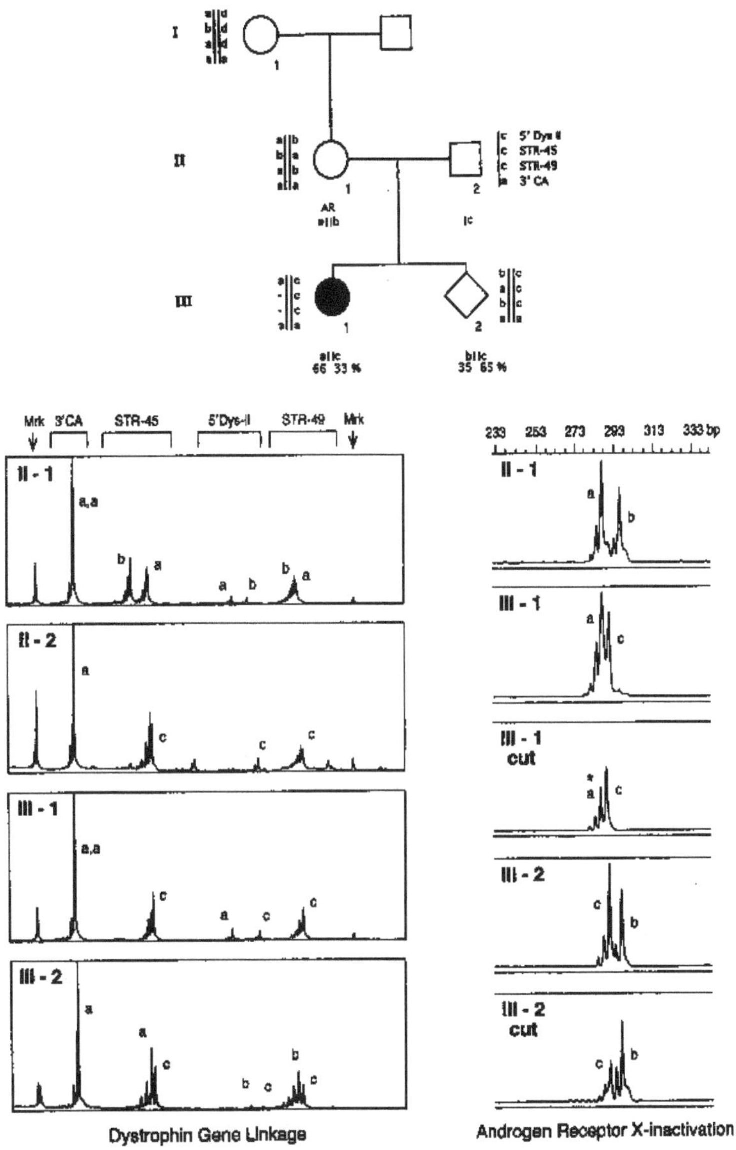

Fig. 3. Counseling of the family of an isolated symptomatic girl carrier reveals a maternally derived *de novo* mutation, and a normal female pregnancy (family 2). Shown is the pedigree of the proband (III-1), with dystrophin gene haplotypes and androgen receptor results summarized below tested individuals. The proband shows preferential activation of the maternal X chr (right panels; “a” allele with asterisk). The close spacing of the AR alleles made quantitation difficult, but the maternal allele was approximated to be active in 66% of cells. The maternally derived dystrophin gene was found to contain a *de novo* deletion mutation encompassing CA repeat loci STR-45 and STR-49. This was not inherited by the female fetus, who was deemed to be a normal female. Experimental data is shown for a subset of individuals, with all results summarized on the pedigree. Reprinted with permission from **ref. *10***.

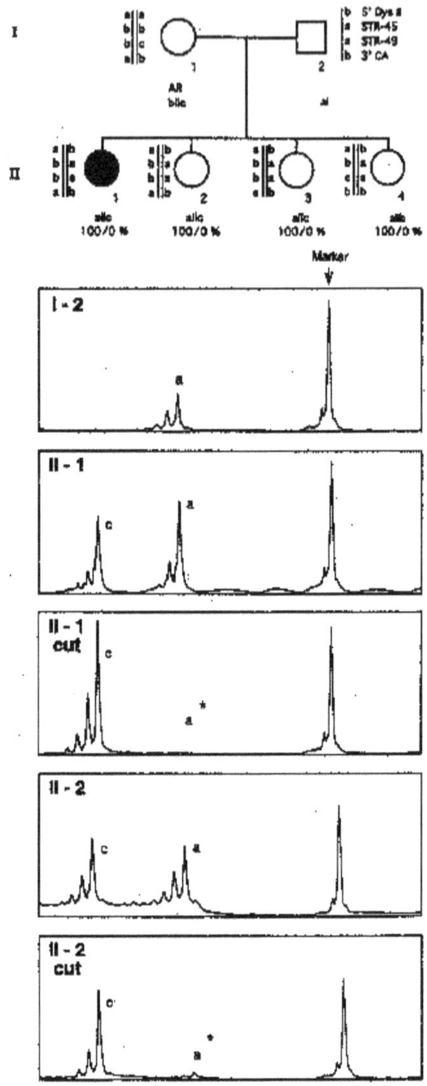

Fig. 4. Paternally derived *de novo* dystrophin gene mutation in a proband (II-1) is probably not inherited by female sibs, based on correlation of X-inactivation patterns and CPK data. Shown is the pedigree of a symptomatic isolated female carrier of DMD (II-1), with dystrophin gene haplotypes and androgen receptor X-inactivation data shown near each individual. The proband is using the paternal X chr in 100% of cells, and shows marked dystrophin deficiency in muscle. This indicates a paternally derived new mutation. The *a priori* risk to her three female siblings for carrier status is the gonadal mosaicism risk to the father, or approx 15%. However, each of the three sibs shows usage of the paternal X in nearly 100% of cells. If any of the three were in fact carriers, then they should show grossly elevated CKs and muscle symptoms. Because all three had normal CPK, it was concluded that they were not carriers. Experimental data is shown for a subset of individuals, with all results summarized on the pedigree. Reprinted with permission from **ref. *10***.

2. Materials

2.1. Immunostaining of Muscle Biopsies

1. Muscle biopsy (100–200 mg) flash-frozen in isopentane cooled in liquid nitrogen.
2. Antidystrophin antibodies (Ab) (60 kd, d10 sheep polyclonals).
3. Anti-α-sarcoglycan Ab (Novocastro monoclonal).
4. Blocking and dilution solution: 10% horse serum in phosphate-buffered saline.
5. Secondary Abs (Cy3-conjugated species-specific Abs; Jackson Immunochemicals).
6. Aqueous mounting media.

2.2. X-inactivation Studies

1. Genomic DNA (prepared by salt extraction).
2. *Cfo*I and *Hpa*II restriction enzymes and SuRE/Cut Buffer L (Boehringer Mannheim).
3. Phenol:chloroform (50:50, equilibrated with Tris, pH 8.0).
4. Ether.
5. *Taq* polymerase and appropriate 10X polymerase chain reaction (PCR) buffer (Perkin-Elmer).
6. Nucleotide precursors (GeneAmp deoxyribonucleoside triphosphate [dNTP]s, Perkin-Elmer).
7. Fluorescently labeled primers (forward primer is flourescently labeled).
8. Met-F (forward primer sequence): 5'-TCCAGAATCTGTTCCAGAGCGTGC-3'.
9. Met-R (reverse primer sequence): 5'-GCTGTGAAGGTTGCTGTTCCTCAT-3'.
10. ABI Sequencer with genescan analysis software.

2.3. Dystrophin Gene Linkage Studies

1. Genomic DNA (prepared by salt extraction).
2. Nucleotide precursors (GeneAmp dNTPs, Perkin-Elmer).
3. AmpliTaq polymerase, and appropriate 10X PCR buffer (Perkin-Elmer)
4. T4 polynucleotide kinase (PNK) and appropriate PNK buffer (New England Biolabs, Beverly, MA).
5. [γ-^{32}P] adenosine triphosphate (ATP) (ICN).
6. Primers.

2.4. Markers Generally Used (Primers)

1.	5'DYSII forward	5'-TAGCTAAAATGTATGAGTA-3'
2.	5'DYSII reverse	5'-AATAGTGTTTTCCTAAGGG-3'
3.	STR45 forward	5'-GAGGCTATAATTCTTTAACTTTGGC-3'
4.	STR45 reverse	5'-CTCTTTCCCTCTTTATTCATGTTAC-3'
5.	STR49 forward	5'-CGTTTACCAGCTCAAAATCTCAAC-3'
6.	STR49 reverse	5'-CATATGATACGATTCGTGTTTTGC-3'
7.	3'CA forward	5'-GAAAGATTGTAAACTAAAGTGTGC-3'
8.	3'CA reverse	5'-GGAAGTCTTATCTTTAATATGC-3'

2.4.1. Additional Markers if Others Are Uninformative

1. 5'DYSIII forward 5'-TTTTTTAGGTATAACTTACATACAATAAACC-3'
2. 5'DYSIII reverse 5'-GTGACAATAAGCATATCAGTGGCTGCC-3'
3. 5'DYSI forward 5'-ACTGTAAATGAAATTGTTTTCTAAGTGCC-3'
4. 5'DYSI reverse 5'-GTTAACAAAATGTCCTTCAGTTCTATCC-3'
5. STR44 forward 5'-TCCAACATTGGAAATCACATTTCAA-3'
6. STR44 reverse 5'-TCATCACAAATAGATGTTTCACAG-3'
7. STR50 forward 5'-UAAGGTTCCTCCAGTAACAGATTTGG-3'
8. STR50 reverse 5'-TATGCTACATAGTATGTCCTCAGAC-3'
9. 6% Acrylamide gel and vertical gel box.
10. X-ray film.

3. Method

3.1. Diagnosis of Isolated Female Carriers by Muscle Biopsy

Indications for consideration of an isolated female carrier diagnosis are any isolated female patient who has been found to have a proximal MD with elevated SCK levels; facial weakness, myotonia, nerve conduction defects, and normal SCK levels each argue for alternative diagnoses. Rare carriers have more complex phenotypes, but many of these have chromosomal abnormalities involving the dystrophin gene: Female patients presenting at very young ages with complex phenotypes and markedly elevated SCK levels should be tested for cytogenetic abnormalities, and biopsied if any abnormality of Xp21 is detected.

The authors have the most success with well-preserved (frozen in isopentane cooled in liquid nitrogen), open biopsies containing more than 2000 muscle fibers (100–200 mg). The authors cryosection biopsies in cross-section at 4 μ, and immunostain with sheep polyclonal Abs directed against both the amino-terminal region of the rod domain (60 kDa) ***(14)***, and cysteine-rich carboxyl-terminal domain (d10) ***(15)***.

3.2. X-Inactivation Studies to Identify the Mutant Dystrophin Gene

For manifesting carriers, blood DNA will invariably show X-inactivation skewing, in which the X chr harboring the mutant dystrophin gene is used in the majority of cells, and the normal X is used in the minority. This is an important point, because the identification of the more active X chr establishes phase and origin of the mutation. An example of this type of analysis is shown in **Figs. 2–4**. The isolated manifesting female carrier shown was detected by mosaicism of dystrophin expression on muscle biopsy. X-inactivation assays of her peripheral blood clearly show one X more active than the other. Because her muscle shows dystrophin deficiency, and she shows clinical symptoms, her more active X chr must be the one harboring the mutant dystrophin gene.

To determine the parental origin of the more active, at-risk X chr, one or both parents must be genotyped for the autosomal recessive (AR) locus in parallel. The parents' DNA does not need to be cut with methylase sensitive restriction enzymes, because it is generally not important to test for X inactivation patterns in the parents.

3.2.1. Methylation-sensitive Restriction Endonuclease Digest

1. Combine 10.5 µL water, 2.5 µL buffer, 1.0 µL *Cfo*I, 1.0 µL *Hpa*II, and 10 µL genomic DNA of the manifesting carrier (~100 ng) in a micro-Eppendorf tube (.75 mL).
2. Incubate at 37°C for 2 h.

3.2.2. Phenol–chloroform Extraction

This step should be completed under a hood.

1. Add 60 µL phenol–chloroform to digested sample tubes; vortex.
2. Spin in microcentrifuge at 4°C for 3 min.
3. Carefully pipet off the top phase (the DNA), and transfer to a new tube.
4. Add 60 µL ether; vortex.
5. Spin in microcentrifuge at 4°C for 3 min.
6. Pipet bottom layer (DNA) carefully, and transfer to a new tube.
7. Repeat steps 4–6.
8. Discard phenol–chloroform/ether, and use digested (cut) product in PCR.

3.2.3. Polymerase Chain Reaction

Uncut and cut samples must be used in separate PCR reactions.

1. Prepare four different PCR reactions:
   a. Reaction A. 5 µL restriction enzyme cut DNA sample from the carrier.
   b. Reaction B. 2 µL (100 ng) genomic DNA (undigested) from the carrier.
   c. Reaction C. 2 µL (100 ng) genomic DNA (undigested) from the mother of the carrier.
   d. Reaction D. 2 µL (100 ng) genomic DNA (undigested) from the father of the carrier.
2. Set up PCR reactions:
   a. DNA (above) + water to 20 µL.
   b. 2.5 µL 10X PCR buffer.
   c. 2.0 µL dNTP precursors (2.5 m*M* each).
   d. 0.5 µL of each forward/reverse primer (forward is fluorescently labeled), 50 ng/µL 0.2 µL Amplitaq DNA polymerase.

3. PCR conditions: Run on a Perkin-Elmer DNA Thermal Cycler: 1 cycle, 95°C, 5 min.; 28 cycles, 96°C, 45 s, 60°C, 30 s, 72°C, 30 s.

3.3. ABI Genescan

Load the cut and uncut PCR products beside each other, for each sample, separately. Be sure to run a size marker to ensure correct PCR product size (approx. 275–310 bp).

Calculate the relative percentage of each X that is active in the manifesting carrier.

1. Each sample will have two peaks, corresponding to the two X chrs, if the patient is heterozygote; approx 95% of individuals are heterozygote for the AR locus. Identify peaks as 1 and 2 in both the digested and undigested lanes.
2. First, derive a normalization factor for unequal amplification of peaks:

   (Undigested peak 2 area) (y) / (Undigested peak 1 area) = 1

   Solve for (y), and use in formula below.
3. Then, solve for relative X inactivation patterns

   (Digested peak 2 area) (y) x 100 / (Digested peak 1 area) = z

   (100) – z % cells with chr 2 active
   z = % cells with chr 1 active
4. For manifesting carriers, the more active X chr will harbor the dystrophin gene mutation (at-risk X chr).
5. The parental origin of the at-risk (more active) X chr is determined by whether the AR allele on the at-risk X was inherited from the mother or the father.

3.4. Methods Notes

1. A control sample that is highly skewed should be used to as a positive control.
2. The phenol–chloroform extraction may result in loss of cut sample.
3. If digestion appears to fail, using the positive-control sample, check the restriction endonucleases. Restriction enzymes may have expired or need a longer incubation period.

4. Linkage Analysis PCR

Radiation shielding should be used throughout this entire process.

4.1. Labeling Forward primers with [γ-^{32}P] ATP

1. Combine the reagents, 9 µL distilled H_2O, 1.5 µL 10X PNK buffer, 1 µL PNK, 1 µL [γ-^{32}P] ATP, and 2.5 µL forward primer (20 µ*M*), mix, and incubate for 30 min, at 37°C.
2. The labeled primers can be kept at –20°C for up to 2 wk.

4.2. Polymerase Chain Reaction

1. Combine the PCR reagents, 7.95 µL H_2O, 1.25 µL 10X PCR Buffer, 1.0 µL dNTPs, 1.0 µL of the ^{32}P-labeled forward primer, 0.2 µL reverse primer (20 µ*M*),

and 0.1 µL Amplitaq DNA polymerase. It is suggested to make a master mix, and aliquot out for each sample.
2. Add the DNA template (1.0 µL, 50 ng/µL conc.) to the PCR mix in a 96-well microtiter PCR plate.
3. PCR conditions (run on a PTC-100, thermocycler [MJ Research]): 1 cycle, 94°C, 3 min; 28 cycles, 94°C, 30 s, 53°C, 30 s, 65°C, 4 min; 1 cycle, 65°C, 7 min.
4. Load samples onto a 6% acrylamide gel. Run at 50 W or less.
5. Expose gel on X-ray film, and develop.
6. Interpret results and alleles from the film.
7. Derive haplotypes.

5. Notes

1. Specific markers used may prove uninformative. Additional markers are listed in Materials.
2. Insufficient intensity of bands corresponding to alleles. Longer exposures or use of an intensifying screen may result in greater intensity, but can give poor resolution. Consider using new, high-specific-activity γ-labeled ATP or new polynucleotide kinase enzyme.
3. Primer and DNA concentrations may also be changed to optimize conditions.

References

1. Politano, L., Nigro, V., Nigro, G., Petretta, V. R., Passamano, L., Papparella, S., Di Somma, S., and Comi, L. I. (1996) Development of cardiomyopathy in female carriers of Duchenne and Becker muscular dystrophies. *JAMA* **275,** 1335–1338
2. Kinoshita, H., Goto, Y., Ishikawa, M., Uemura, T., Matsumoto, K., Hayashi, Y. K., Arahata, K., and Nonaka, I. (1995) A carrier of Duchenne muscular dystrophy with dilated cardiomyopathy but no skeletal muscle symptom. *Brain Dev.* **17,** 202–205.
3. Mirabella, M., Servidei, S., Manfredi, G., Ricci, E., Frustaci, A., Bertini, E., Rana, M., and Tonali, P. (1993) Cardiomyopathy may be the only clinical manifestation in female carriers of Duchenne muscular dystrophy. *Neurology* **43,** 2342–2345.
4. Hoffman et al. (1992)
5. Bushby, K. M., Goodship, J. A., Nicholson, L. V., Johnson, M. A., Haggerty, I. D., and Gardner-Medwin, D. (1993) Variability in clinical, genetic and protein abnormalities in manifesting carriers of Duchenne and Becker muscular dystrophy. *Neuromusc. Disord.* **3,** 57–64.
6. Azofeifa, J., Voit, T., Hubner, C., Cremer, M. (1995) X-chromosome methylation in manifesting and healthy carriers of dystrophinopathies: concordance of activation ratios among first degree female relatives and skewed inactivation as cause of the affected phenotypes. *Hum. Genet.* **96,** 167–176.
7. Matthews, P. M., Benjamin, D., Van Bakel, I., Squier, M. V., Nicholson, L. V., Sewry, C., et al. (1995) Muscle X-inactivation patterns and dystrophin expression in Duchenne muscular dystrophy carriers. *Neuromusc. Disord.* **5,** 209–220.

8. Bonilla, E., Younger, D. S., Chang, H. W., Tantravahi, U., Miranda, A. F., Medori, R., et al. (1990) Partial dystrophin deficiency in monozygous twin carriers of the Duchenne gene discordant for clinical myopathy. *Neurology* **40,** 1267–1270.
9. Sumita, D. R., Vainzof, M., Campiotto, S., Cerqueira, A. M., Canovas, M., Otto, P. A., Passos-Bueno, M. R., and Zatz, M. (1998) Absence of correlation between skewed X inactivation in blood and serum creatine-kinase levels in Duchenne/Becker female carriers. *Am. J. Med. Genet.* **80,** 356–361.
10. Hoffman, E. P., Pegoraro, E., Scacheri, P., Burns, R. G., Taber, J. W., Weiss, L., Spiro, A., and Blattner, P. (1996) Genetic counseling of isolated carriers of Duchenne muscular dystrophy. *Am. J. Med. Genet.* **63,** 573–580.
11. Pegoraro, E., Schimke, R. N., Garcia, C., Stern, H., Cadaldini, M., Angelini, C., et al. (1995) Genetic and biochemical normalization in female carriers of Duchenne muscular dystrophy: evidence for failure of dystrophin production in dystrophin competent myonuclei. *Neurology* **45,** 677–690.
12. Pegoraro, E., Schimke, R. N., Arahata, K., Hayashi, Y., Stern, H., Marks, H., et al. (1994) Dystrophinopathy in females: paternal inheritance and genetic counseling. *Am. J. Hum. Genet.* **54,** 989–1003.
13. Pegoraro, E., Whitaker, J., Mowery-Rushton, P., Surti, U., Lanasa, M., and Hoffman, E. P. (1997) Familial skewed X-inactivation: a molecular trait associated with high spontaneous abortion rate maps to Xq28. *Am. J. Hum. Genet.* **61,** 160–170.
14. Hoffman, E. P., Brown, R. H., and Kunkel, L. M. (1987) Dystrophin: the protein product of the Duchenne muscular dystrophy locus. *Cell* **51,** 919–928.
15. Koenig, M., and Kunkel, L. M. (1990) Detailed analysis of the repeat domain of dystrophin reveals 4 potential hinge regions that may confer flexibility. *J. Biol. Chem.* **265,** 4560–4566.

11

Mutation Analysis of X-Linked Emery-Dreifuss Muscular Dystrophy Gene

Daniela Toniolo

1. Introduction

Emery-Dreifuss muscular dystrophy (EDMD) is an X-linked muscular disease first described in the early 1960s in a family from Virginia *(1)*. The disease is characterized by the triad of early contractures of the elbows, Achilles tendons, and postcervical muscles; slowly progressing muscle wasting and weakness, with humeroperoneal distribution in the early stages of the disease; and a cardiomyopathy usually presenting as heart block *(2–5)*. The cardiomyopathy manifests around the age of 20 yr as a cardiac conduction defect, and the associated heart block is a frequent cause of death. Provided that diagnosis is made sufficiently early, the insertion of a cardiac pacemaker can be lifesaving. In no case has mental retardation or an intellectual defect been described. Families in which EDMD is inherited as an autosomal dominant or recessive trait have been reported *(6)*, but the majority of the EDMD cases are inherited as an X-linked recessive trait. Clinically, the three forms are very similar. For this reason, the term "Emery-Dreifuss syndrome" was proposed for the triad of symptoms *(6)*. Molecular diagnosis is therefore very important for an early diagnosis, and to distinguish X-linked EDMD from the autosomal forms, as well as from different MDs presenting with contractures.

The EDMD gene is very small, only about 2 kb long, and it is interrupted by five small introns (*7,8*; **Fig. 1**): Sequence analysis of the gene, and of 700 bp of 5'-flanking DNA, established the structure of the gene and confirmed the presence of the predicted CpG island at the 5' end of the gene embedding the first exon *(8)*. Moreover, the 5' region of the gene, from nt -722 to nt 300, is very rich in recognition sites for ubiquitous transcription factors usually found in promoters for housekeeping genes. Accordingly, the EDMD gene encodes a

From: *Methods in Molecular Medicine, vol. 43: Muscular Dystrophy: Methods and Protocols*
Edited by: K. M. D. Bushby and L. V. B. Anderson © Humana Press Inc., Totowa, NJ

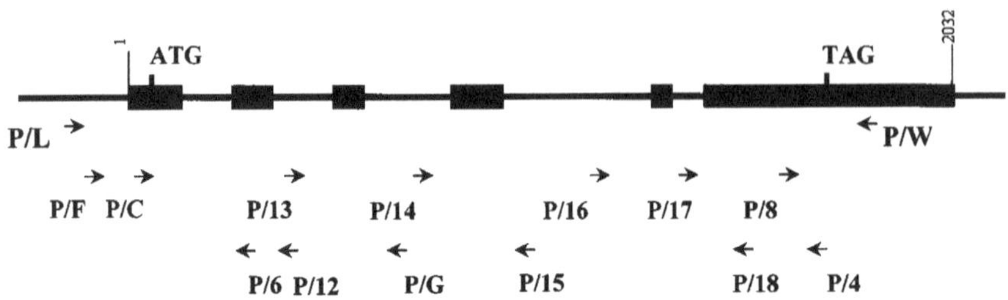

Fig. 1. Schematic representation of the structure of the EDMD gene and the position of the primers. Arrows indicate the orientation of the primers. Blacked in boxes are exons.

mRNA of 1.3 kb, ubiquitously expressed in different cell types, and, in the mouse, early during development *(9)*. The gene is unique, and it encodes a small protein, emerin, 254 amino acids long, of unknown function.

1.1. Strategy

Different approaches have been used to detect mutations in the EDMD gene. In some studies, single-strand conformational polymorphism *(10)* or heteroduplex analysis *(11)* were used. Because of the small size of the gene, however, direct sequencing of exon and exon–intron junctions in genomic DNA *(8,12,13)*, or of the entire coding region, prepared by reverse transcription of RNA *(7,14,15)*, were preferred. So far, >55 mutations have been reported in the EDMD mutation Database, at online Mendelian inheritance in man (OMIM) (www.ncbi.nlm.mih.gov/omin).

The mutations are distributed along the gene, with no evidence of mutation hot spots. Point mutations (47.3%), or small deletions (32.8%), or insertions (10.9%) are the most common. Most mutations introduce premature Stops in the open reading frame. Six mutations occurred in the starting codon (ATG): Such mutations, usually quite rare, are highly represented in EDMD (10.9% of cases). In the remaining cases, mutations are in splice junctions. Rare are large deletions or gene rearrangements. In one case, a complex rearrangement, with a deletion of 429 bases, and an insertion of 103 bases was found *(8)*. In four cases, large deletions, involving the entire gene, were reported. Recently, Small et al. *(16)* reported a case in which the deletion of the entire EDMD gene was caused by a complex rearrangement related to the presence of two very large (11.3 kb) inverted repeats flanking the EDMD and the *FLN1* gene *(17)*. This finding suggested that several types of rearrangements could be produced: Southern blot analysis of 85 individuals demonstrated that 19% of males (12/64) and 33% of females (7 heterozygotes of 21) carried an inversion involving the two genes flanked by the repeats.

The study of mutations in EDMD patients has demonstrated genetic heterogeneity of the disorders. However, in the vast majority of X-linked EDMDs, emerin was completely absent, as a result of these different kinds of mutations. Therefore, protein screening using anti-emerin antibodies ***(14,18,19)*** in muscle or skin biopsy ***(19,20)***, or in buccal smear ***(21)***, should be the first diagnostic tool for EDMD. Direct mutation detection can then identify the specific change at the DNA level.

1.2. Mutation Analysis of EDMD *Gene*

Because of the small size of the *EDMD* gene, only two primers are required for polymerase chain reaction (PCR) amplification of the entire gene from total genomic DNA (**Table 1**). Thirteen primers are sufficient to sequence all exons and exon–intron junctions from both strands, and they are shown in **Fig. 1**. Their sequence is listed in **Table 1**. Sequencing from both strands is especially important for carrier diagnosis, because heterozygotes are not always very well detected by sequencing from only one strand.

2. Materials

2.1. PCR Amplification

1. PCR: XL PCR Kit from Perkin Elmer (PE N808-0182); the kit contains enzymes, buffer, and deoxyribonucleoside triphosphates.
2. Primers (P/L) and (P/W) (*see* **Table 1**), 25 m*M* in water. Primers can be purchased from different companies, and do not need purification.
3. Agarose: any brand of ordinary electrophoresis-grade agarose.
4. Tris-borate–EDTA (TBE) electrophoresis buffer: 5X stock solution contains 0.45 *M* Tris-base, 0.0125 *M* Na-EDTA, 0.45 *M* boric acid. The resulting pH is 8.1.
5. 10X gel loading buffer: 10X TBE, 50% glycerol, 0.25% bromphenol blue, 0.25% xylene cyanol, 10 m*M* Na-EDTA.
6. Bio-Rad (Hercules, CA) Wide MiniSub Cell electrophoresis apparatus.

2.2. Purification of PCR Products

1. Low-melting Sea Plaque Agarose (FMC 50104).
2. Bio-Rad Wide MiniSub Cell electrophoresis apparatus.
3. Water-saturated phenol: Molecular-biology-grade crystallized phenol (Merck) is melted at 65°C, and mixed with water until saturated. It can be stored at 4°C, when protected from light, for about 1 mo.
4. Chloroform:isoamyl alcohol, 24:1.
5. 5 *M* NaCl, 96%, and 70% EtOH.

2.3. Sequencing Reactions

1. Sequencing kit: ABI Prism Dye Terminator Cycle Sequencing Core Kit with Amplitaq DNA polymerase FS.

Table 1
Sequencing Primers

P/L	-106	5'-CTCCCGCGGTTAGGTCCCGCCC-3'	-85
P/W	1984	5'-GGCAGGGGGAGCAAGCACTACTCTG-3'	1960
P/F	-66	5'-GCGGCCGTGACGCGACAACG-3'	-47
P/C	91	5'-CGCCTGAGCCCGCACCCGC-3'	109
P/6	336	5'-CGTAAAGCCTACGAGTTGATCC-3'	315
P/13	457	5'-GGGAGGATGGGGTCGCGAGG-3'	476
P/12	514	5'-TTCTCCAGTGCCGCTCTCGAC-3'	494
P/14	783	5'-TGGGATTCAGATTAGGGCCATCAG-3'	806
P/G	767	5'-CAGTTTCTCCCTCCTAAGGCTGC-3'	745
P/15	1089	5'-CCACCATTTGTACCCAGTGCC-3'	1069
P/16	1192	5'-GCATGAGCACAAGTGGCAAGGC-3'	1213
P/17	1447	5'-CAGGGACGGGCTGGTTCTGGG-3'	1467
P/18	1558	5'-TAGTGCGTGATGCTCTGGTAGG-3'	1537
P/8	1705	5'-GGCTGGGCCAGGATCGCCAG-3'	1724
P/4	1786	5'-TAAATGAAGAAGAGGACGATCAC-3'	1764

2. 3.2 m*M* Oligonucleotide primers in water. Primers can be purchased from different companies, and do not need purification.
3. Purified PCR product: 100 ng/reaction.
4. GeneAMP 9600-9700 PCR system (Perkin-Elmer).
5. 3 *M* NaAc, 96% and 70% EtOH.
6. 40% Acrylamide stock: 38% acrylamide-2% *bis*-acrylamide, filtered through a 0.22-µm filter.
7. TEMED and 10% ammonium persulfate (APS) stock. The APS can be stored in small aliquots (400 mL), at –20°C. Should be thawed only once.
8. Loading buffer: Na-EDTA 50 m*M*: deionized formmamide, 1:5. Use 3 mL for reaction.
9. Applied Biosystem automated sequencing apparatus.

2.4. Mutation Analysis

Software: Perkin-Elmer SeqEd and Sequence Navigator.

3. Methods

3.1. PCR Amplification of EDMD Gene

1. 100 ng genomic DNA is PCR amplified from the primer PL and PW (**Table 1**) in a reaction of 50 mL. 2–4 50 mL reactions are usually required to produce enough DNA for sequencing the whole gene (*see* **Note 1** and **2**).
2. Prepare a master mix under the conditions suggested by the supplier for a 50-mL reaction. Do not add DNA or Taq polymerase (*see* **Note 3**).

3. Aliquot 40 mL master mix into 0.5-mL thin-walled Eppendorf tubes, keeping 10 mL/reaction to dilute the *Taq* polymerase.
4. Add the DNA (100 ng).
5. Add one drop of paraffin oil (Sigma).
6. Hot start: heat at 96°C for 5 min (*see* **Note 4**).
7. Keeping the tubes in the PCR machine, add the *Taq* polymerase diluted in 10 mL master mix. PCR conditions: 96°C for 1 min, 70°C for 3 min, for 40 cycles. Final cycle: 70°C for 7 min. Then keep at 4°C.
8. Add 5 mL gel loading buffer.
9. Run 5 mL of the reaction in 1% agarose gel in TBE containing 0.5 mg/mL of ethidium bromide. Electrophorese at 100 V for about 1 h, until the band is well separated. The band is 2090 bp (*see* **Note 5** and **6**).
10. Photograph the gel on a UV transilluminator.

3.2. DNA Purification

1. Load the whole PCR reaction into 1 lane (1.1 × 0.1 × 0.5 mm) of 1% low-melting agarose gel in TBE. Run at 50 V, at room temperature (RT).
2. Once the separation is complete (about 1 h), transfer the gel on a UV transilluminator and cut the band with a razorblade. Do not expose the gel too long to the UV light, because UV light causes DNA breaks that may interfere with sequencing reactions, by producing nonspecific primers.
3. Transfer the band to a 2-mL Eppendorf tube, melt at 65°C and add 1 vol Tris-EDTA (TE).
4. Add 1 vol phenol saturated with water and 0.1 vol 2 *M* Tris-HCl, pH 8.0, to neutralize the phenol (*see* **Note 8**).
5. Vortex, and spin for 5 min in a microcentrifuge, at RT.
6. Transfer the aqueous phase to a clean tube, and extract the phenol with 100 mL of TE.
7. Mix the two aqueous phases, and extract once with 1 vol chloroform:isoamylalcohol.
8. Precipitate EtOH, and resuspend in 15 mL water.
9. Check the concentration by loading 1 mL on a 1% agarose gel. Compare with serial dilutions of a DNA of known concentration. The DNA should be 30–100 ng/mL.

3.3. DNA Sequencing

1. Prepare 0.2 mL thin-wall PCR tubes in a Perkin-Elmer tube rack for the 9600/9700 Thermal cycler (*see* **Note 9**).
2. Add 1 mL 3.2 m*M* oligonucleotide primers, 1–3 mL DNA to sequence, and 8–10 mL water, to reach a final volume of 12 mL.
3. Prepare, each time, a master mix sufficient for the reaction, following the instructions of the producer. Add 8 mL mix to each tube. Pipet up and down, avoiding direct illumination. The dye terminators are light-sensitive. Do not add oil.
4. Spin briefly using a centrifuge with adapters for microtiter plates, and transfer to a 9600-9700 Perkin-Elmer Thermal cycler. The Thermal cycler should be at 90–96°C.
5. Leave 10 s at 96°C, before starting the cycle sequencing: 96°C for 1 min, 60°C for 4 min, for 25 cycles. Keep at 4°C.

6. Spin briefly, as above, and transfer to 1.5-mL Eppendorf tubes. Add 2 mL 3 *M* NaAc and 50 mL, 96% EtOH.
7. Mix, and keep in ice for not longer than 10 min (*see* **Note 10**).
8. Spin for 20 min in a microcentrifuge, at RT. Wash the pellet, which is not visible, with 70% EtOH, and dry well.
9. Keep dry at –20° until ready for sequencing. Just before use, resuspend in 3 mL loading buffer.
10. Denature at 95°C for 2 min, and transfer immediately to ice.
11. Load on a 4.75% acrylamide gel in TBE, and run on a automated sequencing apparatus (*see* **Note 11**).

3.4. Analysis of Gel

At the end of the run, the sequences should be analyzed using SeqEd, and the portion containing ambiguities should be eliminated. The newly determined sequences should be aligned to the consensus sequence and to themselves. All the ambiguities and differences between the samples and the control DNAs must be checked on the chromatogram.

4. Notes

1. Because the gene is very rich in GC, for an efficient synthesis high temperatures of annealing and synthesis, are required. A long-range *Taq* polymerase system, which allows high temperature of synthesis, is therefore required to get consistent amplification and high amounts of genomic DNA.
2. The genomic DNA should be of high mol wt. Long-range amplification of broken DNA is much less efficient.
3. Great care should be taken to avoid contamination of the PCR reaction by external sources of DNA, especially genomic DNAs other than the one under study. To avoid contamination, use separate pipets and pipet tips with filters, to assemble the reaction. Do not spin PCR reactions after assembling: just mix up and down with the pipet tip. Always perform a control reaction without DNA: If any product is seen in the control, all the reactions should be discarded, and fresh solutions or dilutions should be made.
4. Hot start should be long and at high temperature, because of the high GC content.
5. Under the PCR conditions described, a high amount of only one band of 2 kb should be produced. In case more bands are seen, discard the reactions, and try to set the PCR conditions. Thermal cyclers are not identical.
6. In the original paper *(8)*, a different primer was used, PL instead of PW. It was discovered that PL contained a polymorphic sequence and would not amplify some DNAs. The polymorphism is a CT, instead of GT, at position 1882–1883. The primer PL could still be used, but it may not work.
7. Pour the gel in the cold (4°C), and leave at 4°C for 15–30 min.
8. Do not use phenol–chloroform in this step, but phenol only.
9. Since the sequence reactions should not be done in the presence of oil, the thermal cycle must allow cycling under those conditions.

10. This step is very critical, to get rid of the excess of dye terminators that could interfere with the gel run and reading.
11. Always run a sequence reaction of a normal DNA under the same conditions to control for differences caused by sequence artifacts.

Acknowledgments

The author thanks collaborators and students for establishing the methodology, and specially Silvia Bione and Patrizia D'Adamo, for help with the manuscript. This work was made possible by grants from CNR and Telethon Italy.

References

1. Emery, A. E. H. and Dreifuss, F. E. (1966) Unusual type of benign X-linked muscular dystrophy. *J. Neurol. Neurosurg. Psychiatry* **29,** 338–342.
2. Emery, A. E. H. (1993) Emery-Dreifuss syndrome. *J. Med. Genet.* **26,** 637–641.
3. Toniolo, D., Bione, S., and Arahata, K. (1998) Emery-Dreifuss muscular dystrophy, in *Neuromuscular Disorders: Clinical and Molecular Genetics.* (Emery, A. E. H., ed.), Wiley, London, pp. 87–103.
4. Yates, J. R. W. (1991) European workshop on Emery-Dreifuss muscular dystrophy 1991. *Neuromusc. Disord.* **1,** 393–396.
5. Yates, J. R. W. (1997) 43rd ENMC International Workshop on Emery-Dreifuss muscular dystrophy. *Neuromusc. Disord.* **7,** 67–69.
6. Emery, A. E. H. (1987) X-linked muscular dystrophy with early contractures and cardiomyopathy (Emery-Dreifuss type). *Clin. Genet.* **32,** 360–376.
7. Bione, S., Maestrini, E., Rivella, S., Mancini, M., Regis, S., Romeo, G., and Toniolo, D. (1994) Identification of a novel X-linked gene responsible for Emery-Dreifuss muscular dystrophy. *Nat. Genet.* **8,** 323–327.
8. Bione, S., Small, K., Aksmanovic, V. M. A., D'Urso, M., Ciccodicola, A., Merlini, L., et al. (1995) Identification of new mutations in the Emery-Dreifuss muscular dystrophy gene and evidence for genetic heterogeneity of the disease. *Hum. Mol. Genet.* **4,** 1859–1863.
9. Bione, S., Tamanini, F., Maestrini, E., Tribioli, C., Poustka, A., Torri, G., Rivella, S., and Toniolo, D. (1993) Transcriptional organization of a 450-kb region of the human X chromosome in Xq28. *Proc. Natl. Acad. Sci. USA* **90,** 10,977–10,981.
10. Nigro, V., Bruni, P., Ciccodicola, A., Politano, L., Nigro, G., Piluso, G., et al. (1995) SSCP detection of novel mutations in patients with Emery-Dreifuss muscular dystrophy: definition of a small C-terminal region required for emerin function. *Hum. Mol. Genet.* **4,** 2003–2004.
11. Wulff, K., Ebener, U., Wehnert, C. S., Ward, P. A., Reuner, U., Hiebsch, W., Herrmann, and Wehnert, M. (1997) Direct molecular genetic diagnosis and heterozygote identification in X-linked Emery-Dreifuss muscular dystrophy hy heteroduplex analysis. *Dis. Markers* **13,** 77–86.
12. Yamada, T. and Kobayashi, T. (1996) A novel emerin mutation in a Japanese patient with Emery-Dreifuss muscular dystrophy. *Hum. Genet.* **97,** 693–694.

13. Nagano, A., Koga, R., Ogawa, M., Kurano, Y., Kawada, J., Okada, R., et al. (1996) Emerin deficiency at the nuclear membrane in patients with Emery-Dreifuss muscular dystrophy. *Nat. Genet.* **12,** 254–259.
14. Klauck, S. M., Wilgenbus, P., Yates, J. R. W., Muller, C. R., and Poustka, A. Identification of novel mutations in three families with Emery-Dreifuss muscular dystrophy. *Hum. Mol. Genet.* **4,** 1853–1857.
15. Small, K., Iber, J., and Warren, S. T. (1997) Emerin deletion reveals a common X-chromosome inversion mediated by inverted repeats. *Nat. Genet.* **16,** 96–99.
16. Chen, E. Y., Zollo, M., Mazzarella, R., Ciccodicola, A., Chen, C., Zuo, L., et al. (1996) Long-range sequence analysis in Xq28: thirteen known and six candidate genes in 219.4 kb of high GC DNA between the RCP/GCP and G6PD loci. *Hum. Mol. Genet.* **5,** 659–668.
17. Manilal, S., Nguyen, T. M., Sewry, C. A., and Morris, G. E. (1996) The Emery-Dreifuss muscular dystrophy protein, emerin, is a nuclear membrane protein. *Hum. Mol. Genet.* **5,** 801–808.
18. Mora, M., Cartegni, L., Di Blasi, C., Barresi, R., Bione, S., Raffaele di Barletta, M., et al. (1997) X-linked Emery-Dreifuss muscular dystrophy can be diagnosed from skin biopsy or blood sample. *Ann. Neurol.* **42,** 249–253.
19. Manilal, S., Sewry, C. A., Nguyen, T. M., Muntoni, F., and Morris, G. E. (1997) Diagnosis of X-linked Emery-Dreifuss muscular dystrophy by protein analysis of leukocytes and skin with monoclonal antibodies. *Neuromusc. Disord.* **7,** 63–66.
20. Sabatelli P., Squarzoni S., Petrini S., Capanni C., Ognibene A,. Cartegni, L., et al. (1998) Oral exfoliative cytology for the non invasive diagnosis in X-linked EDMD patients and carriers. *Neuromusc. Disord.* **8,** 67–71.

II

The Molecular Approach

B. Genetics: *Autosomal Recessive Muscular Dystrophies*

12

Analysis of *LAMA2* Gene in Merosin-Deficient Congenital Dystrophy

Anne Helbling-Leclerc and Pascale Guicheney

1. Introduction

1.1. Congenital Muscular Dystrophies

Congenital muscular dystrophies (CMDs) are a clinically and genetically heterogenous group of muscle disorders, with onset in early infancy, and autosomal recessive inheritance *(1–3)*. Several forms have been identified: classical or occidental CMD with normal or subnormal intelligence; Fukuyama's CMD (FEND), prevalent in Japan, characterized by severe mental retardation and major structural brain abnormalities *(4)*; and the Walker-Warburg syndrome and muscle–eye–brain disease, both of which are associated with muscle, eye, and brain abnormalities *(5–7)*.

A major breakthrough in the understanding of CMDs was the finding that the laminin α_2-chain was absent in the skeletal muscle in about 50% of patients with classical CMD *(8)*. This permitted the identification of a subgroup of CMDs, referred to as "merosin-deficient" CMD, or "laminin α2-chain-deficient" CMD *(8)*, which was further shown to result from mutations in the laminin α_2-chain gene (*LAMA2* gene) *(9)*. The merosin-deficient CMD patients present hypotonia, contractures, and motor development delay, which are generally more severe than in merosin nondeficient CMD patients *(10)*. In addition, white matter changes have been constantly found by brain-imaging techniques in these patients *(11)*, even if sometimes they are difficult to assess in the early stages of the disease *(12)*.

The laminin-2 (merosin) and the laminin-4 (s-merosin) isoforms, which have molecular formulas α_2-β_1-γ_1 and α_2–β_2-γ_1, respectively, are characteristically enriched in basement membranes surrounding skeletal muscle fibers *(13)*. The

From: *Methods in Molecular Medicine, vol. 43: Muscular Dystrophy: Methods and Protocols*
Edited by: K. M. D. Bushby and L. V. B. Anderson

high tissue specificity of these isoforms is provided only by the α_2-chain, because the other component chains of the laminin isoforms, the β_1- or β_2- and γ_1-chains, are ubiquitous.

1.2. Identification of Mutations in LAMA2 Gene

Analysis of *LAMA2* gene is made difficult by the size and the structure of the gene, which is over 260,000 bp long, and contains 64 exons encoding a 9.5-kb mRNA transcript ***(14,15)***. The size of the exons varies between 87 and 270 bp, except for exons 43 and 52, which are unusually small, with 6 and 12 bp, respectively. The size of the introns varies from 150 to >15 kb ***(15)***. Deletions or insertions of several bp, and deletions of one or several exons, caused by splice-site mutations, can be detected by using reverse transcriptase-polymerase chain reaction (RT-PCR) analysis of illegitimate transcripts of the *LAMA2* gene in peripheral blood lymphocytes ***(16)***. Of course, if a muscle biopsy, immediately frozen and stored in liquid nitrogen, is available, legitimate transcripts can be even more easily analyzed. One- or two-bp deletions or insertions, and most of the point mutations, can be identified on genomic DNA by single-strand conformational polymorphism (SSCP) analysis, followed by sequencing ***(17)***.

CMD with complete laminin α_2-chain deficiency, evidenced by the commercial antibody (Chemicon, El Segundo, CA) directed against the C-terminal G globular domain, is caused by *LAMA2* mutations, leading to the synthesis of truncated laminin α_2-chains lacking part or the whole G domain. Different types of mutations have been identified: splice-site mutations ***(9,18)***, nonsense mutations ***(9,18,19)***, 1-bp deletions ***(18,20)***, 2-bp deletions ***(18,19)***, or deletions of more than two bases ***(20)***. Most of these mutations result in putative truncation in one of the domains forming the short arm of the laminin α_2-chain. These mRNAs may be unstable, but, even if some polypeptides are formed, they will lack the C-terminal G domain and domains I and II of the long arm of the laminin α_2-chain, and, therefore, will not participate in the formation of normal laminin heterotrimers. Hence, no laminin-2 (α_2-, β_1-, γ_1-chains) nor laminin-4 (α_2-, β_2-, γ_1-chains) molecules will be formed. Others mutations ***(18,19)*** should allow synthesis of the laminin α_2-chain with domains I and II, but lacking G–G5 repeats of the C-terminal G domain. The sequence essential for heterotrimer formation and stability (the critical 25-amino-acid sequence at the C terminus of domain I ***[21]***) is maintained in both cases. Trimeric laminin molecules may be formed. Nevertheless, such proteins are probably very unstable, and cannot associate with sarcolemmal constituents, such as α-dystroglycan.

Mutations causing partial laminin α_2-chain deficiency are missense mutations ***(22)***, in-frame deletions ***(23)***, or splice-site mutations leading to in-frame deletion *(24)*. All the mutations induce the formation of abnormal heterotrimer muscle-specific laminins, which probably dramatically disturb the assembly and stability of the laminin network, which implies a weaker linkage of the cytoskeleton to the extracellular matrix, and leads to muscle cell degeneration.

1.3. Prenatal Diagnosis

Prenatal diagnoses of at-risk fetuses have been done by direct trophoblast staining from chorionic villous samples with the commercial antibody (Chemicon), or by genotype analysis and determination of at-risk haplotypes. The chromosome (chr) 6q2 microsatellite markers flanking the *LAMA2* gene, D6S407 and D6S1620 *(25–27)*, and various intragenic polymorphisms, can be used for this purpose. In some cases, additional markers may be useful to get more informativity (**Table 1**). The four *LAMA2* polymorphisms located in exons 12, 19, 37, and 42 (**Table 2**) have been selected, at least two of them are informative in the majority of the families, the most useful being the 5551A/G polymorphism of exon 37 *(18,20)*. They must be used when a recombination has occurred between the markers, D6S1620 and D6S407, to determine whether the mutated gene has been transmitted to the fetus. The 2848A/G polymorphism in exon 19 does not induce the creation or the loss of a restriction site, but it can easily be detected by SSCP. Examples of prenatal diagnoses are represented in **Fig. 1**.

The reliability of prenatal diagnosis by microsatellite analysis is dependent on the absence of locus heterogeneity for the disease. Concerning families with a CMD child having complete merosin deficiency and white matter hypodensity determined by brain imaging, such analysis can be used for prenatal diagnosis with or without a direct assessment of the laminin α_2-chain in fetal chorionic villous biopsies, both in consanguineous and nonconsanguineous families *(26,28,29)*. In contrast, partial merosin deficiency is heterogenous. A secondary reduction of the muscle laminin α_2-chain occurs in F/CMD, which is linked to chr 9q31–33 *(30,31)*, as well as in some patients with mental retardation *(32)*. Thus, microsatellite and haplotype analysis can give reliable information only in consanguineous or informative families. An alternative is to identify the laminin α_2-chain gene defects causing partial laminin α_2-chain deficiency, in order to perform prenatal diagnoses by direct mutation analysis in nonconsanguineous CMD families *(19)*.

2. Materials

2.1. Microsatellite Analysis

1. 10X PCR buffer: 500 m*M* KCl, 100 m*M* Tris-HCl (pH 8.3), 15 m*M* $MgCl_2$ (Boehringer Mannheim, Mannheim, Germany). Store at –20°C.

Table 1
Primer Sequences of Five Chr 6q2 Microsatellite Markers for Linkage Analysis in Laminin α2-chain-Deficient CMD Patients

Markers	Forward primer (5'–3')	Reverse primer (5'–3')	Allele size (bp)	Allele size for M134702
D6S1715	AATCACCAGCAGTGGG	AATGTCTTTTGTAAACTCTCCTAAC	179-201	187-193
D6S407	AAAAGTACCTCCCGCCC	GATGACACCAAGTCACCCA	174-200	174-194
D6S1620	CAAAGAGTAACAATCCTAAGCAAC	TCATCCTAAGTTAATGCACAGC	215-225	219-225
D6S1705	TTGTTTGAGGGATTTTCCAA	GTGACTGGGCATGTCTAGGT	156-172	156-164
D6S1572	CCTGAAATCATCCTGCAA	TTCTCTACAGTGACCAGCC	102-124	110-112

Genetic distances between the markers are the following (from centromer to telomer): D6S1715—1 cM—D6S407—3 cM—D6S1620—0 cM—D6S1705—1 cM—D6S1572. The distances are given in centiMorgans (cM). *LAMA2* gene is located between D6S407 and D6S1620. M124702 is the Généthon's DNA standard.

Adapted with permission from **refs.** ***25*** and ***34***.

Table 2
***LAMA2* Polymorphisms Used for Prenatal Diagnosis**

Exons	Nucleotides	Amino-acid residues	Frequency	Restriction site	SSCP conditions	Ref.
12	1905 G→A	619 CGT(Arg)→CAT(His)	18%	Loss *MaeII*	7°C	***16***
19	2848 A→G	933 CAA(Gln)→CAG(gln)	24%	No change	7°C, 20°C	***16***
37	5551 A→G	1834 GAA(Gln)→GAG(Glu)	38%	New *MnlI*	7°C	***16***
42	6286 G→A	2079 ACG(Thr)→ACA(Thr)	16%	Loss *BsmI*	20°C	***6,18***

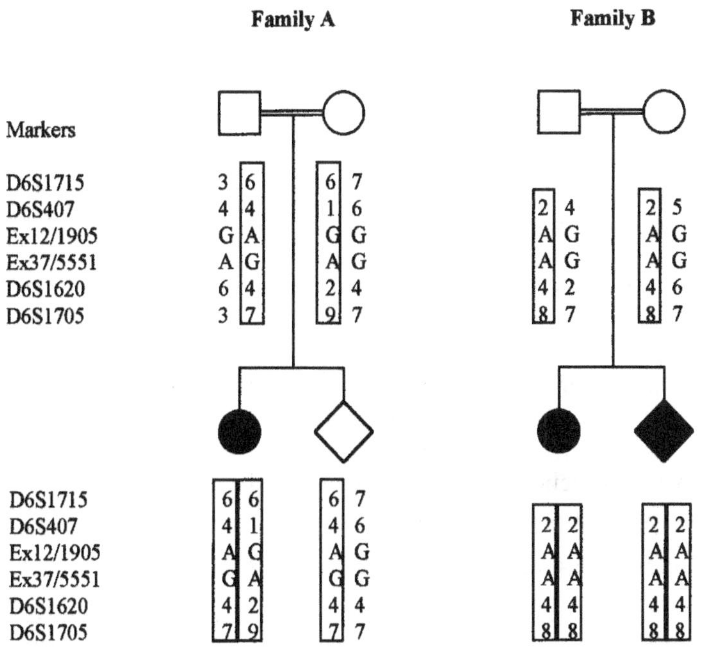

Fig. 1. Prenatal diagnosis by determination of at-risk hplotypes using microsatellites flanking the *LAMA*2 gene and two intragenic polymorphisms in exon 12 and 37. **(A)** Illustrates a nonaffected fetus and **(B)** illustrates a homozygous affected fetus. Affected subjects are represented by black symbols and fetuses by diamonds.

2. Deoxynucleoside triphosphates (dNTPs): Stock at 100 m*M* from Amersham-Pharmacia Biotech. Dilute each dNTP to prepare an equimolar solution of dNTPs at a concentration of 1 m*M* each in sterile dH_2O. Store 500-µL aliquots at –20°C.
3. Oligonucleotide (oligo-nt) primers: Primers to amplify the microsatellite markers (D6S1715, D6S407, D6S1620, D6S1705, D6S1572, and $[CA]_{15}$) (**Table 1**) are synthesized by Eurogentec (Seraing, Belgium). Prepare working solutions at 10 µ*M*, which can be stored at –20°C.

4. Taq polymerase: The authors preferentially use 5 UI/µL from Boehringer Mannheim for microsatellite analysis.
5. Agarose: Use standard agarose, molecular biology grade (Eurobio, les Ulis, France). DNA mol-wt marker XIV (Boehringer Mannheim). Add 1 µg in a separate lane of each agarose gel, to check the size of the PCR products.
6. Tris-borate–EDTA (TBE) electrophoresis buffer: Use a 10X stock solution (Eurobio) at 0.89 *M* Tris, 0.89 *M* boric acid, and 0.02 *M* EDTA (pH 8.0). Store at room temperature (RT).
7. Acrylamide (6%)–urea (50%) gel: 255 g urea (Sigma), 76.5 mL acrylamide 40% of 19:1 acrylamide–*bis*-acrylamide mix (Amresco, Solon, OH), 51 mL 10X TBE, and dH_2O for a final volume of 510 mL. Filtrate on 0.2-µm filter, and store at 4°C in a dark bottle.
8. Ammonium persulfate: Prepare a 10% (w/v) solution, store 1-mL aliquots at –20°C.
9. Agarose gel loading buffer: 250 mg xylene cyanol, 100 mg bromophenol blue, 40 g sucrose, and 3 g sodium dodecyl sulfate and dH_2O for a final volume of 100 mL. Store at +4°C.
10. Formamide gel loading buffer: 20 mg xylene cyanol, 10 mg bromophenol blue, 40 mL formamide, and dH_2O for a final volume of 50 mL. Store 1-mL aliquots at –20°C.
11. Agarose electrophoresis equipment: Wide subcell system (Bio-Rad, Hercules, CA).
12. Polyacrylamide electrophoresis equipment: Sequi-gen GT sequencing cell (Bio-Rad).
13. Nitrocellulose membranes: Hybond N^+ membranes (Amersham Pharmacia Biotech).
14. Standard sodium citrate (SSC) washing buffer: Use a 10X stock solution (Eurobio) at 1.5 *M* NaCl and 1.5 *M* sodium citrate (pH 7.0). Store at RT.
15. Terminal transferase (Boehringer Mannheim).
16. Peroxydase detection system: Use enhanced chemiluminescence detection system (Amersham, kit RPN 3000).

2.2. Mutation Analysis

1. RNA extraction: Use RNA Plus kit from Bioprobe Systems (Montreuil-sous-Bois, France).
2. cDNA synthesis: Use First-Strand cDNA Synthesis Kit from Pharmacia.
3. PCR: Use the same PCR materials as in subheading 2.1., except: 50 m*M* $MgCl_2$, 10X PCR buffer: 670 m*M* Tris-HCl (pH 8.8), 160 m*M* $(NH_4)_2SO_4$, 0.1% Tween-20, and 5 UI/µL *Taq* polymerase from Eurobio. Store at –20°C.
4. Polyacrylamide gel (10%): Use a 37.5:1 acrylamide–*bis*-acrylamide mix. The authors use a 40% ready-mixed solution (Amresco), stored at +4°C.
5. Polyacrylamide electrophoresis equipment: Mighty Small gel electrophoresis unit (Hoefer, San Francisco, CA).
6. Silver (Ag) staining: Use Silver Stain Plus Kit from Bio-Rad. The Fixative Enhancer Concentrate and the Silver Complex Solution can be stored at RT.
7. Fixative Enhancer Solution: 50% isopropanol (reagent-grade), 10% acetic acid (reagent-grade) and 10% Fixative Enhancer Concentrate. The dilution can be kept at RT for several utilizations during the same week.

8. Development accelerator solution reagent: Dissolve 50 g Development Accelerator Solution Reagent slowly in 1 L dH_2O. The development accelerator solution can be stored at +4°C for 3 mo, but must reach ambient temperature before use.
9. Staining solution: Place 35 mL dH_2O into a large beaker or Erlenmeyer flask. Add, in this order: 5 mL Silver Complex Solution, 5 mL Reduction Moderator Solution, and 5 mL Image Development Reagent. Just before use, add 50 mL of the RT Development Accelerator Solution. Mix, and discard after utilization.

3. Methods

3.1. Microsatellite Analyzing

3.1.1. PCR Conditions (see **Note 1**)

1. The final concentrations of the reaction components are: 40 ng genomic DNA, 1 μ*M* each primer, 50 m*M* KCl, 10 m*M* Tris-HCl (pH 8.3), 1.5 m*M* $MgCl_2$, 100 μ*M* each dNTP, 1 U *Taq* polymerase, in a total volume of 50 μL.
2. Use 10 μL DNA at 4 ng/mL solution in 0.5-mL Eppendorf tube or 96-well PCR plate.
3. Add 20 μL mix number 1: 5 μL each oligo-nt primer and 10 μL H_2O.
4. Add one drop of light paraffin oil, and place on a PCR machine.
5. PCR cycling conditions in hot start: Initial denaturation: 94°C for 4 min; hold at 72°C while adding 20 μL mix number 2: 5 μL 10X PCR buffer, 5 μL 1 mM dNTP solution, 9.8 μL H_2O, and 0.2 μL *Taq* polymerase, followed by 35 cycles at 94°C for 1 min, 53°C for 1 min, and 72°C for 1 min. Final synthesis: 72°C for 2.5 min.

3.1.2. Checking Amplification Reaction

1. Mix 5 μL PCR reaction and 5 μL agarose gel loading buffer.
2. Load this mix on a 2% agarose gel, and carry out electrophoresis at 75 mA with ethidium bromide (EtBr), both in the gel and the TBE running buffer (*see* **Note 2**).

3.1.3. Elongation of $(CA)_n$ Probe

1. Mix in a Eppendorf tube stored on ice: 38 μL H_2O; 5 μL oligo-nt $(CA)_{15}$ at 20 μ*M*; 40 μL Na cacodylate at 0.5 *M*, pH 7.6; 2 μL dithiothreitol (DTT) at 5 m*M*; 2 μL each dNTP at 10 m*M*; 4 μL cobalt chloride at 25 m*M* (Boehringer), and 3 μL terminal transferase at 25 UI/μL (Boehringer).
2. Incubate overnight at 37°C.
3. Stop the enzymatic reaction with 4 μL EDTA at 250 m*M*.
4. Purify this solution on Bio-Spin column 300 (Bio-Rad).
5. Estimate the concentration by optical density (OD) at 260 nm.

3.1.4. Microsatellite Analysis

1. Heat at 94°C, 5 μL PCR product with 5 μL formamide loading buffer for 5 min. After denaturation, store on ice.

2. Load 5 µL of this solution onto a 6% polyacrylamide denaturing sequencing gel, previously prerun at 90 W/130 mA during 1 h (*see* **Note 3**).
3. Run the gel until the marker dyes have migrated the desired distances (approx 5 h) (*see* **Note 4**).
4. Transfer passively the PCR products for 1.5 h on Hybond N^+ membrane, previously wet with 1X TBE.
5. Wash the membrane with 5X SSC.
6. Fix DNA on the membrane with UV in a crosslinker (Bio-Rad).
7. Prehybridize the membrane, at 42°C for 10 min, with the previously warmed hybridization solution (kit ECL, RPN 3000, Amersham).
8. Label-elongated $(CA)_n$ with peroxydase: to 300 ng of elongated $(CA)_{15}$, in a final volume of 30 µL dH_2O, add 30 µL peroxydase, then 30 µL glutaraldehyde (kit RPN 3000), mix, incubate for 10 min at 37°C, and use immediately or hold on ice for a short period.
9. Hybridize the membrane with the labeled probe, at 42°C, overnight.
10. Wash the membrane, once with 2X SSC + 0.1% SDS at 42°C for 20 min, and twice with 0.2X SSC at 42°C for 15 min.
11. Revelation by ECL (kit RPN 3000) and exposition on X-Omatic film (Amersham) (for interpretation, *see* **Note 5**).

3.2. Mutation Screening

3.2.1. Study of LAMA2 Gene Transcripts

3.2.1.1. RNA Extraction

RNA extraction is performed with RNA Plus kit, either from lymphoblastoid cell lines or from muscle biopsies.

1. For lymphoblastoid cells, centrifuge 30–50 mL cells at 1500*g* for 10 min, and mix the pellet with 2 mL RNA Plus solution (*see* **Note 6**).
2. For muscle biopsies, homogenize 50 mg tissue in 2 mL RNA Plus solution at +4°C with a Polytron (Polylabo, France), 3× for 10 s on ice.
3. For both cases, add 200 µL chloroform to 1 mL of the mix in a 1.5-mL Eppendorf tube, vortex, and store for 5 min on ice.
4. Centrifuge at 12,000*g* at 4°C for 15 min.
5. Transfer the upper aquous phase to a clean tube.
6. Add 1 vol isopropanol, and store on ice for 30 min.
7. Centrifuge at 12,000*g* at 4°C for 15 min.
8. Wash the pellet with 1.5 mL 75% ethanol at 4°C, and vortex.
9. Recover the RNA by centrifugation at 7500*g* for 10 min at 4°C.
10. Dry the pellet.
11. Redissolve the RNA in 50 µL dH_2O.
12. Estimate the RNA concentration by measuring the OD at 260 nm and 280 nm (*see* **Note 7**).
13. Freeze the samples either at –20°C, in the presence of 0.1 vol 3 *M* NaAc and 2.2 vol ethanol, or at –80°C in dH_2O.

3.2.1.2. cDNA Synthesis

cDNA synthesis is performed using First-Strand cDNA Synthesis Kit from Pharmacia (*see* **Note 8**).

1. Dilute 1 µg RNA (for legitimate transcripts from skeletal muscle) or 4 µg RNA (for illegitimate transcripts from blood lymphocytes) in 8 µL RNase-free water.
2. Heat the RNA solution for 10 min at 65°C, then chill it on ice.
3. Add a mix composed of 5 µL Bulk First-Strand cDNA Reaction Mix, 1 µL DTT solution at 200 m*M*, and 1 µL random hexadeoxynucleosides at 0.2 µg/µL. Pipet up and down several times to mix.
4. Incubate for 1 h at 37°C.
5. Stop the reaction by chilling the tube on ice.

3.2.1.3. *LAMA2* cDNA Analysis

Nested PCRs are used to amplify *LAMA2* cDNA (*see* **Note 9**). The primer sequences are given in **Table 3**. PCR products of 700–900 bp are first amplified with two primer sets and large deletions, usually because of splice-site mutations, can be detected (*see* **Note 10**). Other primers can then be used to amplify 300–500-bp PCR fragments, and allow us to confirm and clarify the deletion. Such fragments can also be analyzed by SSCP (*see* **Subheading 3.2.2.**), and/or sequenced.

1. The final concentrations of the reaction components are: 3.7 µL cDNA, 2 µL 10X PCR buffer, 0.6 µL $MgCl_2$ at 50 m*M*, 1 µ*M* each primer, 300 µ*M* each dNTP, 0.75 U *Taq* polymerase, in a total volume of 20 µL.
2. PCR cycling conditions using the touchdown *(33)*: Initial denaturation: 94°C for 4 min, followed by cycles at 94°C for 1 min, annealing temperature for 1 min, and 72°C for 1.5 min. Final synthesis: 72°C for 2.5 min. The initial and final annealing temperatures were 60 and 52°C, respectively, with decreasing the annealing temperature by 2°C after two cycles and with 30 cycles at 52°C.
3. The second PCR amplification is performed under the same conditions, with 2 µL of the first PCR product as matrix.
4. 5 µL PCR product are mixed with 8 µL agarose gel loading buffer, and loaded on a 2% agarose gel. Electrophoresis is carried out at 75 mA with EtBr in both the gel and the TBE running buffer (*see* **Note 2**).

3.2.2. Study of LAMA2 *Exons by SSCP Analysis*

Sequencing of all 64 exons and their immediate intron boundaries has previously been reported *(15)*. Oligo-nt primers were designed to amplify each *LAMA2* exon, based on the intronic sequences using the OLIGO 4.0 program. The primers were chosen so that at least 30–50 bp of the flanking intron sequences were readable. Sixty-three primer pairs permitted a direct PCR amplification of an exon with the exon–intron boundaries. The sizes of the

Table 3
Overlapping Primers for the Amplification of the cDNA of *LAMA2* Gene

Primer name	Primer sequences (5'–3')	Position within cDNA *(12)*	PCR products	Size (bp)
1F	CTCCTCCTTCTGCTGCTC	71-88	1F/1R	880
1R	GCTGGATCAAGTGGACAA	934-951		
2F	GCAGTCACAGGCACAT	135-151	2F/2R	415
2R	CTGCCAGGGCTTGTATTC	533-550		
3F	TGCTCACAAAGACCCAAG	823-840	3F/3R	1093
3R	GCTGGAGAACACGTTCTG	1899-1916		
4F	ACCCCATTGTCACCAGAA	849-866	4F/4R	1002
4R	TGTCCTCCTACTGCTGGG	1834-1851		
25F	GCACCTGGATCCTGTCAT	1361-1378	25F/4R	409
25R	GTCCGGGTAGCCAGTGTA	1427-1444	4F/25R	595
5F	GGACGACTTGGACTCACC	1723-1740	5F/5R	813
5R	TCCAAGACTCCGGTCTAA	2509-2536		
6F	TGCCGCACAGCTACTACT	1782-1799	6F/6R	662
6R	CTTTAGTAGGCTCGCCAT	2427-2444		
26F	CAGTGCTTGCGAATTTGA	2076-2093	26F/6R	368
26R	AGGATAGGAGACAGCGGA	2168-2185	6F/26R	403
7F	ACACAGGTGGCCCATATT	2385-2402	7F/7R	831
7R	AGTGGTAATGCTGTGGCC	3197-3214		
8F	TTTAGACCGGAGTCTTGG	2518-2535	8F/8R	677
8R	CAGGTATTGGGTGCACAT	3178-3197		
27F	CTTTCTCTGAGGTTTGCC	2823-2840	27F/8R	372
27R	CTCTGACCCTGAACGTTG	2872-2889	8F/27R	371
9F	TGTGCACCCAATACCTGG	3179-3196	9F/9R	993
9R	CAGCTGGAGGAGTCATTG	4155-4172		
10F	GGGCCACAGCATTACCAC	3196-3213	10F/10R	905
10R	TGTCGCATGAAATTTCCA	4084-4101		
28F	GCAGACCATTCTACCCCT	3622-3639	28F/10R	550
28R	CTTGGTGGTCGTGTGCTG	3656-3673	10F/28R	477
11F	GGATGATCCTCGAGTCCA	3994-4011	11F/11R	836
11R	ATGACCATCTGCTCCAGG	4813-4830		
12F	ACCGAGAAGAAGGCCAGT	4784-4801	12F/12R	373
12R	AGGGATTGCCAAATGACT	4428-4445		
29F	AGAGGGGCTGAAATTGTT	4481-4498	29F/12R	366
29R	CACATTCTTGGCAGGAGC	4614-4631	12F/29R	203
13F	ACTGGCCTTCTTCTCGGT	4784-4802	13F/13R	809
13R	TTCATCTGCAAGACGGTT	5576-5593		
14F	CCTGGAGCAGATGGTCAT	4813-4830	14F/14R	767
14R	CGGTTGGCTTCATCGAGT	5563-5580		

(continued)

Table 3 *(continued)*

Primer name	Primer sequences (5'–3')	Position within cDNA *(12)*	PCR products	Size (bp)
30F	GAGACGAGGCCTTTGAGA	5166-5183	30F/14R	414
30R	GGACTCTCCAAACAGCTT	5315-5332	14F/30R	519
15F	GCTAATCGCCTATTTGCA	5447-5464	15F/15R	832
15R	GCGACGCTGTCTGCTAGT	6262-6279		
16F	GGAGAAAAAGAAGGAGGC	5491-5508	16F/16R	761
16R	TTCTTCTTCAGGCCATCG	6235-6252		
31F	GCCTTCAAAGCTTACAGC	5819-5836	31F/16R	433
31R	GGACCTGTTGCCAGTTTT	5908-5925	16F/31R	434
17F	TCCACCAGAACCTCGATG	6222-6239	17F/17R	886
17R	ACGGCTGACCAATGCATA	7091-7108		
18F	CGATGGCCTGAAGAAGAA	6235-6252	18F/18R	798
18R	GCATCCTTTGCAGTCACC	7016-7033		
32F	GGAAGTGCCAAATTTATT	6608-6625	32F/18R	425
32R	TCCAACTCCAGATCCAAC	6677-6694	18F/32R	459
19F	GGTGACTGCAAAGGATGC	7016-7033	19F/19R	829
19R	AGATGCACTTCCAGACGG	7828-7845		
20F	TATGCATTGGTCAGCCGT	7091-7108	20F/20R	737
20R	GCCCCTGTTGAGGAGTAT	7811-7828		
33F	TATATTTTGGTGGCCTGC	7452-7469	33F/20R	376
33R	AATATCTTTGAGGCAGCC	7529-7546	20F/33R	455
21F	GCAGACTGGACAGGCCTA	7786-7803	21F/21R	915
21R	CATTCCCACGACATCCAG	8684-8701		
22F	ATACTCCTCAACAGGGGC	7811-7828	22F/22R	866
22R	GGCTTTTTGGGACTGAT	8660-8677		
34F	CACCCCAGCCTTTCCTAC	8254-8271	34F/22R	423
34R	CTGCAGCACAAGGACCAT	8292-8309	22F/34R	498
23F	ATGTAGATGGGGCTTCCA	8634-8651	23F/23R	767
23R	GATACAGGTTGAACGCCC	9384-9401		
24F	ATCAGTCCCAAAAAAGCC	8660-8677	24F/24R	723
24R	CTCAGTTCCAGGGCCTTG	9366-9383		
35F	AATGGATGGAATGGGTAT	9001-9018	35F/24R	382
36R	AACCCCAGCATCATAGAC	9080-9097	24F/35R	437

Adapted in part from **ref. *9***.

PCR products ranged between 129 and 345 bp, allowing SSCP analysis and direct sequencing (**Table 4**).

3.2.2.1. PCR Conditions

1. The final concentrations of the reaction components are: 50 ng genomic DNA, 2 μL 10X PCR buffer, 0.6 μL $MgCl_2$ at 50 m*M*, 1 μ*M* each primer, 300 μ*M* each dNTP, 0.75 U *Taq* polymerase, in a total volume of 20 μL.
2. PCR cycling conditions using the touchdown *(33)*, with the annealing temperature decreased by 1°C after each two cycles, and stabilized at the lower temperature for 30 cycles. The primer pairs and the initial and final annealing temperatures are given in **Table 4**. Initial denaturation: 94°C for 4 min, followed by cycles at 94°C for 40 s, annealing temperature for 1 min, and 72°C for 1.5 min. Final synthesis: 72°C for 2.5 min.

3.2.2.2. Electrophoresis on Polyacrylamide Gel

1. Denature DNA sample at 95°C for 2 min, and store on ice for at least 5 min.
2. Load 1 μL PCR product mixed with 4 μL formamide loading buffer, onto 10% polyacrylamide gel (8 × 10 cm) previously cooled at 7°C or at 20°C for at least 1 h (*see* **Note 11**).
3. Run with a 8-mA current (per gel). The precise electrophoretic conditions depend on the PCR products being analyzed.
4. When the DNA has migrated the desired distance, Ag-stain the gel.

3.2.2.3. Ag Staining

1. Separate the gel plates, and carefully transfer the gel into a square box (*see* **Notes 12** and **13**).
2. Immerse the gel in 200 mL fixative enhancer solution (this can be reused); shake gently for 20 min.
3. Rinse the gels in 400 mL dH_2O for 10 min, with gentle agitation. After 10 min, decant water, and replace with fresh rinsed water. Rinse for an additional 10 min.
4. Stain with staining solution approx 20 min, or until desired staining intensity is reached (*see* **Note 14**).
5. After the desired staining is reached, place the gels in 5% acetic acid to stop the reaction for at least 15 min.
6. Rinse the gels in high-purity water for at least 5 min.
7. Dry the gel between two sheets of cellophane. For interpretation, *see* **Notes 15–18**.

4. Notes

1. PCR is a very powerful technique, hence contamination of the reaction by even very low levels of DNA from an external source can lead to erroneous results. Great care should be taken to avoid such contamination. The most common source of contamination is by PCR products from previous reactions. One precaution to avoid this is to use separate pipets for setting up the reaction and for analyzing the products. If products are seen in the negative (no DNA) control, then the

Table 4
Oligonucleotide Primers and Conditions for PCR Amplification of *LAMA2* Exons[a]

Exon	Position on cDNA	Exon size (bp)	Location upstream from exon	Forward primer sequence (5'→3')	Reverse primer sequence (5'→3')	Location downstream from exon	PCR product size	PCR conditions
1	50	112	-109	CCTCTTCCCCAGCAGCTG	CCAAGCCCATGCCTCGAC	6	244	53°C
2	162	171	-25	CACCTTCATTTGTCCATC	GCCACACACCTACACACT	12	225	TD 55-50°C
3	333	113	-24	CATATGATGCTGCTAACT	CCACAAACCACTAACTAA	60	214	TD 45-40°C
4	446	243	-22	TGTTGTTGTTATACTTCCCT	TATCAAATGTGCTTAAATGG	19	306	TD 55-50°C
5	689	270	-103	TGGGAGAATGGGAAGTTA	GCAAAACATCATCAAGTCAG	EXONIC	240	TD 55-50°C
6	959	118	-59	GCTTCCTTTATGGTTCTA	ATGACGATATTTTGTTGG	17	211	TD 45-40°C
7	1077	179	-54	TAAATGTATCTGAAATCAAATT	GTTCAACTGTTTACAGTTGC	88	340	TD 55-50°C
8	1256	100	-43	GTTTCTATTCACTTCGTT	AATCATATTTGGCTTTTA	45	205	TD 44-39°C
9	1356	161	-40	TTGTTTTAGAAATGTTGA	TTAXTGGAATAAAXAATG	4	222	TD 44-39°C
10	1517	141	-56	CGCAGCTCATAATGTTGA	GCAGCAAACAGAACCAAA	15	229	TD 50-45°C
11	1658	174	-57	AAAAGCTGCTGATAGATA	TCAGTTAAAGCAGAATAG	23	271	TD 45-40°C
12	1832	102	-50	TGATTTAATAGCCCCATCT	ACATCAGGAAGTAACACG	26	195	TD 45-40°C
13	1934	212	-47	CTCTTTTCAGTTTTACTC	CAAAGTAAATGTGTGAAC	27	303	TD 44-39°C
14	2146	112	-34	ACTTATTCACCATCTCTT	AAGCACTAAGGATACATT	14	177	TD 50-45°C
15	2258	114	-33	CCAAGACTGACTAAAGCC	CCAGGGTAGTAGCTGAAT	65	229	TD 50-45°C
16	2372	128	-49	TGATCCCTGACACCAAAA	GAGCTTATTCATGGGGTA	15	209	TD 50-45°C
17	2500	87	-54	CTTTGTGTATGTCCTTCT	AATCATTTTGCAAGACAG	17	175	TD 45-40°C
18	2587	212	-65	AATATCTAAACATTGCCC	ACATCAATTCTGTCAGGG	23	317	TD 45-40°C
19	2799	107	-27	TGATCACAGGTCTCTCTT	TTATGGGTCAGCCTCTAC	8	159	TD 50-45°C
20	2906	181	-52	ACTTCGAGTTAACTGATT	ATGTAGGACTTAAGTCAT	12	262	TD 44-39°C
21	3087	137	-45	TTTCTATTTTTCCCCTTCTTTG	TATCAATGAGCAAAAAAGTGGT	9	212	TD 55-50°C
22	3224	237	-38	AAAGTTGTTAATGGTTGC	GAAACAGAATTGAGGGAG	33	325	TD 44-39°C
23	3461	144	-79	CTCCCGTTATGCATTCTC	GGCTCAGCAGTTCCCTAC	5	245	TD 50-45°C
24	3605	180	-77	CATGCAGTTCGTAACTTA	GATAAATCTCCAAATGGT	58	332	TD 45-40°C

(continued)

Table 4 *(continued)*

Exon	Position on cDNA	Exon size (bp)	Location upstream from exon	Forward primer sequence (5'→3')	Reverse primer sequence (5'→3')	Location downstream from exon	PCR product size	PCR conditions
25	3785	189	-51	ACCACTTTGGAGAGCTTTATC	CACCAAACAATGACTAACTT	4	263	TD 55-50°C
26	3974	134	-40	CATTCAGTTTTGTCATAG	AAAATAAGAGCTTGAATA	19	210	TD 44-39°C
27	4108	118	-27	ATCTAAGTACATTCTCGC	CAGGTTAGTAGGAGGTAG	6	168	TD 50-45°C
28	4226	135	-85	TGTCTTTGCAGCCACTGA	TTCAAGGAAGGCTCAGAG	7	244	TD 50-45°C
29	4361	125	-29	ACAAACTTCTTCTCCCTT	GTTTCTGATTGGGAAATA	23	194	TD 50-45°C
30	4486	87	-23	CAATCCTTTTCTTTCTGA	TGTGACCCTTTACCATAT	46	173	TD 45-40°C
31	4573	194	-55	TGTGGAGACATGACTTGC	CAGCAAAGCAGTATACGT	3	269	TD 55-50°C
32	4767	143	-54	TCTGCCTGGGATGTTTAG	CTGCCCTGCTTGTGACTG	12	226	TD 50-45°C
33	4910	99	-26	ATGTTTATGGGATGGAAT	TAGGAAGAAGGTGATTTG	81	223	TD 55-50°C
34	5009	112	-25	GTGTTTCCCGAATTTGGT	ATGATGATTAAATGTGAT	13	167	TD 55-50°C
35	5121	163	-47	TGGCATGTTTGTTTACTA	CTGGAAATCTCAGTTTGT	32	259	TD 50-45°C
36	5284	211	-58	ACCCTAAGGCAGTGACAT	CCCAACCTTCTGAGATTA	26	312	TD 44-39°C
37	5495	117	-24	TGTCTTGTTCATAATGGT	TCTCTTTTGAGTTTTACC	11	169	TD 44-39°C
38	5612	164	-25	AAATGCCCTCTTCTCTAC	CCAAAACAAATGACATAC	1	207	TD 55-50°C
39	5776	139	-32	CCCTGCATACTGTTTTTGAAT	GACTTCCATTCCCAGCACAT	18	208	TD 55-50°C
40	5915	103	-21	CATTTGTTTTTCTGTCCAC	TCCAATCGTGTGATAGAA	60	201	TD 55-50°C
41	6018	117	-52	GCTGAGGGATGATAAAAC	GTTGGTAGTGCCTGAATG	6	192	TD 55-50°C
42	6135	183	-54	GCCACTAACTCCACACCC	ACACAATGAAAAAGGAGA	8	262	TD 55-50°C
43	6318	6	-31	TTTGTTTTGCTTCCATGTGA	TTCCTTTTACGCATCTACC	143	197	TD 55-50°C
44	6324	155	-32	ATATACATGCACACTAAT	CAGTTCTGATATGACGAT	14	218	TD 45-40°C
45	6479	144	-51	CAAACTTTCTGAGAGATT	AGCAGCCTAATGAAAAGT	17	229	TD 50-45°C
46	6623	134	-34	TGATATCTCTTGTTTTTG	AATCTTTATTAAGTTGGT	4	189	TD 44-39°C
47	6757	160	-30	TCCCCTTCACTTCAACAC	ACAGGAGGAGGATGAACA	7	214	TD 50-45°C
48	6917	125	-21	TAACGGTATTTCTTTCTG	ACCCTGGGAGAGTTCTCA	12	175	TD 50-45°C
49	7042	163	-52	TGACAGACCGAATAGATA	CACGGAAACTCTGCTATG	15	247	TD 44-39°C
50	7205	145	-29	CCACTGGGGTATGTTTAC	GGCCTATATTGCATTATT	16	207	TD 44-39°C

51	7350	139	-52	ATGTGGTTGATATTGCTC	AACTTAATCCTTAGCTTT	20	228	TD 44-39°C
52	7489	12	-21	TTCCTCTTTCCCGTTATCT	TGGTGTTGCTCTGCTTCTG	78	129	TD 55-50°C
53	7501	121	-33	ATTGCTTTTGCTTTTCAT	AGCAGCCACACTAAGTAA	50	221	TD 50-45°C
54	7622	177	-29	TGTCTACTCTTCCTTTTCCT	TGCATTATCAGCTAGGTGTG	7	234	TD 55-50°C
55	7799	149[b]	-60	CTAAAGCTAAGCCATAAA	GGAAGTTCACCTGAGTTA	31	256	TD 45-40°C
56	7947	177[b]	-51	TGTATTGAATCAGATGTG	GTAGTAGTAATGAGGAGA	10	255	TD 45-40°C
57	8125	169	-27	AAAATCTTATTTATTACA	TCCCTTCTGAAATGACTC	51	264	TD 44-39°C
58	8294	113	-71	TTAGACAGCATCATTACC	TCTTCATTTCTCGGTTCT	28	229	TD 53-48°C
59	8407	190	-70	GATACCGCTCTATTTTAG	GTAATCCCTTAGGGTACT	21	298	TD 45-40°C
60	8597	156	-57	TCTGCATATGTGAAATTT	TCAATAAATGAATCAGCC	38	268	TD 45-40°C
61	8753	154	-86	TACACACATAGAGCACCC	TGGATCTAGCAAGAAGTT	52	309	TD 44-39°C
62	8907	131	-40	ATCCTCTAATCCAAAATA	ATCTACACATCAACAATA	41	229	TD 44-39°C
63	9038	223	-66	TGTGTGAACCATCATGAT	GAAATTGTTGCTGGGGTA	13	319	TD 50-45°C
64	9261	269	-24	GCCCTCTTGCATTGCCTT	TCTGGAGTGTCAATTAGCT	23	334	TD 55-50°C

[a]From **ref. *16***, acknowledgment to the BMJ Publishing Group.

[b]G at position 7947 is the last nucleotide of exon 55 and not the first of the exon 56 as recently published by Zhang et al. (1996). This inducees size changes for exons 55 and 56.

results are invalid, and all working stocks should be discarded and fresh solutions made up.

2. Use of EtBr in the running buffer prevents fading out of the smaller PCR products. Alternatively, the gel can be run without EtBr, then stained when the resolution is complete. The size of each PCR product is checked by using the mol-wt ladder.
3. During the migration, there is always an increase in temperature. It is important to stabilize the inner temperature of the gel before loading samples.
4. The electrophoresis timing depends on the size of the microsatellite studied, determined in Généthon (Evry, France). In a 6% polyacrylamide-urea gel, xylene cyanol migrates at a rate equivalent to 100 bp double-stranded DNA.
5. The sample migration pattern is always compared with a standard pattern corresponding to alleles of known sizes. A control DNA (M134702) can be provided by Généthon. The genotype of this individual for each Généthon marker is given in the Généthon human genetic linkage map ***(34)***, or on www.genethon.fr.
6. The pellet resuspended in RNA Plus can be kept at –80°C.
7. A good extraction of RNA corresponds to a OD ratio (260/280 nm) of approx 2. One OD unit corresponds to 40 µg RNA/mL.
8. All reagents stored at –20°C should be thawed on ice before use. Wear gloves to avoid contamination with ribonucleases from skin.
9. It is necessary to use two controls: genomic DNA as negative control; and control cDNA from trophoblast and from control lymphoblastoid cell lines as positive control.
10. Splicing out of some exons (in particular exons 25, 52, and 54) may occur in absence of any pathological mutation when cDNA is prepared from lymphoblastoid cell lines. Exon 52 is alternatively spliced in skeletal muscle ***(23)***.
11. Temperature is an important parameter in SSCP analysis. The gel system should be assembled and precooled at 7°C for at least 1 h, before loading the samples. The gel should be run as slowly as possible, to avoid any increase in temperature. The exact running conditions depend on the products being analyzed.
12. The Ag staining is only applicable to gels of about 1 mm thickness. Handling a large gel for Ag staining can be difficult. The gel should be gently rolled off the plate into the fixation solution. Staining is then straightforward. After staining, the gel can be trimmed to size before being dried between cellophane.
13. **Caution:** Always wear gloves when using the kit components, and when handling gels.
14. Staining time is dependent on the sample and the quantity loaded. It may take at least 15 min before the bands first become visible.
15. When an abnormal migration pattern is observed by SSCP (**Fig. 2**, track 5), reanalyze the patient sample with the other members of the family, to confirm and determine the transmission of the abnormal profile.
16. After sequencing, if it is a nonsilent nt change, at least 100 chrs of unrelated individuals should be studied to determine if it is a polymorphism or a mutation.
17. If a mutation is found, then an alternative test should be devised to confirm it in the original sample, and in relatives, on new DNA dilutions. This may be a restriction enzyme digestion, if the mutation alters a recognition site. In addition to the

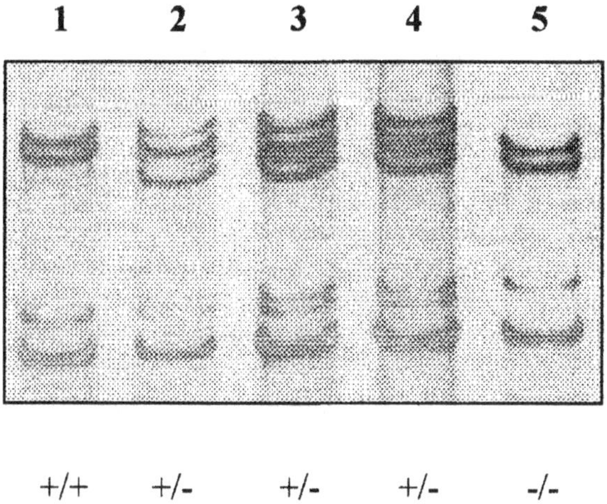

Fig. 2. Detection of *LAMA2* point mutation by SSCP analysis. Analysis of single-stranded PCR products containing exon 31. Track 1 shows the normal migration patter (+/+). Track 5 shows a mutant pattern (–/–). Tracks 2–4 (samples of other family members) display fused patterns of mutated and normal.

obligatory no-DNA control, always use samples that are heterozygous (+/–) and homozygous (+/+) for the restriction site, as controls. The +/+ control sample should always be fully digested. If it is not, the results of the test are invalid. The fragment intensities should be constant in any +/– test samples, compared to the +/– control. Any deviation is indicative of sample-specific partial digestion, and further enzyme should be added to the PCR products, or the analysis should be repeated.

18. The Ag-staining method also stains the proteins present in the PCR reaction. They migrate through the gel as a broad front corresponding to double-stranded DNA of mol wt 140 bp and above.

References

1. Fardeau, M. (1992) Congenital myopathies, in *Skeletal Muscle Pathology* (Mastaglia, F. L., ed.), Churchill-Livingstone, Edinburgh, pp. 237–281.
2. Banker, B. Q. (1994) Congenital muscular dystrophy, in *Myology,* vol. 2 (Engel, A. G. and Franzini-Amstrong, C., eds.), McGraw-Hill, New York, pp. 1275–1289.
3. Dubowitz, V. (1995) Congenital muscular dystrophy, in *Muscle Disorders Childhood* (Dubowitz, V., ed.), Saunders, London, pp. 93–105.
4. Fukuyama, Y., Osawa, M., and Suzuki, H. (1981) Congenital progressive muscular dystrophy of the Fukuyama type: clinical, genetic, and pathological considerations. *Brain Dev.* **3,** 1–29.
5. Donner, M., Rapola, J., and Somer, H. (1975) Congenital muscular dystrophy: a clinicopathological and follow-up study of 15 patients. *Neuropädiatrie* **6,** 239–258.

6. Santavuori, P., Leisti, J., and Kruus, S. (1977) Muscle, eye and brain disease: a new syndrome. *Neuropediatrics* **8 (Suppl. 8),** 553.
7. Dobyns, W. B., Pagon, R. A., Armstrong, D., Curry, C. J. R., Greenberg, F., Grix, A., et al. (1989) Diagnosis criteria for Walker-Warburg syndrome. *Am. J. Med. Genet.* **32,** 195–210.
8. Tomé, F. M. S., Evangelista, T., Leclerc, A., Sunada, Y., Manole, E., Estournet, B., et al. (1994) Congenital muscular dystrophy with merosin deficiency. *C. R. Acad. Sci. Paris, Life Sci.* **317,** 351–357.
9. Helbling-Leclerc, A., Zhang, X., Topaloglu, H., Cruaud, C., Tesson, F., Weissenbach, J., et al. (1995) Mutations in the laminin α_2-chain gene (LAMA2) cause merosin-deficient congenital muscular dystrophy. *Nature Genet.* **11,** 216–218.
10. Fardeau, M., Tomé, F. M. S., Helbling-Leclerc, A., Evangelista, T., Ottolini, A., Chevallay, M., et al. (1996) Dystrophie musculaire congénitale avec déficience en mérosine: analyse clinique, histopathologique, immunologique et génétique. *Rev. Neurol.* (Paris), **152,** 11–19.
11. Van der Knapp, M. S., Smit, L. M. E., Barth, P. G., Catsman-Berrevoets, C. E., Brouwer, O. F., Begeer, J. H., de Coo, I. F. M., and Valk, J. (1997) Magnetic resonance imaging in classification of congenital muscular dystrophies with brain abnormalities. *Ann. Neurol.* **42,** 50–59.
12. Mercuri, E., Pennock, J., Goodwin, F., Sewry, C., Cowan, F., Dubowitz, L., Dubowitz, V., and Muntoni, F. (1996) Sequential study of central and peripheral nervous system involvement in an infant with merosin-deficient congenital muscular dystrophy. *Neuromusc. Disord.* **6,** 425–429.
13. Wever, U. M. and Engvall, E. (1996) Merosin/laminin-2 and muscular dystrophy. *Neuromusc. Disord.* **6,** 409–418.
14. Vuolteenaho, R., Nissinen, M., Sainio, K., Byers, M., Eddy, R., Hirvonen, H., et al. (1994) Human laminin M Chain (merosin): complete primary structure, chromosomal assignment, and expression of the M and A chain in human fetal tissues. *J. Cell Biol.* **124,** 381–394.
15. Zhang, X., Vuolteenaho, R., and Tryggvason, K. (1996) Structure of the human laminin α_2-chain gene (LAMA2), which is affected in congenital muscular dystrophy. *J. Biol. Chem.* **271,** 27664–27669.
16. Chelly, J., Concordet, J. P., Kaplan, J. C., and Kahn, A. (1989) Illegitimate transcription: transcription of any gene in any cell type. *Proc. Natl. Acad. Sci. USA* **86,** 2617–2621.
17. Orita, M., Iwahana, H., Kanazawa, H., Hayashi, K., and Sekiya, T. (1989) Detection of polymorphisms of human DNA by gel electrophoresis as single-strand conformation polymorphisms. *Proc. Natl. Acad. Sci. USA* **86,** 2766–2770.
18. Guicheney, P., Vignier, N., Zhang, X., He, Y., Craud, C., Frey, V., et al. (1998) PCR-based mutation screening of the laminin α_2-chain gene (LAMA2): application to prenatal diagnosis and search of founder effects in congenital muscular dystrophy. *J. Med. Genet.* **35,** 211–217.
19. Guicheney, P., Vignier, N., Helbling-Leclerc, A., Nissinen, M., Zhang, X., Cruaud, C., et al. (1997) Genetics of laminin α_2-chain (or merosin) deficient con-

genital muscular dsytrophy: from identification of mutations to prenatal diagnosis. *Neuromusc. Disord.* **7,** 180–186.

20. Pegaro, E., Mancias, P., Swerdlow, S. H., Raikow, R. B., Garcia, C., Marks, H., et al. (1996) Congenital muscular dystrophy with primary laminin α_2 (merosin) deficiency presenting as imflammatory myopathy. *Ann. Neurol.* **40,** 782–791.
21. Utani, A., Nomizu, M., Sugiyama, A., Miyamoto, S., Roller, P. R., and Yamada, Y. (1995) Specific sequence of the laminin α_2-chain critical for the initiation of heterotrimer assembly. *J. Biol. Chem.* **270,** 3292–3298.
22. Nissinen, M., Helbling-Leclerc, A., Zhang, X., Evangelista, T., Topaloglu, H., Cruaud, C., et al. (1996) Substitution of a conserved cysteine-996 in a cysteine-rich motif of the laminin α_2-chain in congenital muscular dystrophy with partial deficiency of the protein. *Am. J. Hum. Genet.* **58,** 1177–1184.
23. Hayashi, Y., Ishihara, T., Domen, K., Hori, H., and Arahata, K. (1997) A benign allelic form of laminin α_2-chain deficient muscular dystrophy. *Lancet* **349,** 1147.
24. Allamand, V., Sunada, Y., Salih, M. A. M., Straub, V., Ozo, C. O., AlTuraiki, M. H. S., et al. (1997) Mild congenital muscular dystrophy in two patients with an internally deleted laminin α_2-chain. *Hum. Mol. Genet.* **6,** 747–752.
25. Naom, I., D'Alessandro, M., Topaloglu, H., Sewry, C., Ferlini, A., Helbling-Leclerc, A., et al. (1997) Refinement of the laminin α_2 chain locus to human chromosome 6q2 in severe and mild merosin deficient congenital muscular dystrophy. *J. Med. Genet.* **34,** 99–104.
26. Naom, I., D'Alessandro, M., Sewry, C., Ferlini, A., Topaloglu, H., Helbling-Leclerc, A., et al. (1997) Role of immunocytochemistry and linkage analysis in the prenatal diagnosis of merosin-deficient congenital muscular dystrophy. *Hum. Genet.* **99,** 535–540.
27. Helbling-Leclerc, A., Topaloglu, H., Tomé, F. M. S., Sewry, C., Gyapay, G., Naom, I., et al. (1995) Readjusting the localization of merosin (laminin α_2-chain) deficient congenital muscular dystrophy locus on chromosome 6q2. *C. R. Acad. Sci. Paris, Life Sci.* **318,** 1245–1252.
28. Voit, T., Fardeau, M., and Tomé, F. M. S. (1994) Prenatal detection of merosin expression in human placenta. *Neuropediatrics* **25,** 332–333.
29. Muntoni, F., Sewry, C., Wilson, L., Angelini, C., Trevisan, C. P., Brambati, B., and Dubowitz, V. (1995) Prenatal diagnosis in congenital muscular dystrophy. *Lancet* **345,** 591.
30. Toda, T., Segawa, M., Nomura, Y., Nonaka, I., Masuda, K., Ishihara, T., Suzuki, M., et al. (1993) Localization of a gene for Fukuyama type congenital muscular dystrophy to chromosome 9q31–33. *Nature Genet.* **5,** 283–286.
31. Toda, T., Ikegawa, S., Okui, K., Kondo, E., Saito, K., Fukuyama, Y., et al. (1994) Refined mapping of a gene responsible for Fukuyama-type congenital muscular dystrophy: evidence for strong linkage disequilibrium. *Am. J. Hum. Genet.* **55,** 946–950.
32. Topaloglu, H., Talim, B., Vignier, N., Helbling-Leclerc, A., Yetük, M., Afsin, E., Caglar, G., and Guicheney, P. (1998) Merosin-deficient congenital muscular dystrophy with severe mental retardation and normal cranial MRI. *Neuromusc. Disord.* **8,** 169–176.

33. Don, R. H., Cox, P. T., Wainwright, B. J., Baker, K., and Mattick, J. S. (1991) 'Touchdown' PCR to circumvent spurious priming during gene amplification. *Nucl. Acids Res.* **19,** 4008.
34. Dib, C., Fauré, S., Fizames, C., Samson, D., Drouot, N., Vignal, A., et al. (1996) A comprehensive genetic map of the human genome based on 5264 microsatellites. *Nature* **380,** 152–154.

13

α-Sarcoglycan Mutations

Frederica Piccolo, C. de Toma, and Marc Jeanpierre

1. Introduction

1.1. Strategy

Genetic defects of the sarcoglycan (SG) complex (sarcoglycanopathies) are found in patients with autosomal recessive muscular dystrophies ***(1–6)***. α-SG (50 kDa dystrophin-associated glycoprotein, adhalin) is involved in LGMD2D, mapped on 17q21 ***(1,7)***. The continuing progress in the identification and characterization of new mutations in the α-*SG* gene increases the need for a method that can rapidly identify point mutations. Among the 10 mutations that have been observed in two or more unrelated families, the R77C mutation is specially frequent (about 40% of patients) ***(5,9–12)***. The large geographic distribution of the R77C mutation is explained by a highly mutable CpG mutation hot spot, and not by a founder effect. Because this mutation can be readily and directly detected by a simple polymerase chain reaction (PCR) amplification, followed by enzyme digestion, a prior screening for this mutation could reduce the number of patients to analyze. Besides taking into account the occurrence of frequent mutations, the clinical presentation could also be taken into account in the mutation-detection strategy. The R284C mutation results in a much less severe disease, because some adult patients are ascertained after discovery of high serum creatine kinase ***(11)***. In R284C homozygotes, α-SG is moderately decreased in muscle, with little secondary impact on γ-sarcoglycan. Because an important proportion of patients are compound heterozygotes, the authors chose denaturing gradient gel electrophoresis (DGGE) of PCR products as the method to screen gene regions, in order to find abnormal migration patterns caused by single base changes in DNA sequence.

From: *Methods in Molecular Medicine, vol. 43: Muscular Dystrophy: Methods and Protocols*
Edited by: K. M. D. Bushby and L. V. B. Anderson © Humana Press Inc., Totowa, NJ

1.2. Denaturing Gradient Gel Electrophoresis

The DGGE method is based on the electrophoretical separation of double-strand DNA fragments, depending on their melting properties. Blocks of DNA sequences, called melting domains, melt out at discrete temperatures (T_m), which are dependent on their nucleotide (nt) composition. Changes in base sequences, as small as a single-base substitution within a melting domain, affect the thermodynamic stability of double helix, and alter the T_m of the domain.

Separation of the DNA fragments is performed in a polyacrylamide gel containing a linearly increased gradient of DNA denaturing agents, such as formamide and urea, from top to bottom. Electrophoresis apparatus is set at a relatively high temperature, usually 60°C. The DNA fragment enters the gel as a double-stranded molecule, and migrates at a linear rate dependent on its mol wt. At the position in the gel where the denaturant concentration combined to the bath temperature equal the T_m of the first melting domain, the DNA fragment undergoes partial denaturation, and its electrophoretic mobility is strongly retarded.

In a correct denaturing gradient, two DNA fragments, differing by a single base substitution, are retarded at different positions in the gel, and will be separated at the end of the run. Base changes at the domain with the highest T_m generally are not detectable, because, as the domain melts, the DNA fragment undergoes complete denaturation. This can be overcome by attaching a high-temperature melting domain (clamp) at one of the 5' ends of the DNA fragment, by PCR primers. The clamp could be a natural clamp, such as a GC-rich sequence or a chemical such as psoralene.

A DNA fragment from an individual either normal or homozygous for a mutation (or polymorphism) will show either a normal or a mutant homoduplex. A DNA fragment from a heterozygous individual results in four bands: two homoduplexes, corresponding to the wild-type and mutant alleles, and two heteroduplexes, formed by reassortment of strands during PCR. The two heteroduplexes, each of which carries a single-base mismatch, are retarded because of the large destabilization in T_m caused by the mismatches. The DGGE system can be used to examine double-strand DNA fragments of about 100–600 bp. The upper limit of size is partially determined by the fact that gel matrix is polyacrylamide, which slows the mobility of DNA fragments larger than 1000 pb, moreover, larger fragments containing several melting domains could not be completely analyzed.

Lerman's Meltmap program *(8)* calculates the melting map of a given DNA sequence. The first eight exons of the α-SG gene (representing, altogether, more than 95% of the coding sequence) and the 20–30-bp-long flanking intronic sequences were separately amplified by PCR from genomic DNA.

DGGE conditions for α-SG gene analysis were chosen according to the Lerman's Meltmap program, and are presented in **Table 1**. PCR products showing an abnormal migration pattern by DGGE analysis were re-amplified (to avoid the possibility of a mistake on the order of samples run) and directly sequenced.

2. Material

2.1. Polymerase Chain Reaction

The following buffers and reagents are needed for performing the PCR reaction described in the next subheading.

1. The authors use PCR buffer and *Taq* DNA polymerase (5 U/mL) from Boehringer Mannheim.
2. Deoxyribonucleoside triphosphate (dNTP) 25 m*M* mix. The concentrated solutions of dNTPs sold by Pharmacia have reproducibly high quality. For 400 mL mix, add the following:

a. 25 m*M* dATP	100 mL of 100 m*M* dATP
b. 25 m*M* dTTP	100 mL of 100 m*M* dTTP
c. 25 m*M* dGTP	100 mL of 100 m*M* dGTP
d. 25 m*M* dCTP	100 mL of 100 m*M* dCTP

   Store at –20°C in small aliquots.
3. Oligo-nt primers should be 20–25 nts in length, to ensure their relative uniqueness in the genome. Store at –20°C in small aliquots at 50 pmol/mL. Pairs of primers are listed in **Table 2**.

2.2. Denaturing Gradient Gel Electrophoresis

The authors use the DGGE system manufactured by CBS Scientific. The system consists of:

1. Reservoir glass tank with platinum electrode, which serves as heated bath and lower electophoresis chamber.
2. Heater-stirrer unit.
3. Peristaltic pump, to continually replace buffer in the small upper chamber from the large lower chamber.
4. Two gel cassettes with platinum electrodes: They hold gel plates in place to create an upper electrophoresis chamber.
5. Glass plates, spacers, combs, and clamps.
6. Gradient maker.
7. Power supply.

2.3. Reagents, Buffer, and Solutions

The authors use buffer and gel solutions developed by Fisher and Lerman.

Table 1
Amplification of the α-SG Gene and DGGE Conditions

Fragment	Sequence of primers	length (pb)	Annealing temperature (°C)	Gradient (%)	Running time (h) at 160 V
Exon 1	1F: CCTGTCTCTGTCACTCACCG 1R: Pso-AATCCTGCCCCCTCAT CCTGG	128	60	40–90	7.5
Exon 2	197 2F: GCCTGTGTGTTTGGGACTTG 2R: Pso-AATACACCCCAGCCC GCCCGCC	60	40–90	6.5	
Exon 3	239 3F: GGGCTCCTGCTGTGACTCGA 3R: Pso-AATGGCCCACCCCTGT GATTTT	58	50–90	9.0	
Exon 4	4F: Pso-AATTTCTCCCCTAACC CACTTC 4R: AAGACTGGCATTGGTGGGGA	162	60	40–90	7.5
Exon 5	311 5F: Pso-AAGCAGGGATGTGGGG AGGAGC 5R: AGTCCTCTAGGGTTGCACAC	58	40–90	13.0	
Exon 6	6F: CTGCCCCCACTCTGCTGACA 6R: Pso-AAGGGAAGGGGGACTG GGATGG	444	59	Lowest melting domain 30–80 Highest melting domain 40–90	8.5 9.0
Exon 7	7F: TGTCCAGCCAGCCACTTCCT 7R: Pso-AATCCCATACAGACA AGTGCCA	339	58	40–90	11.0
Exon 8	8F: Pso-AAGGGCACCTTGGGGCG AAACC 8R: ATAGTTTGGTGGCGGGGTCC	152	60	30–80	6.5

Table 2
Recurrent Mutations in the α-*SG* Gene

nt change[a]	Exon	Amino acid substitution	Restriction site	Remarks
C92T	2	L(31)P	None	
C100T	2	R(34)C	*Hae*III –	CpG hot spot
G101A	2	R(34)H	*Nla*III +	CpG hot spot
C229T	3	R(77)C	*Nla*IV –, *Aci*I –	CpG hot spot
C292T	3	R(98)C	*Mbo*I –	CpG hot spot
G293A	3	R(98)H	*Nla*III +	CpG hot spot
T371C	4	I(124)T	*Bsr*I +	
T518C	5	L(173)P	None	
G739A	6	V(247)M	*Bsr*DI –	
C850T	7	R(284)C	None	CpG hot spot

[a]nt position in the cDNA sequence (Genbank HSU08895) starting from the initial ATG.

1. Acrylamide stock solution: 40% (w/v) Acrylamide-*bis*-acrylamide, 19:1 premixed solution
2. 50X Tris-acetate–EDTA (TAE) gel running buffer. For 1 L, use the following:

2 *M* Tris base	242.3 g Tris base
1 *M* sodium acetate	136.1 g NaAc trihydrate
0.05 *M* EDTA	18.6 g/L Titriplex III Merck
	H_2O to 1 L
pH 7.7	Adjust the pH to 7.7 with acetic acid

3. 90% denaturant acrylamide stock solution. For 500 mL, use

6% acrylamide	75 mL acrylamide stock solution
36% formamide	180 mL deionized formamide
6.3 *M* urea	190 mL ultrapure urea
1X TAE running buffer	10 mL 50X TAE gel running buffer
	H_2O to 500 mL

   Filter through 0.45-mm nylon filters (formamide will dissolve many of the standard filter material), and store at +4°C in dark bottles.
4. 90% denaturant acrylamide stock solution. For 500 mL, use:

6% acrylamide	75 mL acrylamide stock solution
1X TAE running buffer	10 mL 50X TAE gel running buffer
	H_2O to 500 mL

   Store at +4°C in dark bottles.
5. Polymerization catalysts.
   (*N*,*N*,*N*′,*N*′-tetramethylethylenediamine) (TEMED)

10% APS stock solution	1 g ammonium persulphate
	H_2O to 10 mL

   Store TEMED at +4°C; store 10% APS at –20°C in small aliquots for one use only.

6. Neutral loading buffer. For 10 mL:

80% glycerol	8 mL glycerol
10 m*M* Tris-HCl, pH 7.5	100 mL 1 *M* Tris-HCL, pH 7.5
25 m*M* EDTA	500 mL 0.5 *M* EDTA
0.1% bromophenol blue	
0.1% xylene cyanol	
	H_20 to 10 mL

3. Methods

3.1. PCR

1. Combine the following reagents in a microcentrifuge tube: 5 mL 10X PCR buffer, 1 mL dNTP (25 m*M*), 50 pmols of each oligo-nt primer, 1 mL genomic DNA (100 mg/mL), 0.3 mL of Taq DNA polymerase (5 U/mL), and add H_2O to 50 mL
2. Amplification cycles: initial denaturation at 94°C for 4 min; initial annealing at the appropriate temperature for 1 min; 35 cycles: 40 s at 72°C, 40 s at 94°C, 40 s at the appropriate annealing; temperature; final incubation at 72°C for 2 min.
3. PCR reactions are performed in a MJ Research Thermal Cycler.
4. Analyze approx one-tenth of amplified products by agarose gel electrophoresis, to roughly quantitate the amount of the amplified DNA.

3.2. Heteroduplex Formation and DNA Clamping

1. Heteroduplexes are produced by heating PCR products at 94°C for 5 min and incubating at 55°C for 45 min.
2. PCR fragments are clamped after UV irradiation at 365 nm for 25 min.

3.3. DGGE Analysis

1. The CBS apparatus tank requires about 16 L running buffer. The correct level of buffer reaches the underside of the upper reservoir of cassettes. The upper reservoir holds 50 mL buffer. The peristaltic pump ensures the buffer recirculation from tank to the upper chamber. The running buffer may be used 20–30× before it should be changed. Buffer temperature in the tank must be 60°C. Make sure that 60°C is maintained. Before actually running gels, turn on the peristaltic pump and check to be sure buffer is correctly cycling.
2. Glass plate setup: Assemble the two plates with gasket and spacers, clamp bottom and sides of the sandwich assembly with two casting clamps on each side, and stand it on the base of clamps. Place comb.
3. Make up equal volumes of denaturant solutions, corresponding to the two end points of the gradient, by mixing 0 and 90% stocks. Total volume of denaturant solution should equal the volume between plates. The authors' apparatus, with glass plates of 17.7 × 22 cm and 0.75 mm spacers, requires a 26-mL total gel vol: Prepare 13 mL of both denaturant solutions. Chill on ice.
4. Place the gradient maker on a magnetic stirrer with stir bars in both chambers. Fit the outlet of gradient maker with a 0.8-mm tubing, ending with a 20-gage needle

to deliver acrylamide to plate sandwich. Connect it to a peristaltic pump, and place needle between plates.

5. Pour the denser solution into the downstream chamber, slowly open the valve between the two chambers to fill channel with denaturant solution, close valve, and pour the less-dense solution in the other chamber.
6. Turn on the magnetic stirrer. Add catalysts (11 mL TEMED and 70 mL APS 10%, for 17.7 × 22 cm gel plates), turn on peristaltic pump to start flow, and open the internal valve. Adjust flow so that the gradient pours over a period of 10 min.
7. Allow gel to polymerize for 1.5 h at room temperature.
8. After polymerization, remove gasket and clamps. Tape sides of plate sandwich to prevent perpendicular electrical field from interfering with migration. Remove comb.
9. Fix gel sandwich to cassette with large clamps, fill upper chamber with running buffer, and rinse each well with buffer, to remove urea and formamide.
10. Add one-quarter vol of loading buffer to PCR products. Load samples. Immerse cassette into preheated tank buffer, connect electrodes and recirculating tubes, and turn on peristaltic pump.
11. Switch on power supply at appropriate voltage.
12. When run is completed, switch off power supply and peristaltic pump, disconnect electrodes and recirculating tubes, remove cassettes, and remove glass sandwich from cassettes. Remove tape, and softly separate glass plates. Keep gel adhering to one plate (take care in handling gel).
13. Stain with 0.5 mg/mL ethidium bromide 15 min, and view bands on transilluminator.
14. The presence of two melting domains in exon 6 requires a two-step analysis: The lowest melting domain is directly analyzed in the entire PCR product (heteroduplex formation and clamp); the highest melting domain is investigated after *Mbo*II digestion (**Table 1**).

    To perform *Mbo*II digestion, add: 20 mL PCR product; 3 mL 10X digestion buffer; 0.5 mL *Mbo*II. Put at 37°C for 3 h, before performing hetroduplex formation, and clamp.

3.3. Sequence

The authors use the DyeTerminator method, derived from Sanger's method.

3.4. Direct Detection of Mutation and Restriction Enzyme Analysis

Ten mutations have been observed more than once (**Table 2**). The frequent R77C mutation can be readily detected by a simple PCR amplification, followed by *Nla*IV digestion.

References

1. Roberds, S. L., Leturcq, F., Allamand, V., Piccolo, F., Jeanpierre, M., et al. (1994) Missense mutations in the adhalin gene linked to autosomal recessive muscular dystrophy. *Cell* **78,** 625–633.

2. Noguchi, S., McNally, E., Ben Othmane, K., Hagiwara, Y., Mizuno, Y., et al. (1995) Mutations in the dystrophin-associated protein g-sarcoglycan in chromosome 13 muscular dystrophy. *Science* **270,** 819–822.
3. Bönnemann, C. G., Modi, R., Noguchi, S., Mizuno, Y., Yoshida, M., et al. (1995) β-sarcoglycan (A3b) mutations cause autosomal recessive muscular dystrophy with loss of the sarcoglycan complex. *Nat. Genet.* **11,** 266–273.
4. Lim, L. E., Duclos, F., Broux, O., Bourg, N., Sunada, Y., et al. (1995) β-sarcoglycan: characterization and role in limb-girdle muscular dystrophy linked to 4q12. *Nat. Genet.* **11,** 257–285.
5. Piccolo, F., Roberds, S. L., Jeanpierre, M., Leturcq, F., Azibi, K., et al. (1995) Primary adhalinopathy: a common cause of autosomal recessive muscular dystrophy of variable severity. *Nat. Genet.* **10,** 243–245.
6. Duggan, D. J., Gorospe, J. R., Fanin, M., Hoffman, E. P., and Angelini, C. (1997) Mutations in the sarcoglycan genes in patients with myopathy. *N. Engl. J. Med.* **336,** 618–624.
7. McNally, E. M., Yoshida, M., Mizuno, Y., Ozawa, E., and Kunkel, L. M. (1994) Human adhalin is alternatively spliced and the gene is located on chromosome 17q21. *Proc. Natl. Acad. Sci. USA* **91,** 9690–9694.
8. Abrams, E. S., Murdaugh, S. E., and Lerman, L. S. (1995) Intramolecular DNA melting between stable helical segments: melting theory and metastable states. *Nucleic Acids Res.* **23,** 2775–2783.
9. Passos Bueno, M. R., Moreira, E., Vainzof, M., Chamberlain, J., Marie, S. K., et al. (1995) Common missense mutation in the adhalin gene in three unrelated Brazilian families with a relatively mild form of autosomal recessive limb-girdle muscular dystrophy. *Human Mol. Genet.* **4,** 1163–1167.
10. Fanin, M., Duggan, D. J., Mostacciuolo, M. L., Martinello, F., Freda, M. P., et al. (1997) Genetic epidemiology of muscular dystrophies resulting from sarcoglycan gene mutations. *J. Med. Genet.* **34,** 973–977.
11. Carrie, A., Piccolo, F., Leturcq, F., de, T. C., Azibi, K., et al. (1997) Mutational diversity and hot spots in the α-SG gene in autosomal recessive muscular dystrophy (LGMD2D). *J. Med. Genet.* **34,** 470–475.
12. Higuchi, I., Iwaki, H., Kawai, H., Endo, T., Kunishige, M., et al. (1997) New missense mutation in the α-SG gene in a Japanese patient with severe childhood autosomal recessive muscular dystrophy with incomplete α-SG deficiency. *J. Neurol. Sci.* **153,** 100–105.

14

Mutation Detection in β- and γ-Sarcoglycan (LGMD2E and LGMD2C)

Carsten G. Bönnemann and Louis M. Kunkel

1. Introduction

1.1 General Introduction

Direct mutation analysis in the genes for β- and γ- sarcoglycan (SG) is performed in a patient in whom a type of autosomal recessive limb-girdle muscular dystrophy (LGMD) affecting the SG complex is suspected. Ideally, this suspicion should have been substantiated by analysis of the SG complex using immunohistochemical (IHC) methods and/or Westernblot analysis of a muscle biopsy specimen from the patient before proceeding to the actual mutation analysis (*see* Chapter 15). In addition, the IHC results may directly suggest the primary *SG* gene involved (*see* subheading), thus potentially streamlining the search for the underlying mutation, which otherwise may have to cover all four currently known *SG* genes.

The analysis of the β- and γ-*SG* genes in this laboratory is mostly based on polymerase chain reaction–single stranded conformation polymorphism analysis (PCR-SSCPA) performed on genomic DNA isolated from the patient's blood lymphocytes. SSCPA was developed following the observation that single-stranded DNA molecules of the same length may assume different conformations, based on their exact nucleotide (nt) composition when separated under nondenaturing conditions, following an initial step of denaturation ***(1,2)***. These single-strand secondary structures are dependant on the formation of intrastrand hydrogen bonds and base stacking, so that a single nt difference may directly influence the conformation of the single strand, reflected in altered migration of the molecule in a nondenaturing gel matrix. The system thus allows the separation of DNA strands, based on single nt differences.

From: *Methods in Molecular Medicine, vol. 43: Muscular Dystrophy: Methods and Protocols*
Edited by: K. M. D. Bushby and L. V. B. Anderson © Humana Press Inc., Totowa, NJ

The templates used for the SSCPA are single exons amplified by PCR from the patient's genomic DNA, using primers located in the introns, up- and downstream from the individual exon. The splice donor and acceptor sites are thus included in the analysis, as well.

It is difficult to arrive at precise predictions about the sensitivity of SSCPA, because it depends on the exact nt composition in the vicinity of the mutation, the length of the fragment, and the exact conditions under which the assay is performed *(3–9)*. In particular, the composition of the gel matrix, including presence or absence of glycerol, temperature and power at which the separation is performed, and salt concentration in the matrix and running buffer, are important, and no single condition may be sufficient to detect all possible mutations. Unfortunately, there are no useful algorithms that predict the influence of each of these factors on the result. Even though the use of at least two different gel conditions will significantly improve the sensitivity of mutation detection, it can be assumed that the mutation detection rate with SSCPA will not reach fully 100%. Another potential pitfall of the technique is that, because single exons are amplified directly from genomic DNA, a deletion of an entire exon on only one allele will not be detected using the SSCPA technique alone, especially since this type of analysis cannot be considered gene-dosage-sensitive.

The clear benefit of SSCPA lies in its ease and robustness of performance. It can be established and performed reliably in a number of different laboratory environments. Because the technique also separates the mutant allele from the wild-type (WT) conformation, it allows for ready isolation, reamplification, and direct sequencing of the mutant fragment. Also, since each allele gives rise to two independent single strands after denaturation, each single-base change has two chances of being detected in this analysis (one for each single strand deriving from the mutant allele).

This laboratory performs the gel analysis under two different conditions for each reaction, using the 0.5X MDE (Mutation Detection Enhancing, FMC) acrylamide formulation, with and without the addition of glycerol (*6,9,10* [Bioproducts, BMA, Rockland, ME]). The authors tend to use 5% glycerol, but have used up to 10% successfully. Electrophoresis is performed at 6–7 watts for 10–18 h in 0.6X Tris-borate–EDTA (TBE) at room temperature (RT). Nonradioactive SSCPA can also be used with silver (Ag) staining, as the first-line approach to mutation detection in a new sample, because this technique takes less time, appears to be quite sensitive, and eliminates the hazards of handling radioactivity. Because, in the SG disorders, the expected result in a given patient often will be a novel mutation (for recurrent mutations, *see* **Subheadings 1.2.2.** and **1.3.2.**), optimization of the screening assay is difficult. Once mutations have been identified, these can be used to test new gel conditions for their sensitivity in detecting these known mutations. In cases in which no mutations are detected with the radioactive SSCPA conditions used, but are suspected to a high degree (for instance, on the basis of IHC analysis of the patient's muscle biopsy), the authors either proceed to nonradioactive SSCPA on the Pharmacia Phast system (Amersham Pharmacia Biotech, Piscataway, NJ) with automated Ag staining, or perform direct sequencing on the genomic single-exon PCR products.

All abnormal conformers detected by SSCP analysis need to be further verified by direct sequencing of the excised and amplified fragment. Differentiation of a disease-causing mutation vs a polymorphism is important, especially for novel missense changes (*see* **Subheading 3.7.**). In cases in which a mutation is suspected of affecting splicing, and muscle biopsy tissue is available, reverse transcription (RT)-PCR can be performed to confirm the pathogenic effect of the mutation on mRNA splicing.

1.2. β-Sarcoglycan

Mutations in the β-*SG* gene located on chromosome 4q12 underlie LGMD2E, a form of autosomal recessive (AR) LGMD of variable severity, although the initial presentation often is in childhood, followed by a severe course ***(11–13)***. This type of AR LGMD has now been described in various populations in both sporadic and familial cases with SG-deficient LGMD ***(11–13)***. It coexists with LGMD2A in extensive interrelated pedigrees in the Indiana Amish, in whom it is caused by a homozygous missense mutation (Thr151Arg) ***(12)***.

1.2.1. Gene/Protein Structure

The open reading frame of the β-*SG* gene is encoded on six exons, and spans a genomic distance of approx 18 kb ***(13)***. Exon 1 is embedded in a dense CpG island making its analysis more difficult. Exon 6 includes the stop codon followed by a long 5'-UTR. The expression of the other *SG* genes is restricted to muscle, but the mRNA for β-SG, in addition to skeletal muscle and heart, is also expressed at lower levels in other tissues, such as brain and kidney. There is no current evidence for alternative splice forms involving the coding region. The protein is a type 2 (the N-terminus is within the cell) single transmembrane molecule with three putative extracellular N-linked glycosylation sites (residues 158, 211, and 258) and one putative intracellular serine phosphorylation site with a caseine kinase 2 consensus sequence (residue 21). Four spaced cysteines (Cys), at the extracellular C-terminus, form a motif with some homology to a partial epidermal growth factor (EGF) module, similar to the Cys in the C-terminus of γ- and δ-SG. In addition, there is a single Cys residue in the immediate extracellular domain, potentially involved in intermolecular disulfide bonding. There also is an eight residue polyalanine tract at the N-terminus of the protein, although it is unknown whether it also exists in the processed protein.

The polyalanine tract is encoded by a corresponding number of imperfect GCG triplets. Even though no mutations have been described relating to expansions or contractions of this repeat, it is worthwhile to keep this theoretical possibility in mind, and to include exon 1 in the mutation analysis (*see* **Note 1**).

1.2.2. Mutational Spectrum and Recurrent Mutations

The mutational spectrum reported thus far ***(11–16)*** allows for some preliminary conclusions: Missense, as well as truncating, mutations occur in the gene, with truncating mutations commonly associated with a severe phenotype. The truncating mutations (nonsense mutations, microdeletions, splice-site mutations, duplications) are evenly spread across the gene. The situation is more complicated for the missense mutations, in which, for some, a more variable phenotype has been observed (Arg91Leu, Ser114Phe, Thr151Arg, Tyr184Cys); others are associated with a severity that is indistinguishable from the truncating mutations (Arg91Pro, Met100Lys, Leu108Arg). There also appears to be a cluster of missense mutations in the immediate extracellular domain, encoded on exon 3 of the *β-SG* gene, including some of the missense mutations with a severe phenotype. A few mutations have been seen more than once, including an 8-bp duplication in exon 3 ***(14)*** and Tyr184X in Italian patients (unpublished observations), Thr151Arg in the Indiana Amish ***(12)***, and Ser114Phe in Europe and the United States (***14,15***; Bönnemann and Kunkel, unpublished observations). Some residues are affected more than once, although by different mutations: Gln11 ***(14)***, Arg91 (***13***; and *see* ref. ***36***), and Tyr184 (***11,16***; Bönnemann and Kunkel, unpublished).

1.2.3. Analysis

Absence of the entire sarcoglycan complex is quite frequently observed in cases with β-sarcoglycan mutations (***11–13,17***); In contrast, the pattern may look different in primary γ- or α-SG mutations (*see* Chapter 22), so that, in cases of total absence of all SGs, IHC analyzes the *β-SG* gene first (although δ-SG mutations may show a similar pattern ***[17,18]***). Primers for the amplification of all six exons directly from genomic DNA are available and are listed in **Table 1**. Because of the high CG content of exon 1, separate procedures must be followed to allow for successful amplification (*see* **Subheading 3.9.1.**). Protocols for radioactive SSCPA, as well as for nonradioactive SSCPA, with Ag staining using the Pharmacia PhastSystem, are described. Abnormal conformers detected on the SSCP analysis are further analyzed by reamplification and sequencing. In addition, a protocol is provided for multiplexing the PCR reactions for β-SG exons 2–6, which may be useful if higher sample throughput is required for screening purposes.

Table 1
β-Sarcoglycan Genomic Primer Set

N	M
3 μL (= 45 ng genomic DNA.	->
0.5 μL l common primer	->
0.5 μL WT primer	–
–	0.5 μL mutant primer
0.3 μL control primer A	->
0.3 μL control primer B	->
0.75 μL $MgCl_2$	->
2.5 μL buffer	->
2.0 μL 2.5 m*M* each dNTP	->
0.25 μL Pt *Taq* polymerase (5 U/μL)	->
14.9 μL H_2O	->
Total 25 μL	

1.3. γ-Sarcoglycan

Primary γ-SG mutations underlie AR LGMD) type 2C. The first comprehensive description of this phenotype (initially referred to as "severe childhood autosomal recessive muscular dystrophy") was reported by Ben Hamida et al. ***(19)***. Linkage was established to 13q12 in the Tunisian population ***(20)***, before the *γ-SG* gene was cloned by Noguchi et al. ***(21)*** and mapped to the same genomic region. A common deletion of a single thymidine residue from a five-thy track (corresponding to cDNA positions 521–525), in exon 6 of the γ-SG gene, underlies most of the cases of recessive MD seen in northern Africa and the Maghrebian ***(21)***. However, LGMD 2C is not restricted to the northern African/mediterranean populations: It has now been reported from a number of populations around the world ***(14,21–25)***. Subsequently, it has become apparent that there can be considerable variability in the severity of the clinical phenotype, with milder manifestations even within the same family or between families carrying the same mutation ***(23,26)***. This variability may also be seen in the other sarcoglycanopathies.

1.3.1. Gene/protein Structure

The *γ-SG* gene consists of eight exons spanning a relatively large genomic distance of over 200 kb ***(23)***. The initiation codon is located in exon 2, so that exon 1 contains 5-UTR only. Single exons can be amplified from genomic DNA, with primer pairs situated in flanking intronic sequences. Like β-SG, this protein also is a type 2 single transmembrane protein with the N-terminus within the cell. There is one putative N-linked glycosylation site in the extracellular domain (residue 110), and a putative threonine phosphorylation site on the intracellular site (residue 7). In addition, there are four intracellular tyrosines, the phosphorylation status of which also is not known. Again, similar to β- and δ-SG, there are four spaced Cys residues at the C-terminus with some homology to partial EGF modules in addition to a single Cys residue close to the membrane.

1.3.2. Mutational Spectrum and Recurrent Mutations

The mutational spectrum is notable for the relatively wide geographic distribution of the del521T mutation, especially in families whose origins can be traced back to northern Africa or the mediterranean countries. Although the mutation in northern Africa occurs in linkage disequilibrium, with a 122-bp allele of the intragenic marker D13S232, in other populations, this association is not necessarily seen ***(22)***. In addition, it appears that truncating mutations arising from deletions are more common than are missense mutations. Very few missense mutations have been described so far, most importantly an A to G transition causing a substitution of a highly conserved Cys for a Tyr at position 283. This mutation is mostly prevalent in Romano Gypsy pedigrees ***(24)***, but can be seen outside of this genetic context (Bönnemann et al., submitted). Other missense mutations are rarely found, for example, Leu90Thr (Bönnemann et al., submitted). Large-scale genomic deletions of the entire gene and adjacent genomic regions need to be considered as well (Bönnemann et al., submitted). Partial or complete deletions of the gene will not be picked up by SSCP analysis, and may suggest homozygosity for a mutations that, in fact, is hemizygous. Similarly, a deletion on one allele, affecting only a part of the gene, may leave a point mutation on the other allele in a heterozygous state, if the point mutation lies in the nondeleted part of the gene. Therefore, one disease-causing allele may appear undetectable, unless the partial deletion is recognized. Analysis of the parents, loss of heterozygosity studies, quantitative Southern blotting, or dosage sensitive PCR studies may be warranted.

1.3.3. Analysis

Although SG mutations tend to cause concomitant secondary IHC reductions in the other components of the SG complex, more specific patterns of reduction have recently become apparent ***(17,22,25)***. In particular, absence of γ-SG immunoreactivity with reduced but preserved immunoreactivity for α-, β-, and, in particular, δ-SG, appears to be predictive of primary γ-SG mutations, irrespective of the type of mutation (Bönnemann et al., submitted). Antibodies (Abs) against α-, β-, γ-, and δ-SG are currently available as mouse monoclonal Abs, and can be used easily for this purpose. Thus, IHC analysis of the muscle biopsy with these Abs, before proceeding to genetic analysis, is highly recommended (*see* Chapter 22). Other factors, such as disease progression and general preservation of the muscle sarcolemma, may play additional roles in determining the actual IHC picture. The total loss of all SG components, as judged by IHC does not necessarily rule out the presence of γ-SG mutations, although it would make a primary β- or δ-SG mutation more likely.

The primary screening tool for mutations in the δ-SG gene used in this laboratory, again is based on SSCPA, using at least two different conditions for gel electrophoresis to maximize the chance for mutation detection. The primer pairs for the amplification of all eight exons of γ-SG directly from genomic DNA are listed in **Table 2**. Protocols for radioactive SSCPA, as well as for nonradioactive SSCP with Ag staining, using the Pharmacia Phast system, are described. Abnormal conformers detected on the SSCP analysis are again further analyzed by reamplification and sequencing. In addition, the authors also provide a protocol for multiplexing the PCR reactions, allowing for analysis of the entire gene in three lanes per patient.

In cases in which there is an appearance of homozygosity for a mutation in the patient, but apparent lack of a carrier status in one of the parents, the question of a larger genomic deletion on one allele is raised. In these cases, loss of heterozygosity studies using polymorphisms in the gene, as well as quantitative Southern blot and PCR analysis, need to be performed.

2. Materials and Solutions (*see* Note 2)

2.1. General Materials

1. Genomic DNA at a concentration of 15 ng/μL in water or Tris-EDTA (TE), stored at +4°C (*see* **Note 3**).
2. *Taq* polymerase (Boehringer Mannheim).
3. 10X PCR buffer (Boehringer Mannheim): 100 m*M* Tris-HCl (pH 8.3), 15 m*M* $MgCl_2$, 500 m*M* KCl, or equivalent *Taq* polymerase and buffer recommended for that enzyme.
4. PCR primers at a concentration of 10 pmol/μL (10 μ*M*). Store in small aliquots at –20°C in H_2O or TE.
5. Deoxyribonucleoside triphosphate (dNTP) mix at 2.5 m*M* each, store in small aliquots at –20°C, to avoid repeated freeze–thaw cycles.
6. MDE gel mix (FMC Bioproducts).
7. 50% Glycerol stock solution.
8. SSCP stop solution: 95% formamide, 20 m*M* EDTA, pH 8.0, 0.05% each bromephenol blue/xylene cyanol.

Table 2
γ-Sarcoglycan Genomic Primer Set

Exon/Size of product	Forward (5' -> 3')	Reverse (5' -> 3')
1 (396 bp)	cta tca tgc ttt agg gtt taa atg	tct aag tta aaa ctg agc act t
2 (267 bp)	ctc tct cct ctc gtg aac aca ctc	caa aac aag aac atg ctt acc ag
3 (162) bp	tac gca ttg tct ctt ttt ttt ttt taa c	aaa gca caa att att tgt ctt aac
4 (148 bp)	cag cac cta ttt tgc aaa ttt tat aaa tc	gca cca tga tga agc tgg act c
5 (226 bp)	gtt gac gtg gca tgt gta aaa	gtt gtg ttt ttc tcg agt tag tac
6 (195 bp)	tgg tgt cac tta ttt tac ttc tgc	cta aca tta ttc cag cac ata cc
7 (178 bp)	ttt tgt gct tct ttt cct cat ctc	cag tag gag gct gat ctg tga
8 (319 bp)	cct taa ctc ttc gtc tcc cat ctt	gcg ttt acg tcc cat cca cgc tgc c

9. 1 TBE (make 10X stock): 89 m*M* Tris-borate, pH 8.3, 2 m*M* Na_2EDTA.
10. 1 Tris-acetate–EDTA (make 50X stock): 40 m*M* Tris-acetate pH 8.1, 1 m*M* Na_2EDTA.
11. N'-tetramethylethylenediamine (TEMED).
12. 10% Ammonium persulfate.
13. Agarose for analytical and preparative (low melting point) gel electrophoresis.
14. Ethidium bromide (EtBr) stock solution (10 mg/mL).
15. PCR product purification system (i.e., Promega Wizzard PCR Preps DNA purification system or a similar system).
16. Restriction endonuclease *Rsa*I with appropriate buffer (usually included with the enzyme).

2.2. β-SG Exon 1 Amplification

1. 5 *M* Betaine (Aldrich no. 21,906-1).
2. Dimethylsulfoxide (DMSO).
3. Optional: platinum (PT) *Taq* polymerase (Gibco-BRL) with 10X buffer and 50 m*M* $MgCl_2$.

2.3. RNA Isolation/RT-PCR

1. Trizol (Gibco-BRL).
2. Chloroform.
3. Isopropanol.
4. 70% Ethanol.
5. $pd(N)_6$ random primers at 200 ng/μL (Pharmacia).
6. Gibco-BRL Superscript II plus proprietary first-strand buffer.
7. RNase H (Gibco-BRL).
8. 0.2 *M* dithiothreitol (DTT), included with Gibco-BRL Superscript II.

2.4. Equipment

1. Aerosol plugged plastic pipet tips.
2. Thermocycler capable of multiwell format.
3. Electrophoresis power supply (suitable for sequencing gel electrophoresis).
4. Upright acrylamide gel apparatus (sequencing gel), with glass gel plates and 0.4-mm spacers and sharktooth combs.
5. Gel dryer.
6. Agarose gel apparatus.
7. Centrifuge (e.g., Sorvall).
8. Swinging bucket centrifuge.
9. Polytron tissue homogenizer.
10. ABI sequencer or sequencing setup for manual double-stranded PCR product cycle sequencing.
11. Autoradiogram film and film cassette.
12. Appropriate plastic shielding for radioactive work.
13. RAD tape or similar autoradiogram marker.
14. Nonobligatory (for nonradioactive SSCP): Pharmacia PhastSystem with development unit, Phast DNA Ag staining kit, 12.5% homogenous Phast Gels, and native buffer strips.

3. Methods

3.1. Standard SSCPA Protocol

1. Set up the following reaction for each patient and each primer pair, taking appropriate precautions for handling radioactivity. Use of a multiwell PCR setup is recommended.
2. Make an appropriate master mix for each exon. In setting up the reaction, always include a negative (H_2O only) and a wild-type control. In cases in which the analysis is directed at the detection of a known mutation, a sample known to contain this particular mutation should be included as a positive control (*see* **Note 4**). α-SG exon 1 requires special conditions (*see* **Subheading 3.9.1.**): 2 μL 15 ng/μL DNA (= 30 ng DNA), 0.5 μL each of forward and reverse primer at 10 pmol/μL (10 μ*M*) = 5 pmol each, 1 μL 10X PCR buffer (Boehringer), 0.8 μL 2.5 m*M* each dNTP, 0.1 μL [^{32}P]-deoxycytidine triphosphate (dCTP), 0.1 μL *Taq* polymerase (Boehringer) 5 U/μL, and 5.5 μL H_2O, to a total of 10 μL.
3. Overlay the reactions with a drop of mineral oil (this is not necessary if a cycler with a heated lid is used).
4. Spin down briefly in a swinging bucket centrifuge.
5. The cycling parameters include: initial denaturation at 94°C for 2.5 min, annealing at 55°C (β-SG) or 58°C (γ-SG) for 0:40 min, extension at 72°C for 0:40 s, denaturation at 94°C for 0:40 min, for a total of 35 cycles, followed by final annealing at 55/58°C for 2 min, and final extension at 72°C for 5 min.

3.2. SSCPA Gel Electrophoresis

1. While the PCR reactions are in progress, prepare two large sequencing gels with 0.4-mm spacers and sharktooth combs (*see* **Note 5**). Several ways and setups to ensure leak-free gels are now available, including taping (make sure to double-tape the lower edges of the gel), rubber clamps, and horizontal gel-pouring stations.
2. Prepare two 0.5X MDE gels, with and without the addition of 5% glycerol. For a 75-mL gel mix, combine the following components in a beaker on a stir plate (one at a time): 51.75 mL H_2O (44.25 mL H_2O + 7.5 mL 50% glycerol for the 5% glycerol gel), 18.75 mL 2X MDE (FMC) (= 0.5% final), and 4.5 mL 10X TBE (= 0.6X TBE final).
3. Add approx 30 µL TEMED and 300 µL freshly prepared 10% APS. With the addition of these reagents, the gel is now starting to polymerize, and must be poured immediately.
4. Use a 60-mL syringe with a filter attached, to carefully pour the gel, avoiding bubbles. Insert the inverted sharktooth comb, and clamp the top of the gel with three binder clips.
6. Allow 45–60 min for the gels to polymerize completely.
7. Rinse off excess polyacrylamide from the gel plates, and examine the gel carefully for bubbles and impurities. Mark such regions and avoid the corresponding lanes when loading the gel, to avoid distortion of the bands (*see* **Note 6**).
8. Attach the gel to the electrophoresis apparatus, and fill upper and lower chamber with 0.6X TBE. Carefully examine the setup for leaks; mark the buffer level in the upper chamber to detect slow leaks.
9. The gel can now be prerun at the same settings used in the final electrophoresis, to help equalize potential temperature gradients across the matrix.
10. Transfer 2 µL of each PCR reaction into 8 µL stop solution in a new multiwell plate, and spin down briefly.
11. In the thermocycler, heat the samples to 95°C for 5 min, quench on ice slush, and load 2 µL sample per lane on the two gels for each sample. All samples amplified with the same primer pairs should be assayed in adjacent lanes, to allow for easy comparison of the bands between lanes (*see* **Note 7**).
12. Electrophoresis is performed at constant wattage (6–7 W per gel) at RT for 12–16 h in 0.6X TBE (*see* **Note 8**).
13. After completion of electrophoresis, the gels are transferred onto Whatman paper, and dried using a vacuum gel drier at 80°C for 60 min.
14. Before exposure to X-ray film, it is very important to unambiguously label the dried gel with either radioactive ink or a nonradioactive marker, such as RAD tape. This will allow for later precise alignment of the film with the gel, in order to cut abnormal bands of interest from the dried gel for reamplification.
15. The gel is exposed to film overnight at RT, or for a few hours at –80°C with an intensifying screen. Exposure at RT is preferable, because the bands tend to appear sharper.

Table 3
β-Sarcoglycan Genomic Multiplexed Primer Set

Set 1	Exon **2** F+R with Exon **3** F+R and Exon **4** F+R
Set 2	Exon **5** F+R and Exon **6** F+R

Table 4
γ-Sarcoglycan Genomic Multiplexed Primer Set

Set 1	Exon **1** F+R with Exon **2** F+R and Exon **7** F+R
Set 2	Exon **3** F+R with Exon **5** F+R and Exon **8** F+R
Set 2	Exon **4** F+R and Exon **6** F+R

3.3. Nonradioactive SSCPA

1. An alternative SSCPA protocol that avoids the use of radioactivity, and is considerably faster to perform, utilizes the Pharmacia PhastSystem automated gel electrophoresis system. It also compares favorably in sensitivity for mutation detection with other gel conditions *(27)*. One disadvantage is the limited number of samples that can be conveniently analyzed per electrophoresis (16 on two parallel gels).
2. The PCR reactions are performed with the same primers and conditions as given for the standard SSCPA PCR, but radioactivity is omitted.
3. Scaling-up of the individual reaction, to a total of 25 μL, may increase the yield and therefore visibility on the gel.
4. After completion of the PCR, 3 μL of the reaction is mixed with 3 μL stop solution.
5. The samples are denatured for 5 min at 95°C, quenched on ice slush, and 1 μL is loaded in each lane, using the appropriate loading comb.
6. The samples are separated on native 12.5% PhastGels, using native buffer strips, and the following electrophoresis parameters (programmed per gel): 1.1: 400 V, 5 mA, 1 W, 15°C, 100 Volts × hours (Vh); 1.2: 25 V, 5 mA, 1 W, 15°C, 2 Vh; 1.3: 400 V, 5 mA, 1 W, 15°C, 150–200 Vh; sample applicator down at 1.2 0 Vh, and up at 1.3 0 Vh.
7. The gels are stained using the Pharmacia PhastGel DNA Ag staining kit, using the protocol supplied by the manufacturer.
8. With the help of a magnifying glass, abnormal conformers can also be excised, eluted, and reamplified.
9. If the analysis is stopped before the xylene cyanol has left the gel, heteroduplex formation can be assessed in addition, although the SSCP portion of the gel will appear more compressed.

3.4. Multiplexed SSCPA

1. To multiplex reactions so that multiple exons can be examined in the same lane, the primer sets given in **Table 3** for β-SG, and in **Table 4** for γ-SG, are

prepared by adding equal volumes of the 10 μ*M* primer stocks at , and mixing thoroughly.

2. The PCR reactions are then set up as described previously, but, instead of the individual primers, the appropriate primer mix is now added. The volume of the individual reaction should be scaled up to 25 μL. Under multiplexed conditions, 7.5 pmol of each individual primer is used per 25-μL reaction. Thus, for a two-exon assay (four combined primers), use 3 μL and, for a three-exon assay (six combined primers), 4.5 μL of the corresponding primer mixes, and adjust the added water appropriately, for a reaction volume of 25 μL. Thus, the reaction mix per sample is: 5 μL 15 ng/μL DNA (= 30 ng DNA); 3 μL/4.5 μL for a two- and three-exon mix, respectively; 2.5 μL 10X PCR buffer (Boehringer); 2 μL 2.5 m*M* each dNTP; 0.25 μL [^{32}P]-dCTP; 0.25 μL *Taq* polymerase (Boehringer) 5 U/μL; 12 μL/10.5 μL H_2O for a two and for a three exon mix, respectively, to a total of 25 μL.
3. Cycling conditions and gel conditions are identical to the single-exon conditions (*see* **Note 9**).
4. The order of exons on the multiplexed gel can be deduced from their relative sizes given in **Tables 1** and **3** (*see also* **Fig. 1**; **Note 10**).

3.5. Analysis of Results

1. Upon autoradiography, conformers for the known normal samples are compared to the patient lanes.
2. Bands migrating differently from the normal patterns are indicative of changes in the sequence of the patient DNA sample.
3. One or more abnormal bands, *in addition* to the WT configuration, is indicative of a heterozygous state for the change (**Fig. 2A**; *see* **Note 11**).
4. The presence of abnormal bands, in the absence of one or more of the WT bands, indicates homozygosity for the change (**Fig. 2B**).
5. Even though two bands are usually expected for each allele (one for each single strand; *see*, e.g., **Fig. 2**), two single strands may co-migrate at the same position, resulting in only one additional band on the autoradiogram (as in **Fig. 1A**).
6. Likewise, a given single strand may assume more than one conformation, so that the banding pattern may appear considerably more complex.
7. In the heterozygous state, the coexisting WT and mutant bands often will be of lesser intensity, compared to the homozygous WT bands in the controls (*see* **Fig. 1A**).
8. Since the gel matrix containing glycerol significantly retards the migration of the DNA molecules within the gel, the faster-migrating double-stranded DNA in the sample is retained in the gel, and will be visible on the autoradiogram. This can be of advantage, because it will show the formation of heteroduplex molecules that may form when WT and mutant strands reanneal to each other. These heteroduplex molecules often will migrate differently from the WT or mutant double-strands, and thus be visible in the double-stranded portion of the gel (**Fig. 3**; *6,10*).

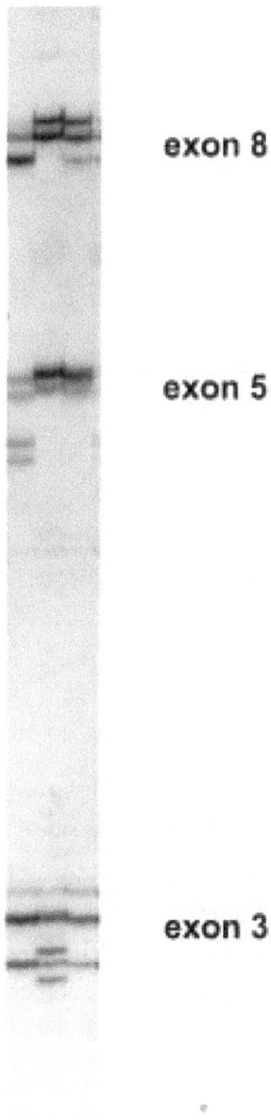

Fig 1. Examples of SSCP patterns in β-SG exon 3. **(A)** demonstrates a heterozygous change in the second and third lane (Leu108Arg); **(B)** shows a homozygous mutation in lane 1 (Arg91Pro).

3.6. Sequence Analysis of an Abnormal Conformer

1. To retrieve an abnormally migrating band from the gel for reamplification and direct sequencing, carefully align the film with the gel over a light box, and tape the film to the dried gel, then turn both over.
2. Outline the band of interest with a pencil on the back of the gel.
3. Remove the film from the gel, and, with a razorblade or scalpel, excise the outlined band, making sure that the dried gel matrix is still attached to the Whatman paper.

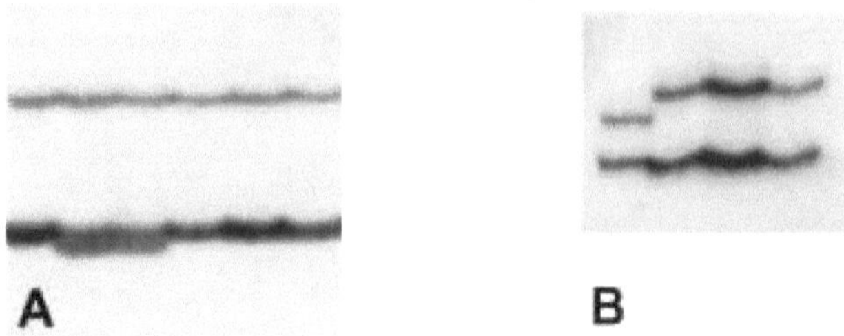

Fig 2. Example of a multiplexed set (γ-SG exons 3, 5, and 8) separated on a 0.5X MDE gel without glycerol. Not the polymorphisms apparent in all three exons (compare to **Table 7**).

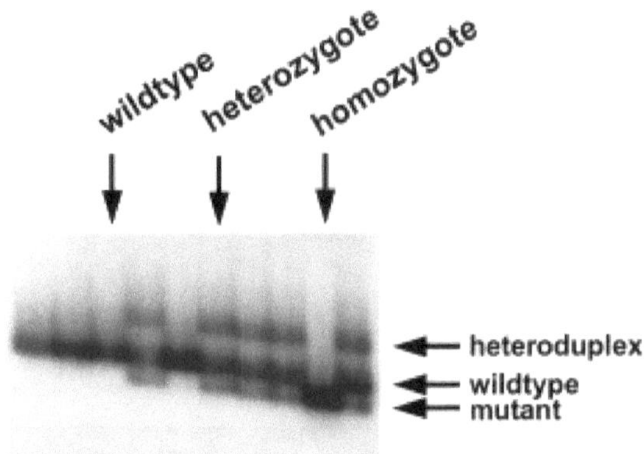

Fig 3. The three possible genotypes resulting from the ARMS analysis for the Leu91Arg mutation in β-SG. The upper band (control amplification) serves as a positive control for the PCR reaction. Each proband has an N = normal and M = mutant lane; the genotypes can be read directly, depending on the presence or absence of a specific product in the respective lanes.

4. Drop the slice into 50 µL ddH_2O in a 500-µL PCR tube.
5. Elute the DNA by incubating the gel slice at 37°C over night, cool to RT, and recollect the water at the bottom of the tube with brief centrifugation (*see* **Note 12**).
6. Reamplify the DNA fragment in a 50-µL PCR reaction, using the original primer pair, and 3 µL of the eluate, using the original cycling conditions for a total of 30 cycles.
7. The annealing temperature corresponds to the temperature used in the original amplification, and, of course, the radioactivity is omitted, and all reagents are scaled-up by a factor of 5 for the 50-µL reaction.
8. A 5-µL aliquot of the PCR product is separated by electrophoresis in a 2% analytical agarose gel containing 1 µL 10 mg/mL EtBr per 100 mL gel, and the reaction product is examined for purity.

9. If, in addition to the expected band, any additional weaker bands are detected, the entire reaction should be separated on a 2% preparative low-melt agarose gel containing 1 μL 10 mg/mL EtBr per 100 mL gel. The correct band excised, melted, and purified (i.e., Promega Wizzard PCR Preps DNA purification system, or a similar system).
10. If the reaction appears pure, with only a single band of the expected size, the PCR reaction can be purified directly (i.e., Promega Wizzard PCR Preps DNA purification system, or a similar system), avoiding the preparative gel electrophoresis step.
11. An aliquot is submitted to sequencing with the original forward and reverse primer, to sequence both strands of the DNA fragment. Any protocol allowing for direct sequencing of double-stranded PCR products is suitable; this laboratory uses an automated cycle-sequencing protocol on an ABI 377 (Applied Biosystems) sequencer, utilizing dRhodamine chemistry (*see* **Note 13**).
12. In cases in which the analysis of the autoradiogram suggests the presence of a homozygous change, a PCR product, generated directly from genomic DNA (60–90 ng of genomic DNA as starting material in a 50-μL reaction, followed by gel purification of the PCR product), can also be directly analyzed for the presence of a mutation.
13. The sequence is now compared to the CDNA reference sequence (Genbank accession number U31116 for β-sarcoglycan and 434976 for γ-sarcoglycan). Intron/exon border sequences are given in **Table 5** (β-sarcoglycan) and **Table 6** (γ-sarcogycan).

3.7. Confirmation of Mutations

1. After a novel change has been positively identified by sequence analysis, its status as a disease-causing mutation must be confirmed by a number of approaches. First, the presence of the mutation in the probands genomic DNA needs to be demonstrated in an independent assay. This is done to rule out the possibility that a mutation was introduced by the *Taq* polymerase early in the PCR reaction performed for the original SSCPA (*see* **Note 13**). Direct sequencing of an independently generated PCR product from the patient's genomic DNA will provide the necessary information. Homozygous mutations are easily seen in the sequence, and heterozygous deletions will be apparent, in that the sequence will degenerate into two nonsynchronous tracings following the change. Heterozygous single-base-pair changes can be seen as double peaks in the chromatogram, or as double bands on the sequencing gel.
2. If the mutation generates or abolishes a restriction enzyme cut site at that position, this can be used to assay for the mutation in an independent amplification.
3. An assay based on a mutation specific vs WT specific oligo-nt such as the amplification-resistant mutation detection system (ARMS) PCR *(28,29)*, can be used as well.
4. The inheritance of the mutation(s) from both parents should be demonstrated by showing the expected heterozygosity in the parents, using one of the methods discussed (SSCPA, sequencing, or alteration of a restriction site).

Table 5
β-Sarcoglycan Intron/Exon Borders

		exon 1	intron 1
		– GCTGCAGAACAG	gtctgtgagtac -
		A. . A . . E . . Q . .	
		11	
intron 1	**exon 2**	**exon 2**	intron 2
- tttcatttttag	CAAAGTTCCAAT -	- ATCAATTTAATA	gtgagtatttgt -
	Q . . S . . S . . N. .	I . . N . . L . . I . .	
	12	81	
intron 2	**exon 3**	**exon 3**	intron 3
- gttctttttcag	ATAACACTTGTT -	- AACAACCAGCCT	gtaagttgccac -
	I . . T. . L . .V. .	N . . N . . Q . . P. .	
	82	143	
intron 3	**exon 4**	**exon 4**	intron 4
- tttttttgaag	ATTGTTTTTCAG -	- TCTACTGAAAGG	gtatgatttatt -
	I . .V. . F. . Q . .	S . .T. . E . . R . .	
	144	207	
intron 4	**exon 5**	**exon 5**	intron 5
- ttaaattttcag	ATTACCAGCAAT -	- GAGTTAAAGGCGA	gtgagtattctt -
	I . .T. . S . . N . .	E . . L . .K . . A . .	
	208	251	
intron 5	**exon 6**		
- ttctcctaatag	GAAAACAGTAAT -		
	E . . N . . S . . I . .		
	252		

The GenBank accession number for the cDNA sequence is U31116 and GenBank accession numbers for exons 1-6 are U63796-U63801

5. If the patient appears to be homozygous for a given change, but the mutation occurs in heterozygous form in only one of the parents, and the other parent shows WT configuration, one must suspect the presence of a larger deletion in the parental allele showing the WT configuration the parent carrying the deleted allele in heterozygous form only shows the WT conformers on SSCPA. The patient, on the background of a deleted allele, would thus appear to be homozygous for the mutation on the nondeleted allele, but in fact is hemizygous. Obviously, sample mixup and questions about parentship need to be ruled out, as well.
6. Furthermore, especially in cases of missense mutations and intronic mutations without knowledge of effects on splicing (*see* **Subheading 3.8.**), a normal control population needs to be examined for the presence or absence of the change in question to rule out a polymorphism.

Table 6
γ-Sarcoglycan Intron/Exon Borders

intron 1	**exon 2**	**exon 2**	intron 2
- acactccgtggc	AGATGGTGCGTG -	- TGGTTTTCTCCA	gtaagtatcatt -
	M . . V. . R . . E . .	W. . F. . S . . P. .	
	1	65	
intron 2	**exon 3**	**exon 3**	intron 3
- tttttttaacag	GCAGGAATGGGC -	- CACTCCAGAGTG	gtaagaaaatgt -
	A . . G . . M . . G . .	R . . L . . K . .V. .	
	66	99	
intron 3	**exon 4**	**exon 4**	intron 4
- atctctttctag	GACTCATCTCTG -	- GGTTAAAAGTCG	gtgagtccagct -
	D . . S . . S . . L . .	. . L . . K . . B . . G	
	100	129	
intron 4	**exon 5**	**exon 5**	intron 5
- ttaattcttcag	GTCCCAAAATGG -	- TTCGAGTAACTG	gtatgtactaac -
	. . P. . K . . M . .V	. . R . .V. . T. . G	
	130	169	
intron 5	**exon 6**	**exon 6**	intron 6
- ttttttgtttag	GGCCTGAAGGGG -	- TCAAGACCTTAG	gtaagaattttt -
	. . P. . E . . G . . A	. Q . . D . . L . . R	
	170	193	
intron 6	**exon 7**	**exon 7**	intron 7
- tcctcatctcag	ATTAGAATCCCC -	- AGTGATGGAATG	gtgagttcattc -
	. . L . . E . . S . . P.	S . . D . . G . . M . .	
	194	234	
intron 7	**exon 8**		
- tctcccaaccag	CTTGTGCTTGAT -		
	L . .V. . L . . D . .		
	235		

The GenBank accession number for the cDNA sequence is U34976 and GenBank accession numbers for exons 1-8 are U63388-U63395

3.8. RNA Isolation and RT-PCR (see Note 14)

Intronic mutations, which potentially affect splicing by altering the consensus splice donor and acceptor sites, can be further analyzed by RT-PCR on RNA isolated from muscle. In this way, the presence of abnormal splicing can be confirmed. Very small pieces, or even microtome slivers, are usually sufficient to generate adequate amounts of template for the PCR. The following protocol follows in general the recommendations given by Gibco-BRL for use of the Trizol reagent.

1. Homogenize the small piece of tissue directly in 3 cc Trizol (Gibco-BRL), using a Polytron tissue homogenizer, until the Trizol solution appears clear without visible debris.
2. Spin the homogenate at 12,000*g* for 10 min at 4°C, and transfer to a new tube.
3. Leave 5 min at RT, add 0.6 mL chloroform, shake vigorously by hand, and incubate another 2–3 min at RT.
4. Spin the sample at 12,000*g* for 10 min at 4°C, and carefully transfer the upper aqueous phase to a new tube.
5. Precipitate the RNA with 3 mL isopropanol; incubate 10 min at RT.
6. Spin at 12,000*g* for 10 min at 4°C, decant the isopropanol, and wash the RNA pellet by adding 3 mL 75% EtOH kept at –20°C.
7. Vortex, and spin again at 7500*g* for 5 min at RT.
8. Briefly air-dry the RNA pellet, and resuspend the RNA up in 25 µL diethylpyrocarbonate (DEPC) H_2O (*see* **Note 15**).
9. Store at –80°C, if not processed immediately (*see* **Note 16**).
10. For the RT-PCR, use up to 11 µL total RNA in the reverse transcriptase reaction, and add 1 µL pd$(N)_6$ random primer at 200 ng/mL (Pharmacia). Add DEPC ddH_2O to 12 µL, if less RNA is used. Alternatively, 1 µL oligodeoxythymidine 500 ng/mL may be used.
11. Heat the mix to 70°C for 10 min to denature RNA secondary structure; cool on ice.
12. Add: 4 µL 5X reverse transcriptase buffer (Gibco-BRL Superscript II), 2 µL 0.1 *M* DTT, and 1 µL 10 m*M* dNTPs.
13. Incubate the reaction at 25°C for 10 min, to allow for annealing of the pd$(N)_6$ random primers, then raise the temperature to incubate at 42°C for 2 min.
14. Add 1 µL reverse transcriptase (Gibco-BRL superscript II) = 200 U = 20 µL total volume.
15. Incubate at 42°C for 1–2 h. At the end of this incubation, 2U RNaseH can be added to digest RNA in DNA/RNA hybrids: incubate at 37°C for 20 min; finally heat-inactivate the reaction for 5 min at 95°C, and chill on ice (*see* **Note 17**).
16. Dilute the sample to 40 µL with H_2O. The reaction is now ready for use as a template in the PCR; the remainder can be stored at –20°C.
17. For the PCR, use 1 µL undiluted cDNA, but also try dilutions, such as 1:20 and 1:50, because residual RNA in the reaction may inhibit the PCR.
18. To demonstrate abnormal splicing, design primers located on exons adjacent to the exon presumably affected by the splicing defect.
19. Annealing temperatures depend on the cDNA primers chosen to demonstrate the abnormal splicing. It is advised to use 35 cycles in the thermocycling program. Always include a cDNA sample from a normal muscle specimen as a control.
20. Products are resolved on a 3% agarose containing EtBr, and compared to the WT sample processed in parallel. The abnormally spliced product will be recognizable by a change in size. An entire exon may be skipped in splicing, or an alternative splice site may be used, also giving rise to an abnormally sized product.
21. The PCR product can also be purified on a low melting agarose gel and the product analyzed by sequencing.

3.9 Specific Protocols for β-SG

3.9.1. Amplification of β-SG Exon 1

1. Because of the very high CG content in the 5' region of the gene, the amplification conditions for exon 1 of β-SG are different. The authors found the use of 1 *M* betaine, in combination with 5% DMSO, to generate the clearest result.
2. The authors also use for this reaction an Ab-coupled *Taq* polymerase (platinum *Taq* polymerase, Gibco-BRL) for an automated hot start, but manual hot start can be used as well.
3. The higher reaction volume (25 μL) also helps in the consistency of this reaction.
4. The authors provide two forward primers (I and II), of which II generates a larger product, incorporating more sequence 5' of the transcriptional start site, and producing slightly higher yields in the amplification.
5. Set up the following reaction for each sample to be analyzed (make master mix, to minimize pipeting errors): 3 μL DNA (15 ng/μL), 0.5 μL each primer 1 and primer 2 at 10 pmol/μL, 2.5 μL 10X Pt *Taq* buffer (Gibco-BRL), 0.75 μL 50 m*M* $MgCl_2$, 5 μL 5 *M* betaine (=1 *M* final concentration), 1.25 μL DMSO, 2 μL 2.5 m*M* each dNTP, 0.25 μL [^{32}P]-dCTP, 0.25 μL PlatinumTaq polymerase (Gibco-BRL), and 9 μL H_2O, to a total of 25 μL.
6. The cycling parameters for β-SG exon 1 include: initial denaturation at 94°C for 3 min, annealing at 60°C for 0:40 min, extension at 72°C for 0:40 s, denaturation at 94°C for .5 min, for a total of 35 cycles, followed by final annealing at 60°C for 3 min, and final extension at 72°C for 7 min.
7. The reactions are analyzed under the same gel conditions as outlined in the general protocols.
8. Sequencing of exon 1 amplimers will also require the addition of betaine to the sequencing reaction, as well.

3.9.2. Screening for Specific Mutations in β-SG

3.9.2.1. Thr151Arg

For assessment for the Thr151Arg mutation found in the Indiana Amish population, the laboratory of Beckmann at Généthon in Evry, France has developed an allele specific touchdown PCR test. This test has not been used in this laboratory: the authors must refer to the reference describing it ***(12)***.

3.9.2.2. Arg91Leu

An additional mutation that may be of interest for a single mutation screening tool is a β-SG mutation initially identified in the North African population of Tunisia, Arg91Leu (*see* ref. ***36***). The authors have developed an ARMS assay for this mutations, which may be useful for prescreening other patients from this region who are found not to carry the del521T in γ-SG. The ARMS assay *(28,29)* is based on two PCR reactions per patient, both of which contain primers to amplify an unrelated genomic region as a positive control for the reaction as well as a common primer located in intron 2 of the β-SG gene. In addition one reaction contains a WT allele-specific primers that will not amplify from the mutant allele, and the other a mutant specific primer that will not amplify from the WT allele. The ultimate 3' base in each primer corresponds to the base position that is mutated; in the penultimate 3' base in both primers is deliberately mismatched, to further destabilize primer annealing and prevent amplification in case of a mismatch at the ultimate position. This way, the genotype at the mutated base in a given sample can be read directly from the presence or absence of the WT and mutant products, given that the internal control primers show normal amplification. The utilization of an automatic or manual hot start of the PCR reaction is essential for the absolute specificity of the reaction. The authors had good luck with the Pt *Taq* polymerase with Ab-mediated hot start (Gibco-BRL), but have also used manual hot start successfully.

1. Primers (all at 10 pmol/µL):

   control primer A: ccc acc ttc ccc tct ctc cag gca aat ggg

   control primer B: ggg cct cag tcc caa cat ggc taa gag gtg

   These primers generate a 360-bp fragment from exon III of the 1-antitrypsin gene *(29)* as a control from an unrelated genomic locus.

   common primer: tgg tga taa tat ttt cta ctt gtt ttc caa tta c (intron 2)

   WT-specific primer: act cca tac tat cac agc cat ttg gtc caa tac

   mutation-specific primer: act cca tac tat cac agc cat ttg gtc caa taa

2. The following protocol uses the Ab-tagged Pt *Taq* polymerase (Gibco-BRL) as a means for a convenient hot start of the reaction (a requirement to achieve the necessary specificity), but a manual hot start can be used as well. Make two master mixes, one for normal (N), one for mutant (M), as in **Table 1**.
3. If a manual hot start is to be used, a mix of 1X PCR buffer and 1.25 U polymerase per 5 µL is prepared, and the reaction mix adjusted to 20 µL (with 1X buffer concentration). The reaction without the polymerase is held at 95°C for 2–3 min; 5 µL each of the enzyme mix is added to the individual tubes, and the regular amplification program is started.
4. The program for the thermocycler includes: initial denaturation at 94°C for 3 min, annealing at 60°C for 1 min, extension at 72°C for 0:40 s, denaturation at 94°C for 0:40 min, for a total of 35 cycles, followed by final annealing at 60°C for 3 min, and final extension at 72°C for 7 min.
5. For analysis of the assay, separate 12.5 µL PCR reaction by electrophoresis on a 3% agarose gel containing EtBr. Include negative water control, wild-type, and,

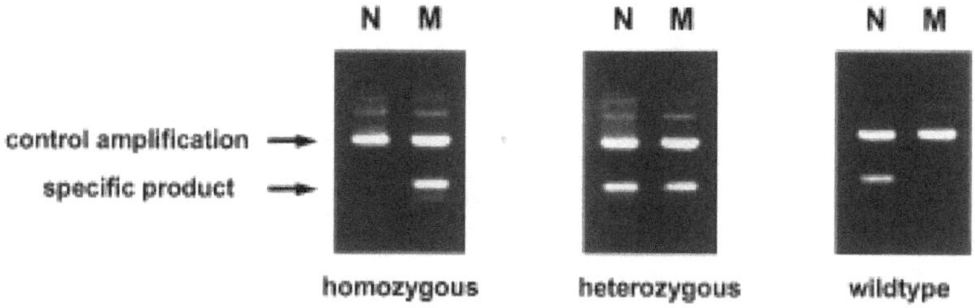

Fig 4. Heteroduplex portion of the γ-SG exon 6 amplicon separated on a 0.5X MDE–5% glycerol gel. Shown is the Δ521T mutation in various combinations. In the heterozygote case, a heteroduplex is formed between the WT and mutant products.

if available, mutant control in each run. Only if the larger control reaction product is seen in each lane is the absence or presence of an allele-specific band meaningful (*see* **Fig. 4**).

3.10. Specific Protocols for γ-SG

3.10.1. Screening for Specific Mutations in γ-SG

3.10.1.1. DEL 521 T

This mutation, commonly seen in northern African regions, but also around the mediterranean and in other countries, is best seen in heteroduplex portion of the 5% glycerol/0.5X MDE gel. This is seen at the bottom of the gel after a maximal 13 h run at 7 W at constant RT. The homozygous mutant pattern corresponds to a band migrating faster, compared to the WT, whereas the heterozygote pattern consists of three bands: WT, mutant, and the heteroduplex (*see* **Fig. 4**).

3.10.1.2. CYS283TYR

This mutation is almost exclusively seen in Romano-Gypsy populations ***(24)***, but can also rarely be seen outside of a clear Gypsy context (Bönnemann et al., submitted). The assay for this mutation is based on the novel introduction of an *Rsa*I site in exon 8 of γ-SG by this mutation.

1. Exon 8 is amplified directly from 60 ng genomic DNA using the primer pair given in **Table 3** for exon 8, the PCR reaction purified with a Promega Wizzard PCR Preps DNA purification system, or an equivalent method, and half of the product is digested with 1–5 U *Rsa*I in the appropriate buffer condition.
2. The reaction is analyzed by electrophoresis in an EtBr-stained 4% agarose gel with parallel processed WT, homozygous, and heterozygous mutant samples (if available).

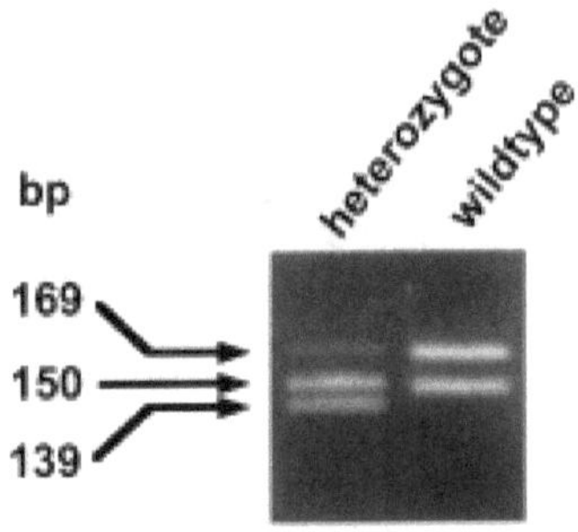

Fig 5. *Rsa*I digest of γ-SG exon 8 for the Cys283Tyr mutation. Note the appearance of a 139-bp fragment resulting from the new *Rsa*I site in the 169-bp band.

3. An internal *Rsa*I site in the γ-SG exon 8 amplicon serves as an internal positive control for the digest, resulting in 169- and 150-bp fragments in the normal case. Introduction of the novel *Rsa*I site by the mutation allows digestion of the 169 bp fragment into 139- and 30-bp fragments. Presence of the mutation therefore is indicated by the appearance of the 139-bp fragment, with the 30-bp fragment not clearly seen on every gel (**Fig. 5**).

3.10.2. Analysis for Larger Deletions in the γ-SG Gene

As discussed in **Subheading 3.7.**, a deletion encompassing a large proportion of the γ-*SG* gene or the entire locus must be suspected in cases in which the proband shows apparent homozygosity for the mutant allele, but only one of the parents is heterozygous for the change. Three methods may be used to look for the presence of larger deletions, based on loss of heterzygosity:

1. Loss of heterozygosity analysis, using polymorphisms within the gene, can be performed by SSCPA to confirm this suspicion. Some of the polymorphisms listed in **Table 7** may be present and hopefully informative in the family under analysis. If a larger proportion of the γ-*SG* gene was lost on one parent's allele, lack of parental contribution may be evident for some of these polymorphisms, as well. The same type of analysis can be performed using linkage analysis with some of the polymorphic repeat markers in the vicinity of the gene, such as the intragenic marker, D13S232 ***(30)***, as well as the marker D13S787, for instance.
2. To further assess the γ-*SG* gene for larger deletions, quantitative Southern blot analysis can be performed using standard procedures ***(31)***. 2.5 µg genomic DNA is digested with the appropriate enzyme.
   a. The DNA is carefully quantified again following the digest (using DAPI fluorometry or another DNA-specific fluorometer, such as the Dynaquant by Hoefer, Arcade, NY), to ensure equal loading on the gel.
   b. 2 µg are loaded onto a 0.8% agarose gel.

Table 7
Polymorphisms in the γ-Sarcoglycan Gene

Exon	Base pair changed	Codon/base	Amino acid
2	114	TTG -> TTC	L38L
3	228	GAT -> GAC	D76D
4	312	CTG -> CTT	L104L
4	347	CGC -> CAC	R116H
5	410	AGT -> AAT	S137N
8	830	CTT -> CTC	L235L
8	860	AAC -> AGC	S287N
1 (5' UTR)	88 upstream of intron 1	G -> A	
5 (intron 4)	- 30	A -> G	
7 (intron 6)	- 18	(T) n variable	
8 (31 UTR)	911-912	Ins G	
8 (31 UTR)	889	C -> T	
8 (31 UTR)	940	G -> A	
8 (31 UTR)	942	C -> G	

c. Electrophoresis, EtBr staining, photography, and Southern blotting onto a suitable membrane are performed according to routine procedures ***(31)***.

d. As a probe, a full-length, γ-SG, cDNA-labeled by PCR amplification with the incorporation of [α-^{32}P]dCTP, should be used. The cDNA template and primer sequences can be obtained from the author's laboratory.

e. Enzymes used have included *Eco*RI, which results in two assessable bands (a number of the hybridizing exons are too small to be satisfactorily visible on the autoradiograph); *Hind*III and *Taq*I, in addition, show restriction fragment-length polymorphisms, which are also potentially useful for loss of heterozygosity assessment in the proband (*see* **Note 18**).

3. The authors have also developed a semiquantitative PCR assay to analyze a proband for loss of individual exons in the γ-*SG* gene, since smaller deletions may not be seen on the Southern blot analysis (*see* **Note 16**).

   a. For this assay, individual exons (exons 2–8) are multiplexed with a pair of control primers, amplifying an independent genomic locus in the same reaction. This allows comparison of quantity of product within the same sample, as well as between samples.

   b. Amplification is performed for a total of 25 cycles only, still within the linear range of the reaction.

   c. The authors again use the same control primers given for the β-SG ARMS assay, amplifying a 360-bp fragment from exon III of the α_1-antitrypsin gene ***(29)***, at 10 pmol/μL working stock.

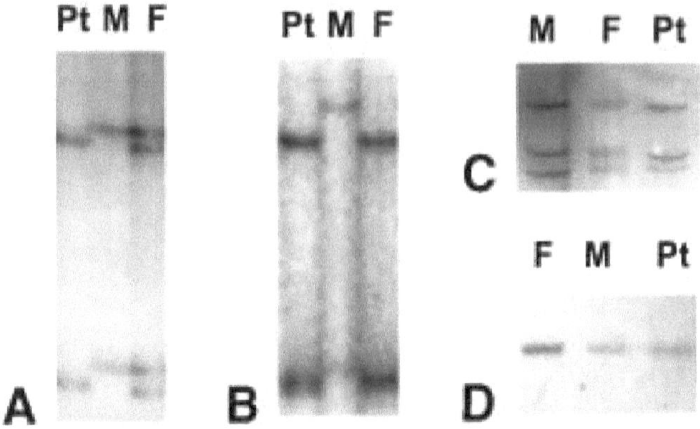

Fig 6. Example for a large deletion of the γ-SG gene locus on the maternal allele. (**A**) The patient (Pt) appears homozygous for a mutation affecting the splice donor site of intron 2, but only the father (F) is heterozygote for the change; the mother (M) shows only the WT configuration. (**B**) Lack of a maternal contribution is confirmed by analyzing a polymorphism on exon 8, where the only maternal allele seen is not inherited to the patient, who shows only the paternal allele. (**C**) The same constellation can also be seen on a Ag-stained SSCP gel for exon 2. (**D**) Confirmation is further obtained by quantitative Southern blotting (*Eco*RI digest); the band for mother and patient is half as intense, compared to the band in the father.

control primer A: ccc acc ttc ccc tct ctc cag gca aat ggg

control primer B: ggg cct cag tcc caa cat ggc taa gag gtg

d. For each γ-SG exon 2–8 and each proband, as well as normal DNA and water control, set up the following reaction: 6 µL 15 ng/µL DNA, 1 µL each of forward and reverse primer at 10 pmol/µL (10 µ*M*), 1 µL each of control primer A and B at 10 pmol/µL (10 µM), 5 µL 10X PCR buffer (Boehringer), 4 µL 2.5 m*M* each dNTP, 0.5 µL *Taq* polymerase (Boehringer) 5 U/µL, and 30.5 µL H_2O, to a total of 50 µL.
e. Cycling conditions include: initial denaturation at 94°C for 2.5 min, annealing at 58°C for 0:40 min, extension at 72°C for 0:40 min, denaturation at 94°C for 0:45 s, for a total of 25 cycles, followed by final annealing at 58°C for 2 min, and final extension at 72°C for 5 min.
f. Resolve the products on a 4% agarose gel stained with EtBr. The upper band, at 360 bp corresponds to the control amplification from the unrelated genomic locus, and corresponds to a normal gene dosage, the lower band corresponds to the γ-SG exon analyzed. Its intensity is compared to the control band and to the amplification product in the normal sample. A heterozygous deletion on one allele will be indicated be approx one-half intensity of the lower band, a homozygous deletion by its total absence.

4. Notes

1. Polyalanine tract mutations have so far only been described in three autosomal dominant conditions: syn/polydactylie Hox D13 *(32)*, cleidocranial dysplasia *(33)*, and oculopharyngeal MD *(34)*. In oculopharyngeal MD, there is evidence that a small increase in the number of alanine residues may act as a recessive; the higher numbers confer a dominant phenotype *(34)*.
2. Keep patient DNA samples and reagents used in the PCR physically separate in the laboratory from where the results are analyzed and fragments are isolated and sequenced, to avoid contamination of the patient material and reagents with amplified products. Separate sets of pipetors should also be used for the same reason. Keeping reagents in small aliquots also allows for easier replacement should contaminations occur. It also avoids repeated freeze–thaw cycles.
3. It is important for the reproducibility of the genomic PCR amplifications to accurately quantitate the genomic DNA stocks. Also, a separately stored aliquot should be kept, in case contamination of the sample occurs, or if questions about the identity of a sample arise in the course of the analysis.
4. When setting up the assays for single exons for the first time, it is helpful to try the amplification without the addition of radioactivity first, and resolve the results on a 3% ethidium-stained acrylamide gel. The pilot reactions should be carried out in the same reaction volume (10 μL) and the same thermal cycler as the eventual radioactive reactions.
5. Sharktooth combs have the advantage of allowing comparisons of adjacent lanes, without intervening spaces. This can make the recognition of subtle shifts and alterations from one lane to the next easier.
6. Imperfections in the gel matrix may lead to distortion of the bands, making interpretation of the results difficult.
7. In general, it is useful to analyze as many samples as possible for the same exon in adjacent lanes. Since most of the samples will show wild-type conformers, or, potentially, also common polymorphisms, true mutations will be easier to distinguish.
8. Exact electrophoresis run times should be evaluated and determined for each laboratory as the conditions are set up. They depend primarily on the wattage used, the presence or absence of glycerol, as well as on the fragment size analyzed, but there also is some variability dependent on the electrophoretic setup.
9. Before multiplexing the reactions in a radioactive reaction, it is worthwhile to initially test the conditions on a few samples in a cold reaction, and separate the reactions on a 3–4% EtBr-stained agarose gel. In case the amplification is not complete for all exons, the authors would first change the final $MgCl_2$ concentration in the reaction, from the 1.5 m*M* in the standard buffer, to 2 m*M*.
10. Denser multiplexing of more exons is possible, but can make clear interpretation of the gels more difficult, because of the increasingly complex banding pattern. Also, the compression on the glycerol-containing gels can preclude proper separation of the individual exons, if the sizes are too densely spaced. In general, it is also possible to perform the single exon reactions separately first, and mix aliquots of each reaction only for the denaturation and gel separation.

11. If an abnormal conformer is suspected, but not clearly seen, the same sample can be rerun on a different gel condition, such as a 10% glycerol–0.5X MDE, or on a 49:1 acrylamide:bisacrylamide gel at 4°C/35 W for 4 h. Unconvincing or faint looking abnormal bands can also be reconfirmed by repeating the SSCPA. Spurious bands are usually not reproducible, but a true abnormal conformer may show more convincingly.
12. Shorter incubation times at higher temperatures have been used, e.g., 3 min at 80°C *(35)*.
13. For sequencing of reamplified gel fragments or direct genomic amplification products, direct sequencing protocols are preferred over subcloning of the PCR products into plasmid vectors for sequencing, because rare PCR-introduced mutations, which occurred later in the amplification, tend to dilute out in the bulk of the PCR products; they could show up at random in the subcloned single molecules. Therefore, if subcloning must be done, a sufficient number of clones should be sequenced. For direct sequencing of the PCR products, it is important to sequence in both directions, using the forward and reverse primers. This will help to resolve sequencing ambiguities, especially in direct genomic PCR amplifications, in which a heterozygote change must be identified.
14. All solutions and materials need to be handled with the usual RNase precautions, water needs to be treated with DEPC.
15. If there was very little starting material, the pellet may not be clearly visible, so proceed nonetheless with the following steps.
16. RNA isolated this way is not very clean, and should probably be used as soon as possible.
17. RNaseH treatment, in general, is useful if the amplified segment is long, and, in general, to improve the yield of the RT-PCR. For the purpose of the mutation confirmation, it is not really necessary.
18. Since the exons in γ-SG are small, not many bands are seen on the blot (a number escape detection, because of the faintness of the resulting hybridization signal), so that this assay may only be useful in deletions encompassing the entire gene. The semiquantitative PCR assay should then be used to assay for single-exon deletions.

References

1. Orita, M., Suzuki, Y., Sekiya, and Hayashi, K. (1989) Rapid and sensitive detection of point mutations and DNA polymorphisms using polymerase chian reaction. *Genomics* **5,** 874–879.
2. Hayashi, K. (1991) PCR-SSCP: A simple and sensitive method for detection of mutations in the genomic DNA. *PCR Methods Applications* **1,** 34–38.
3. Hayashi, K. and Yandell, D. W. (1993) How sensitive is PCR-SSCP? *Human Mutat.* **2,** 338–346.
4. Sarkar, G., Yoon HS and Sommer, S. S. (1992) Screening for mutations by RNA single-strand conformation polymorphism (rSSCP): comparison with DNA-SSCP. *Nucleic Acids Res.* **20,** 871–878.

5. Sheffield, V. C., Beck, J. S., Kwitek, A. E., Sandstrom, D. W., and Stone, E. M. (1993) The sensitivity of single-strand conformation polymorphism analysis for the detection of single base substitutions. *Genomics* **16,** 325–332.
6. Ravnik-Glavac, M., Glavac, D., and Dean, M. (1994) Sensitivity of single-strand conformation polymorphism and heteroduplex method for mutation detection in the cystic fibrosis gene. *Hum. Mol. Genet.* **3,** 801–807.
7. Leren, T. P., Solberg, K., Rodningen, O. K., Ose, L., Tonstad, S., and Berg, K. (1993) Evaluation of running conditions for SSCP analysis: application of SSCP for detection of point mutations in the LDL receptor gene. *PCR Methods Applications* **3,** 159–162.
8. Glavac, D. and Dean, M. (1993) Optimization of the single-strand conformation polymorphism (SSCP) technique for detection of point mutations. *Human Mutat.* **2,** 404–414.
9. Liu, Q. and Sommer, S. S. (1994) Parameters affecting the sensitivities of dideoxy fingerprinting and SSCP. *PCR Methods Applications* **4,** 97–108.
10. Keen, J., Lester, D., Inglehearn, C., Curtis, A., and Bhattacharya, S. (1991) Rapid detection of single base mismatches as heteroduplexes on Hydrolink gels. *Trends Genet.* **7,** 5.
11. Bönnemann, C. G., Modi, R., Noguchi, S., Mizuno, Y., Yoshida, M., Gussoni, E., et al. (1995) β-sarcoglycan (A3b) mutations cause autosomal recessive muscular dystrophy with loss of the sarcoglycan complex. *Nature Genet.* **11,** 266–273.
12. Lim, L. E., Duclos, F., Broux, O., Bourg, N., Sunada, Y., Allamand, V., et al. (1995) β-sarcoglycan (43 DAG): Characterization and involvement in a recessive form of limb-girdle muscular dystrophy linked to chromosome 4q12. *Nature Genet.* **11,** 257–265.
13. Bönnemann, C. G., Passos-Bueno, R., McNally, E. M., Vainzoff, M., de Sá Moreira, E., S. K. Marie, et al. (1996) Genomic screening for β-sarcoglycan mutations: Missense mutations may cause severe limb-girdle muscular dystrophy type 2E (LGMD 2E). *Hum. Mol. Genet.* **5,** 1953–1961.
14. Duggan, D. J., Gorospe, J. R., Fanin, M., Hoffman, E. P., and Angelini, C. (1997) Mutations in the sarcoglycan genes in patients with myopathy. *N. Engl. J. Med.* **336,** 618–624.
15. Ginjaar, H. B., vander Kooi, A., Ceelie, H., Kneppers, A. L. J., Barth, P. G., Busch, H. F. M., Wokke, J. H. J., et al. (1997) Sarcoglycanopathies in Dutch patients with autosomal recessive limb girdle muscular dystrophies. *Neuromusc. Disord* **7, 440,** GP441B.446.
16. dos Santos, M. R., Rieira, E. M., Jorge, P., Pires, M. M., and Guimarães, A. (1998) Novel mutation (Y184C) in exon 4 of the beta-sarcoglycan gene identified in a portuguese patient. Mutations in brief no. 177. On line. *Hum. Mutat.* **12,** 214–215.
17. Vainzof, M., Passos-Bueno, M. R., Moreira, E. S., Pavanello, R. C. M., Marie, S. K., Anderson, L. V. B., et al. (1996) The sarcoglycan complex in the six autosomal recessive limb-girdle muscular dystrophies. *Hum. Mol. Genet.* **5,** 1963–1969.

18. Nigro, V., de Sa Moriera, E., Piluso, G., Vainzof, M., Belsito, A., Politano, L., et al. (1996) the 5q autosomal recessive limb-girdle muscular dystrophy (LGMD 2F) is caused by a mutation in the δ-sarcoglycan gene. *Nature Genet.* **14,** 195–198.
19. Ben Hamida, M., Attia, N., Chabouni, H., and Fardeau, M. (1983) Autosomal recessive severe, proximal myopathy in children, common in Tunisia. *Rev. Neurol.* **139,** 289–297.
20. Ben Othmane, K., Ben Hamida, M., Pericak-Vance, M. A., Ben Hamida, C., Blel, S., Carter, S. C., et al. (1992) Linkage of Tunisian autosomal recessive Duchenne-like muscular dystrophy to the pericentromeric region of chromosome 13q. *Nature Genet.* **2,** 315–317.
21. Noguchi, S., McNally, E. M., Ben Othmane, K., Hagiwara, Y., Mizuno, Y., Yoshida, M., et al. (1995) Mutations in the dystrophin-associated protein γ-sarcoglycan in chromosome 13 muscular dystrophy. *Science* **270,** 819–822.
22. McNally, E. M., Duggan, D. J., Gorospe, J. R., Bönnemann, C. G., Fanin, M., Lidov, H. G. W., et al. (1996) Mutations in the carboxyl-terminus of γ-sarcoglycan cause muscular dystrophy. *Hum. Mol. Genet.* **5,** 1841–1847.
23. McNally, E. M., Passos-Bueno, R., Bönnemann, C. G., Vainzoff, M., De Sá Moreira, E., Lidov, H. G. W., et al. (1996) Mild and severe muscular dystrophy caused by a single γ-sarcoglycan mutation. *Am. J. Hum. Genet.* **59,** 1040–1047.
24. Piccolo, F., Jeanpierre, M., Leturcq, F., Dode, C., Azibi, K., Toutain, A., et al. (1996) A founder mutation in the gamma-sarcoglycan gene of gypsies possibly predating their migration out of India. *Hum. Mol. Genet.* **5,** 2019–2022.
25. Sewry, C. A., Taylor, J., Anderson, L. V., Ozawa, E., Pogue, R., Piccolo, F., et al. (1996) Abnormalities in alpha-, beta- and gamma-sarcoglycan in patients with limb-girdle muscular dystrophy. *Neuromusc. Disord.* **6,** 467–474.
26. Ben Hamida, M., Ben Hamida, C., Zouari, M., Belal, S. and Hentati, F. (1996) Limb-girdle muscular dystrophy 2C: clinical aspects. *Neuromusc. Disord.* **6,** 493–494.
27. Vidal-Puig, A. and Moller, D. E. (1994) Comparative sensitivity of alternative single-strand conformation polymorphism (SSCP) methods. *Biotechniques* **17,** 490–492, 494, 496.
28. Ferrie, R. M., Schwarz, M. J., Robertson, N. H., Vaudin, S., Super, M., Malone, G., and Little, S. (1992) Development, multiplexing, and application of ARMS tests for common mutations in the CFTR gene. *Am. J. Hum. Genet.* **51,** 251–262.
29. Little, S. (1995) ARMS analysis of point mutations, in *Current Protocols in Human Genetics* (Dracopoli, N. C., et al., eda.), John Wiley, New York, pp. 9.8.1–9.8.12.
30. Ben Othmane, K., Speer, M. C., Stauffer, J., Blel, S., Middleton, L., Ben Hamida, C., et al. (1995) Evidence for linkage disequilibrium in chromosome 13–linked Duchenne-like muscular dystrophy (LGMD2C). *Am. J. Hum. Genet.* **57,** 732–734.
31. Maniatis, T., Fritsch, E. F., and Sambrook, J. (1990) *Molecular Cloning: A Laboratory Manual.* Cold Spring Harbor Laboratory, Cold Spring Harbor, NY.
32. Muragaki, Y., Mundlos, S., Upton, J., and Olsen, B. R. (1996) Altered growth and branching patterns in synpolydactyly caused by mutations in HOXD13. *Science* **272,** 548–551.

33. Mundlos, S., Otto, F., Mundlos, C., Mulliken, J. B., Aylsworth, A. S., Albright, S., et al. (1997) Mutations involving the transcription factor CBFA1 cause cleidocranial dysplasia. *Cell* **89,** 773–779.
34. Brais, B., Bouchard, J-P, Xie, Y. G., Rochefort, D. L., Chrétien, N., Tomé, F. M. S., et al. (1998) Short GCG expansion in the PABP2 gene cause oculo–pharyngeal muscular dystrophy. *Nature Genet.* **18,** 164–167.
35. Hayashi, K. (1996) PCR SSCP: single-strand conformation polymorphism analysis of PCR products, in *Laboratory Protocols for Mutation Detection* (Landegren, U., ed.), Oxford University Press, Oxford, UK, pp. 14–22.
36. Bönnemann, C. G., Wong, J., Ben Hamida, C., Ben Hamida, M., et. al. (1998) LGMD 2E in Tunisia is caused by a missense mutation Arg91Leu in β-sarcoglycan. *Neuromuscular Disorders* **8,** 193–197.

15

Mutation Analysis in δ-Sarcoglycan (LGMD2F)

Vincenzo Nigro

1. Introduction

Limb-girdle muscular dystrophies (LGMDs) constitute a clinically and genetically heterogeneous group of inherited diseases. In the past few years, four autosomal recessive forms have been demonstrated to result from mutations in the genes encoding dystrophin-associated glycoproteins (*1–3*, and references therein). Mutations in α-sarcoglycan (SG) *(4,5)*, β-SG *(6,7)*, γ-SG *(8)*, δ-SG *(9)* cause LGMD2D, LGMD2E, LGMD2C, and LGMD2F, respectively. In these forms, when any SG is missing, the others are also markedly reduced, adding support to the hypothesis that these proteins function as a tetrameric unit, the SG complex *(10)*.

The δ-SG is the fourth and smallest subunit of the SG complex *(11–13)*. It was identified by expressed sequence tag database searching and cDNA library screening for its sequence similarity with the γ-SG. The gene spans at least 100 kb, and is assigned to human chromosome 5q33, close to the markers D5S487 and D5S1439. It is expressed in striated and smooth muscle as an 8-kb transcript, encoding a basic (isoelectric point 9.2) transmembrane glycoprotein of 290 amino acids (35 kDa). δ-SG is a sarcolemmal glycoprotein with a small intracellular domain, a single transmembrane hydrophobic domain (aa 35–59), and a large extracellular C-terminus of 231 amino acids. The extracellular domain of δ-SG contains four closely spaced cysteine residues that are a common feature of all SGs *(11)*.

Mutations in δ-SG are responsible for LGMD2F, the most recently identified disease of the SG complex, characterized by a severe phenotype, with early wheelchair confinement and shortened life-span *(9)*. In Brazil, the LGMD2F is not rare among Duchenne-like MD patients *(14)*. In contrast, Duggan et al. *(15)* identified only two δ-SG mutations (4%) in the screening of

From: *Methods in Molecular Medicine, vol. 43: Muscular Dystrophy: Methods and Protocols*
Edited by: K. M. D. Bushby and L. V. B. Anderson © Humana Press Inc., Totowa, NJ

54 biopsies from U.S. MD patients, selected for the absence or strong reduction of α-SG staining. Discrepancies in the estimation of LGMD2F frequency could depend on differences in selection of patients, ethnic background, and testing sensitivity.

1.1. Testing Strategy

All LGMD2F mutations so far identified are single-nucleotide (nt) substitutions/deletion in the coding sequence. In LGMD2F, deletions involving one or more δ-SG exons have not yet been described, but cannot be ruled out. For example, in the cardiomyopathic Syrian hamster (animal model of δ-SG deficiency), there is a deletion of the promoter and first exon of the gene ***(16)***. Generally, patient samples are screened for mutations following observation of histological α-SG deficiency, or after linkage analysis. However, immunofluorescence data alone often do not address the primary defect, and, in addition, most families, especially in developed countries, are small and not informative for linkage. The following set of guidelines will be useful for screening a large number of LGMD patients for mutations in the δ-SG exons and flanking introns. Although there are mutation-detection techniques that identify the vast majority of DNA sequence differences, they often require dedicated equipment and/or lengthy setup. Other techniques, based on kit usage, are not suitable for large screening projects, because the cost becomes high. The author therefore suggests single-strand conformational polymorphism (SSCP) or heteroduplex analysis (HA), since they use standard sequencing equipment, require no particular optimization time, and are inexpensive.

1.1.1. Polymerase Chain Reaction Design

The *δ-SG* gene is split into at least nine exons, all but the last two separated by huge genomic distances, spanning, altogether, over 100 kb. This situation is comparable to that of the dystrophin and γ-SG genes. In all these cases, multiplex polymerase chain reaction (PCR) of consecutive exons is feasible. In fact, long introns prevent the generation of combined PCR products that interfere with the bands of interest. To seize this opportunity, the author designed genomic PCR primers and optimized conditions for multiplex PCR reactions, and, in particular, developed the special buffer indicated in **Subheading 2.1.** Its preparation may be tedious, but it guarantees advantages in yield and quality (**Fig. 1**). The author chose genomic DNA as PCR template, because DNA can be easily found; frozen-muscle biopsy RNA is often not available.

1.1.2. Single-Strand Conformational Polymorphism

SSCP of PCR products is the simplest and most widely used technique to screen for small mutations. After denaturing DNA fragments, each individual

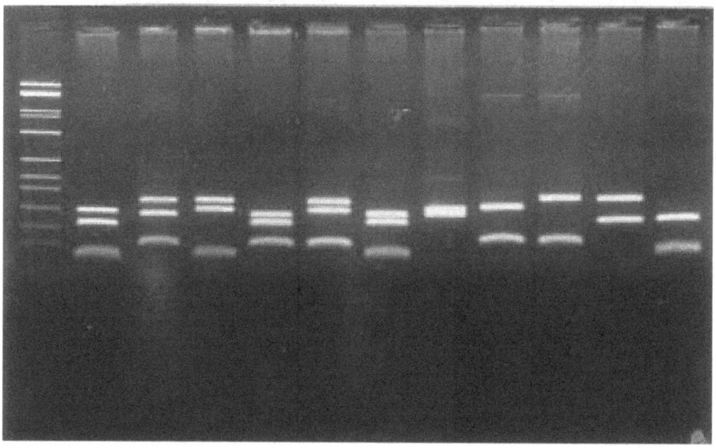

Fig. 1. Multiplex PCR of δ-SG exons (2% agarose gel electrophoresis) Lane 1, Marker; lane 2, ex 4 (206 bp) + ex 6 (111 bp*) + ex 7 (238 bp); lane 3, ex 2 (231 bp*) + ex 3 (135 bp*) + ex 5 (291 bp); lane 4, ex 5 + ex 6 + ex 7; lane 5, ex 2 + ex 3 + ex 4; lane 6, ex 3 + ex 5 + ex 7; lane 7, ex 2 + ex 4 + ex 6; lane 8, ex 2 + ex 7; lane 9, ex 3 + ex 7; lane 10, ex 3 + ex 5; lane 11, ex 4 + ex 5; lane 12, ex 4 + ex 6.

*Product length differs from that reported in Table 2, since some primers were different. Identical results were obtained with all the other primers described (not shown).

strand will form a secondary structure unique to that particular sequence. Under nondenaturing conditions, these conformational differences will cause the DNA strand to migrate differentially within the conformational-sensitive gel matrix. Since SSCP relies on differences in DNA migration, no expensive machinery is required, and the analysis of results is straightforward. Unfortunately, its sensitivity may not be very high (less than 70–80%), if standard conditions are used. The protocol here presented includes some modifications to improve the proportion of mutations that are detected.

1.1.3. Heteroduplex Analysis

HA is dependent on conformational differences in double-stranded (ds) DNA. Briefly, PCR products from wild-type (Ww) and mutant (Mm) DNA samples are mixed in the same tube, and denatured. After incubation at proper temperature, samples reanneal to reconstitute homoduplexes (Ww and Mm), and to form new heteroduplex (Wm and Mw) dsDNA. The mismatch in the heteroduplex DNA generally induces a slower gel mobility. HA is recommended, either in addition or as an alternative to SSCP analysis, for its simplicity

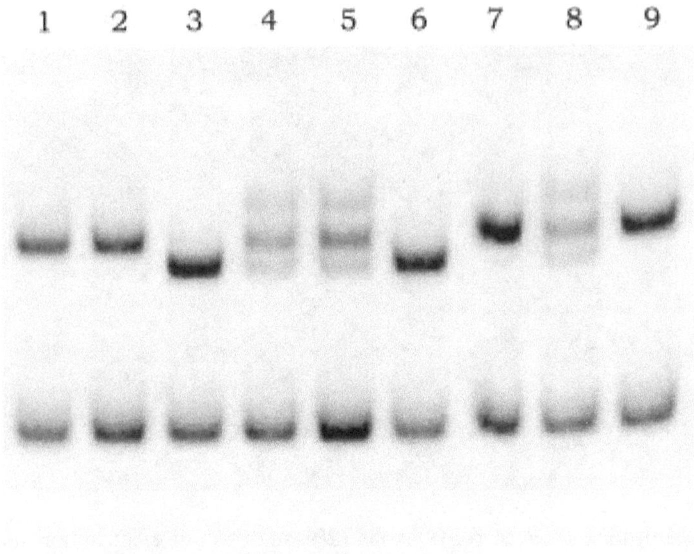

Fig. 2. Multiplex heteroduplex analysis. Exon 4 (206 bp, lower) and exon 7 (238 bp, upper bands) of δ-SG are shown. PCR products include DNA from two LGMD2F individuals with a single-base deletion in exon 7 (del. C 656) of the δ-SG gene. Homozygous samples: lanes 1, 2, 7, and 9, normal homozygous controls; lanes 3 and 6, homozygous MmDNA; in this particular case they have a faster migration with respect to the WwDNA. Heterozygous samples: lanes 4 and 5, mixing of mutant with wild-type samples; lane 7, parent (heterozygous) of patient 6. Heteroduplexes are well evident, since they have retarded migration with respect to all homoduplexes.

and good sensitivity. It was not always very advantageous, but methods have improved. The use of special acrylamide solutions and the careful setup of electrophoretic conditions have overcome most problems. HA represents the first-choice screening method for frame-shift mutations, especially when heterozygous (**Fig. 2**). Because more DNA can be loaded on the HA gel, nonradioactive detection (ethidium bromide [EtBr], silver [Ag] stain) is also used.

1.1.4. Direct Sequencing of PCR Products

When a singularity in migration is seen by SSCP and/or HA, direct sequencing of PCR products should be performed. Cloning of PCR products into plasmids, and subsequent sequencing of plasmids, may be practical only when starting from spurious amplifications. In these cases, however, it is necessary to confirm mutations in several independent clones.

The literature contains reliable sequencing methods (using an automated DNA sequencer, or performing a manual protocol). Given the limited number of samples with candidate mutations in the δ-SG exons, some tips for preparing manual sequencing reactions are described.

2. Materials

2.1. PCR

1. Aerosol Resistant Tips (Molecular BioProducts, MBP). The author recommends ART tips, because they are presterilized and self-sealing barrier tips. Experience has shown that contamination protection with other ordinary filter tips is not reliable.
2. 0.5- (or 0.2) and 1.5-mL microcentrifuge tubes.
3. Water for molecular biology, filtered, diethyl pyrocarbonate-treated and autoclaved. DNase- and RNase-free (Fluka, Buchs, Switzerland, product code 95284). Use for all PCR procedures.
4. 3X DNA polymerase buffer (JF buffer): 90 m*M* Tris, 24 m*M* HEPES (Fluka, product code 54457), 24% glycerol, 3% dimethylsulphoxide (cell culture grade), 6 m*M* dithiothreitol (DTT) (Fluka), 10.5 m*M* $MgCl_2$ (1 *M* solution, Fluka, product code 63069), 60 m*M* potassium L-glutamate (Fluka, product code 49601), 180 m*M* ammonium acetate (5 *M* solution, Fluka, product code 09691), 0.003% acetylated bovine serum albumin (20% solution, Sigma, product code B8894, or equivalent). Do not add HCl or NaOH to adjust pH values. Prepare a 100-mL stock solution using water for molecular biology, and store in small aliquots at –20°C (*see* Note 5).
5. Deoxyribonucleoside triphosphate (dNTP mix (Pharmacia) (join the four 100 m*M* solutions, dilute 10 folds with water for molecular biology, and store in small aliquots at –20°C). Each dNTP now has a concentration of 2.5 m*M*, for a total of 10 m*M*.
6. Primers. See **Table 1** for sequences. The author resuspends or dilutes all the deprotected/desalted oligo-nt primers (Genosys, Genset) at the fixed concentration of 100 μ*M* in water for molecular biology (Fluka). Greater dilution may result in shorter stability. These primary solutions are stored at –20°C. The author observed constant PCR performances, even after 5 yr of storage at –20°C. From primary solution, the author prepares 10 μ*M* working solutions, and store them in ready-to-use aliquots at –20°C.
7. Mineral oil (Sigma, product code *M* 5904): aliquot, and store at room temperature (RT). Be careful to avoid any contamination. Do not expose to UV light, but discard contaminated aliquots.
8. *Taq* DNA polymerase, usually at 5 U/μL (in the order of preference, Perkin-Elmer (Norwalk, CT), Boehringer, Pharmacia), store at –20°C.
9. Agarose, molecular biology grade (FMC Bioproducts, Rockland, ME).
10. Electrophoresis buffer (Tris-tourine–EDTA [TTE]): 1.8 *M* Tris, 0.6 *M* taurine (Fluka, product code 86329), 10 m*M* EDTA. Use as a 20X stock solution and dilute prior to use. Store at RT (*see* **Note 11**).
11. EtBr (10 mg/mL solution): **Caution:** EtBr is a carcinogen. Wear gloves.
12. Glycerol loading dye: 40% glycerol (Fluka), 40 m*M* EDTA, 0.1% bromophenol, and 0.1% cyanol.

Table 1
Composition of PCR Master Mixes

	Component	Starting concentration	Volume per sample (μL)	Final concentration
Master mix 1	Water	–	3[a]	–
	JF buffer	3X	2.5	1X
	dNTP mix	2.5 m*M* each	1	250 μ*M* each
	Forward primer	10 μ*M*	0.5[a]	0.5 μ*M*
	Reverse primer	10 μ*M*	0.5[a]	0.5 μ*M*
	Total volume per sample		7.5	
Master mix 2	Water	–	1.5	–
	JF buffer	3X	0.8	1X
	[α-^{32}P]dATP	10 mCi/mL	0.1	1 μCi/sample
	Taq DNA polymerase	5 U/μL	0.1	0.5 U/sample
	Total volume per sample		2.5	

[a]When multiplexing, multiply the primer volumes by the number of exons and reduce the water volume.

13. Chloroform.
14. Automated thermal cycler, horizontal electrophoresis system, UV transilluminator, sequencing gel apparatus, high-voltage power supply, autoradiography cassettes, shields for β-emitters, and all the other standard laboratory equipment.

2.2. Single-strand Conformational Polymorphism

The same reagent listed in **Subheading 2.1.** In addition:

1. Residue [α-^{32}P]deoxyadenosine triphosphate (dATP) at 400–3000 Ci/mmol (10 mCi /mL) (Amersham, ICN). [α-^{33}P]dATP is more expensive, but its emission is less dangerous and bands are sharper. Store at 4°C up to a month (2 mo for ^{33}P). **Caution:** Use shields, and thoroughly follow safety regulations when using radioisotopes.
2. Glass plates (The author uses the standard size of 40 × 20 × 0.4 cm), 0.4-mm spacers, and sharktooth combs.
3. Dimethylchlorosilane, store at 4°C. Toxic. Work in a fume hood. The nontoxic alternative is Gel Slick solution (FMC Bioproducts, product code 50640).
4. Sticking solution for each plate: Mix 5 mL ethanol, 15 μL acetic acid, and 4 μL γ-methacryloxypropyl-trimethoxysilane (Sigma, product code: M6514). Prepare fresh, and discard if not used.
5. 39.5% acrylamide/0.5% *bis*-acrylamide (80:1 ratio) (Bio-Rad, Hercules, CA), to be used as a 4X stock solution. Dissolve in water for molecular biology and store in a dark bottle at 4°C. **Caution:** Acrylamide is neurotoxic. Always wear gloves when working with the unpolymerized monomer. Follow all precautions reported in the material safety data sheet prior to use.

6. 50% v/v glycerol in water for molecular biology. Store at RT.
7. 10% ammonium persulfate (APS) (Sigma, Bio-Rad): Store at 4°C up to a week.
8. *N,N,N',N'*,-tetramethylethylenediamine (TEMED) (Bio-Rad): Store at 4°C.
9. Formamide loading dye: 95% deionized formamide (Fluka), 20 m*M* EDTA, 0.2% bromophenol and 0.2% cyanol. Store in aliquots at –20°C.
10. 72- or 60-well plastic microwell plates (Terasaki, Nunc).
11. Oven at 160°C.
12. 10% acetic acid in dH_2O. Store at RT.
13. Autoradiography films coated with emulsion on one side (Kodak BioMax MR). This is required for maximum resolution and sensitivity for ^{33}P autoradiography. Use films under safelight conditions recommended by the manufacturer.

2.3. Heteroduplex Analysis

The same reagents listed in **Subheading 2.1.** and **2.2.** In addition:

1. MDE gel solution 2X concentrate (FMC Bioproducts) (optional). Store at RT.
2. Urea (UltraPure, Gibco-BRL, or equivalent).
3. Ethylene glycol (>99%, Fluka).

2.4. Sequencing of PCR Products

1. Quiaquick PCR purification kit (Quiagen, Dorking, UK).
2. Thermo Sequenase ^{33}P-labeled terminator cycle sequencing kit (Amersham).

3. Method

3.1. Polymerase Chain Reaction

Reagents and solutions for PCR procedures should be predispensed in aliquots, using separate pipets, never used for other DNA manipulations (*see* **Note 1**).

3.1.1. PCR Setup

1. Thaw all the components, and place them at RT, with the exception of the enzyme.
2. Mix thoroughly, and spin (15 s).
3. Prepare two reaction master mixes in two separate microcentrifuge tubes, adding the reagents according to the recipes given in Table 1, and in the same order as listed. For agarose gel analysis, the radiolabeled dATP must be omitted. *Taq* polymerase must be added to master mix 2 immediately before use. Calculate volumes for the number of samples plus two (or plus 10%), to allow for inaccuracy of pipeting (*see* **Notes 1–6**).
4. Aliquot 7.5 µL master mix 1 into each of the 0.5-mL (or 0.2-mL) microcentrifuge tubes labeled with the patient identification number.
5. Overlay reaction mixtures with one drop of sterile mineral oil (20–30 µL). Mineral oil can be omitted when using a PCR cycler with heated lid.

6. Add 0.5 µL of each DNA sample (50–200 ng/µL) to the mineral oil. The additional volume of the DNA is not considered, since 5–10% of evaporation of small samples can usually be measured at the end of the PCR amplification.
7. Mix briefly, and spin.
8. Set the tubes into the thermocycler. Program the machine according to manufacturer's instructions, using the following guidelines: denaturation at 95°C for 1 min (once); wait at 85°C for 5–10 min (once).
9. During this time, dispense 2.5 µL master mix 2 into each of the microcentrifuge tubes, beneath the mineral oil. Put the tip through the oil and press pipet button slowly down to first stop (measuring stroke), and wait until no more liquid is emptied. To avoid air bubbles, do not press button down to second stop.
10. Run the program for 30 cycles, using the following steps: denaturation at 95°C for 25 s; annealing and elongation at 63°C for 2–4 min (*see* **Notes 7** and **8**). If the automated thermal cycler is endowed with autoextension function, the annealing-elongation time should be extended from 2 min (first cycle) to 4 min (last cycle) (approx +4 s/cycle).

3.1.2. Analysis of PCR Results

1. Prepare a 2% standard agarose gel in 0.5X TTE. Add 1/10,000 EtBr, and pour the gel. It is important to use thin combs (<0.6 mm) for optimal resolution.
2. When the PCR is completed, bring the tubes to a separate bench, or, better, to a room not used to isolate DNA or to prepare PCR. Add 1 µL 10X glycerol–dye solution to each sample and 80 µL of chloroform, and cap tightly.
3. Vortex, and briefly spin (15 s).
4. Extract the blue sample with a separate pipetor (P-20 or P-100), not used to isolate DNA or to dispense PCR solutions. Change tip for each sample. Put the upper phase in 1.5-mL microcentrifuge tubes labeled with the same numbers as the PCR samples. Samples can now be stored at 4°C for up to 1 mo before analysis.
5. Electrophorese 5 µL from each reaction on the agarose gel run in 0.5X TTE at 8 V/cm, until the bromophenol dye has reached 50% of the total length of the gel.
6. Visualize under UV light.
7. Clean carefully the post-PCR area.

An example of multiplex PCR amplification of exons 2–7 is shown (**Fig. 1**). It is critical to use PCR conditions that minimize unwanted byproducts, prior to carrying out mutation-detection screening in a much larger number of DNA samples. There should only be one single, clear band for each primer pair (in the case of unsatisfactory results [i.e., fuzzy or very faint bands] *see* **Note 9**).

3.2. Single-Strand Conformational Polymorphism

It is important to set up PCR conditions very carefully, before analyzing the products in SSCP; otherwise, amplifications may result in artifact bands that interfere with the identification of the bands of interest. Multiplexing is necessary to reduce the workload and exposure to radioactivity (**17**). In this case, one control reaction should also be prepared for each primer pair, to facilitate the subsequent identification of the multiple SSCP bands.

1. Prepare the PCR reaction using the same guidelines in **Table 1**, with the inclusion of the radiolabeled nt in master mix 2. Follow safety regulations when using radioisotopes.

3.2.1. SSCP Gel Casting

1. Plate cleaning and treatment can be carried out as usual. Glass plates must be thoroughly cleaned and free of dried gel residues or dust. The author prefers to leave the gel attached to one glass plate, in order to carry out all further manipulations with ease. In this case, the two glass plates must be treated separately. One (always the same) is treated with dimethylchlorosilane or Gel Slick solution, and the other with the sticking solution (*see* **Note 10**).
2. Prepare the gel solution. For a gel of 200 × 400 × 0.4 mm, 40 mL are usually adequate. Thinner gels give better resolution, but it is much more difficult to rinse sample wells. For fragments up to 300 bp, prepare a 10% acrylamide gel (80:1 acrylamide/crosslinker ratio). Mix the following in a sidearm vacuum flask: 2 mL 20X TTE buffer, 10 mL 40% acrylamide solution, 4 mL 50% glycerol solution, 24 mL H_2O.
3. Degas mixture under vacuum for 5 min.
4. Add 35 µL TEMED and 200 µL 10% APS. Mix, and immediately pour the gel solution between the plates, and insert comb. Allow gel to polymerize at RT for at least 60 min.
5. When polymerization of the gel is complete, remove comb, and carefully rinse sample wells. It is crucial to remove all acrylamide fragments (*see* **Notes 11** and **12**).
6. Attach plates to gel electrophoresis apparatus, according to manufacturer's instructions. Fill upper and lower chambers with 1X TTE buffer, so that wells are covered, and rinse them with buffer, using a syringe or a Pasteur pipet, until there are no more bubbles in the wells.
7. Prerun the gel for at least 60 min in cold room (4–6°C) at 500 V in 1X TTE buffer.

3.2.2. SSCP Gel Loading

1. Add 30 µL formamide–dye solution and 150 µL chloroform to each PCR sample, and cap tightly.
2. Vortex, and briefly spin (15 s).
3. Extract the blue sample with a separate pipet (P-20 or P-100), never used to prepare DNA, solutions, or PCR. Change the tip for each sample. Put the upper phase in 1.5-mL microcentrifuge tubes labeled with the same numbers as the PCR samples. Samples can be stored at RT, or at 4°C, for up to a week (if ^{32}P is used). ^{33}P reactions may be stored for up to 2 wk.
4. Put a 5–µL aliquot of each sample into a plastic microwell plate. You should have about 40 µL of each sample, useful for up to eight SSCP gels.

5. Again rinse the wells thoroughly with buffer, using a syringe or a Pasteur pipet, making sure that there are no bubbles.
6. Place the microwell plate for 3 min at 95°C, to denature the samples. Chill on ice, and apply 1.5 µL of each sample immediately to a prerun nondenaturing SSCP gel. It is advisable to discard the remainder of the denatured samples. For additional SSCP analyses, it is better to use a fresh aliquot of the PCR sample each time. Run a nondenatured control on the SSCP gel, as well as one control reaction for each exon alone.
7. Electrophorese for 9–14 h at 950 V (approx 24 V/cm) in 1X TTE buffer at 4–6°C (*see* **Note 13**).
8. After the run is completed, slowly and carefully remove the silanized glass plate, using a blade as a lever. The gel should be perfectly adherent to the other plate. Soak the gel in 1 L 10% acetic acid for at least 35 min (always use fresh solution). Rinse thoroughly in dH_2O.
9. Dry the gel directly onto the glass in a (prewarmed) 160°C oven for at least 25 min. The gel must appear like a film. Otherwise, keep on drying at 160°C.
10. Cool the glass plate at RT.
11. Expose for at least 12–24 h to a Kodak MR film at –20 or –80°C, without using intensifying screens. Do not expose at RT, to prevent rehydration of the gel. If less radioactivity or a decayed isotope is used, expose longer.
12. Develop the autoradiogram.

3.2.3. Analysis of SSCP Results

1. Compare the lanes. Carefully identify and take note of the bands of the different exons, with the aid of control samples. This is the most important and difficult part of the interpretation of results. There are two polymorphisms in the δ-SG gene: C84T (Tyr28Tyr), with frequency 0.20 in exon 2, and G290A (Arg97Gln), with frequency 0.06 in exon 3. When multiplexing, the polymorphic shifts will help to identify these exons (**Table 2**).
2. If too many bands appear in SSCP samples, control the position of the bands of the nondenatured sample.

3.3. Heteroduplex Analysis

3.3.1. HA Gel Casting

1. Multiplex PCR, plate cleaning, and treatment can be carried out as for SSCP (*see* **Notes 10–12**).
2. Prepare the gel solution. For radioactive fragments, use the same gel dimensions as for the SSCP (40 mL solution). For a nonradioactive gel of 40 cm × 20 cm × 1 mm, at least 80 mL solution are necessary (*see* **Note 16**). Mix the following in a side-arm vacuum flask: 2 mL 20X TTE buffer, 16 mL 40% acrylamide solution (alternatively, use 20 mL 2X MDE gel solution [*see* **Note 14**]), 4 mL ethylene glycol, 5 g urea, and H_2O (fill to 40 mL).
3. Degas mixture under vacuum for 5 min.

Table 2
δ-SG Gene: Exons and PCR Primers

Exon	Length bp	5' cDNA position[a]	Codons	Forward primer (5'–3')	Reverse primer (5'–3')	Product size (bp)
1a	97	–137	–	CAGTAGCTGTGAGTCGGTCTGACA	CTCTCTTGTCCGTTTCACAAACCG	280[b]
1b	46	–43	1	–	–	–
2	189	4	2–64	CAGCGGTTTAATGTGAGTGCTTCT	CCGGAAGAAAGCTAAACAAACCTAGA	273
3	102	193	65–98	TCATATCTTCCCTGTTATCTCTGTGT	CAATAATGCCTCCTTCTCTCAGCAG	171
4	88	295	99–128	TCATGTCTTTCTCTTATTTTCTTATTGC	GGTTCATATGGTGTTTCCTTTGACC	206
5	120	383	128–168	GCGATGAGACTAATGGTGTTTTCTCT	TGGGAGGACATATCCTGTTCATAACA	291
6	73	503	168–192	CAGGTGACTCCAGTATCTCCAATCT	GCACAGAGCAAGGCAATAGCCATT	179
7	124	576	192–233	CCTTGAGCATGAACTTCCTTTTGTA	TGGCCTGTTGAAGCTGTAGCTCT	238
8	>7000	700	234–290	TGAATGTCAAGAGAAGAGACGACAGC	GCAGCCAGTGTGTAAAGCCAAAAA	301

[a]Nucleotide positions according to **ref. *11***.
[b]Product contains 186 bp of promoter.

4. Add 35 µL TEMED and 200 µL of 10% APS. Mix, and immediately pour the gel solution between the plates, using the standard procedure. Insert a well-forming comb 5 mm below the top of the short plate. A sharktooth comb is not preferable. Proceed as indicated for SSCP gel.

3.3.2. HA Gel Loading

1. After thermal cycling, add 8 µL formamide-dye solution and 150 µL chloroform to each PCR sample, and cap tightly.
2. Vortex, and briefly spin (15 s).
3. Extract samples as indicated in **Subheading 3.2.2., step 3**.
4. Mix 3 µL of WwDNA and patient DNA in the same microwell (*see* **Note 17**).
5. Denature the samples in the microwell plate for 2 min at 95°C. Incubate the microwell plate at 37°C for 30 min on a block heater (to avoid contaminations, never use a PCR machine), and apply 2 µL of each sample to a prerun HA gel. Rinse the wells with buffer using a syringe or a Pasteur pipet thoroughly, leaving no bubbles. Load at least one lane with a known heteroduplex DNA (it can also be a PCR product derived from an unrelated gene) and one lane with a DNA marker.
6. Electrophorese at 1000 V (approx 25 V/cm) in 1X TTE for 8–14 h at 4–6°C, according to the fragment length.
7. Continue as in **Subheading 3.2.2., steps 8–12**.

3.3.3. Interpretation of HA Results

1. The mutant DNA should produce four bands: two slower-moving (often visible) heteroduplex DNAs and two faster-moving (overlapping) homoduplex DNAs.
2. Identify and take note of the bands of the different exons, with the aid of single-exon PCR. This is easier than in SSCP analysis. Again, the δ-SG polymorphisms can be helpful for identifying the bands and checking the sensitivity of the method.

3.4. Direct Sequencing of PCR Product

When a DNA is suspected of containing either a homozygous or a heterozygous mutation in one exon, sequencing reaction should be 100% reliable, to discover the mutation. In particular, misinterpretation of results may be possible. In order to use sequencing to obtain clear-cut answers, the author advises the following guidelines:

1. Amplify the mutant sample, together with two wild-type samples, as controls.
2. Include only the two primers of the mutated exon in the PCR reaction.
3. Carry out PCR, and check the products for yield and specificity on 2% agarose gel. Further optimize the reaction if the bands are not satisfactory.
4. Clean the PCR product using Quiagen PCR purification kit, according to the manufacturer's instructions.

5. The DNA is ready to be sequenced. The best results are obtained using the ThermoSequenase ^{33}P-labeled terminator cycle sequencing kit, according to manufacturer's instructions (*see* **Notes 18** and **19**).

4. Notes

1. Great care must be taken to avoid cross contamination of PCR reactions. The source of contaminating DNA is generally derived from previous PCR reactions. Pipets are a major medium of contamination. Use a separate set of pipets, dedicated to the setting up of the PCR reactions alone. Use a special area of the lab to set up PCR. The author always prepares PCR under a dedicated airflow cabinet (Genesphere).
2. The use of mechanical Eppendorf 4810-4910 pipet (0.5–10 µL) allows considerable cost savings, because its accuracy permits the scale-down of the reaction volumes.
3. Primer oligo-nt are usually purchased from lead suppliers (Genset, Genosys, Gibco-BRL) and not housemade. The author recommends this choice. Otherwise, check the primer quality on a 15% polyacrylamide denaturing gel.
4. Primers are diluted to a concentration of 100 µ*M* (or higher) in water for molecular biology, and stored at –20°C, since this assures long storage time without degradation. More diluted primers are, in fact, unstable.
5. The use of special JF buffer avoids the generation of spurious products, and allows co-amplifying the exons in any combination, without careful adjustment of PCR temperatures and conditions. When preparing 3X JF buffer, use commercial solutions of $MgCl_2$ and ammonium acetate to avoid mistakes in weighing hygroscopic powders.
6. DNA template preparation. All standard methods to recover DNA are usable. However, problems may be encountered if the EDTA or salt concentration remains high. In this case, the author precipitates the DNA with 2 *M* ammonium acetate and 2 vol 100% ethanol at RT for 20 min, and spins for 10 min.
7. The PCR program here recommended provides the same temperature for annealing and elongation steps. It generally works very well using primers of 20–30 nt. Shorter or A-T-rich primers require a lower annealing temperature and/or longer annealing/elongation times (up to 6 min). To include more than four primer pairs in the multiplex PCR reaction, you must use more concentrated primer solutions (20 µ*M* or more). With this protocol, the author amplifies exons of the different SG genes in sets of three, four, or more exons (up to 18 for some applications). These guidelines are appropriate for all commercially available thermal cyclers. There is no obvious limitation for multiplex SSCP analysis, since exons of the same expected size may migrate very differently in gel. For multiplex HA, it is better to check the products using the same electrophoretic conditions as for mutation screening.
8. It is not necessary to store the PCR product at 4°C. It is also not necessary to add a final overnight step at 4°C, because PCR products are stable at RT.
9. If it is necessary to improve a spurious PCR, try using different EDTA concentrations, without changing temperatures. The author usually adds 0.5 m*M*, 1 m*M*,

1.5 m*M* EDTA (final concentration in the PCR). On the other hand, if no band is visible, set a lower annealing temperature.

10. When glass plates are treated as indicated, the gel fully binds to the nonsilanized glass. All subsequent steps are performed using the glass plate as a stiff support, without the risks of gel breakages and/or distortions. Before using this protocol, be sure that the autoradiographic cassettes are large enough to contain the glass plates. Generally, standard glass plates (20 × 40 × 0.4 cm) are contained in 30 × 40 cm cassettes.
11. The author discourages replacing TTE with Tris-borate–EDTA, since multiplex PCR buffer contains 8% glycerol, and samples will resolve in fuzzy bands, with loss of resolution.
12. Gels can also be poured the day before use. In this case, it is crucial to wet the polymerized gel with dH_2O, and seal with a transparent wrap.
13. Alternative SSCP conditions are: to run the gel at 15°C, and/or to substitute glycerol with 10% sucrose.
14. The addition of about 4 *M* urea to the gel is useful to improve the HA resolution. If you want to improve resolution, replace *bis*-acrylamide with piperazine diacrylamide (Bio-Rad, code 161–0202) using a 80:1 acrylamide/crosslinker ratio. Alternatively, purchase a more expensive 2X MDE gel solution.
15. Many researchers simultaneously examine heteroduplex and SSCP on the same gel. This relies on the finding that if excess DNA is added to denaturation buffer, dsDNA will also form. Even though the advantage of this method is to reduce the workload, chief disadvantages are that conditions are not optimized for both SSCP and HA, and, more important, that either you leave the SSCP near the wells (with loss of resolution) or you risk to lose dsDNA bands, which runs much more rapidly than the single-stranded fragments. It is, however, possible to use differently diluted PCR samples for both HA and SSCP.
16. When using nonradioactive HA, it is advisable to use Ag staining. In fact, with EtBr, bands may appear broader, because more DNA needs to be loaded on the gel. The Ag staining method also shows proteins present in the PCR reaction. After PCR, extract samples with phenol–chloroform.
17. When examining DNA from heterozygous individuals (compound mutations or parents of LGMD2F patients) by HA, two samples do not need to be mixed. Load PCR samples, each for gel lane, without prior denaturation.
18. When using a linear sequencing kit (i.e., Sequenase 2.0), you have first to reamplify 0.5 µL unpurified PCR products, using two separate reactions, the first one containing only the forward primer and the second one only the reverse primer. For this second PCR, you can also scale up volumes to 50 µL, but do not change reagent concentrations or temperatures. Do not cycle for more than 15×. Purify the product using Quiagen or equivalent kit, according to manufacturer's instructions. After the final elution with Tris-EDTA, precipitate the DNA, adding 0.1 vol sodium acetate and 3 vol of 100% ethanol. Mix, and incubate for 10 min at RT. Centrifuge, discard the supernatant, and wash the pellet with 70% ethanol, then dry. Do not denature DNA any more. Add the primer not used for

the second PCR (antiparallel to the single-stranded product). Now the DNA is ready to be sequenced.

19. Always carry out sequencing reactions on both strands, and in parallel with wild-type controls. There are many examples of false mutations resulting from strong compressions.

Acknowledgments

The author thanks B. Moncharmont, A.A. Puca, and J. Sepe for helpful suggestions on the manuscript. The financial support of Telethon, Italy (Grant 899), is gratefully acknowledged.

References

1. Bönnemann, C. G., McNally, E. M., and Kunkel, L. M. (1996) Beyond dystrophin: current progress in the muscular dystrophies. *Curr. Opin. Pediatr.* **8,** 569–582.
2. Beckmann, J. S. and Bushby, K. M. (1996) Advances in the molecular genetics of the limb-girdle type of autosomal recessive progressive muscular dystrophy. *Curr. Opin. Neurol.* **9,** 389–393.
3. Straub, V. and Campbell, K. P. (1997) Muscular dystrophies and the dystrophin-glycoprotein complex. *Curr. Opin. Neurol.* **10,** 168–175.
4. Roberds, S. L., Leturcq, F., Allamand, V., Piccolo, F., Jeanpierre, M., Anderson, R. D., et al. (1994) Missense mutations in the adhalin gene linked to autosomal recessive muscular dystrophy. *Cell* **78,** 625–633.
5. Piccolo, F., Roberds, S. L., Jeanpierre, M., Leturcq, F., Azibi, K., Beldjord, C., et al. (1995) Primary adhalinopathy: a common cause of autosomal recessive muscular dystrophy of variable severity. *Nature Genet.* **10,** 243–245.
6. Bönnemann, C. G., Modi, R., Noguchi, S., Mizuno, Y., Yoshida, M., Gussoni, E., et al. (1995) β-sarcoglycan (A3b) mutations cause autosomal recessive muscular dystrophy with loss of the sarcoglycan complex. *Nature Genet.* **11,** 266–272.
7. Lim L. E., Duclos, F., Broux, O., Bourg, N., Sunada, Y., Allamand, V., et al. (1995) β-sarcoglycan: characterization and role in limb-girdle muscular dystrophy linked to 4q12. *Nature Genet.* **11,** 257–265.
8. Noguchi, S., McNally E. M., Ben Othmane, K., Hagiwara, Y., Mizuno, Y., Yoshida, M., et al. (1995) Mutations in the dystrophin-associated protein γ-sarcoglycan in chromosome 13 muscular dystrophy. *Science* **270,** 819–822.
9. Nigro, V., Moreira, E., Piluso, G., Vainzof, M., Belsito, A., Politano, L., et al. (1996) Autosomal recessive limb-girdle muscular dystrophy, LGMD2F, is caused by a mutation in the δ-sarcoglycan gene. *Nature Genet.* **14,** 195–198.
10. Ozawa, E., Noguchi, S., Mizuno, Y., Hagiwara, Y., and Yoshida, M. (1998) From dystrophinopathy to sarcoglycanopathy: evolution of a concept of muscular dystrophy. *Muscle Nerve* **21,** 421–438.
11. Nigro, V., Piluso, G., Belsito, A., Politano, L., Puca, A. A., Papparella, S., et al. (1996) Identification of a novel sarcoglycan gene at 5q33 encoding a sarcolemmal 35kDa glycoprotein. *Hum. Mol. Genet.* **5,** 1179–1186.

12. Jung, D., Duclos, F., Apostol, B., Straub V., Lee, J. C., Allamand, V., et al. (1996) Characterization of delta-sarcoglycan, a novel component of the oligomeric sarcoglycan complex involved in limb-girdle muscular dystrophy. *J. Biol. Chem.* **271,** 32,321–32,329.
13. Yoshida, M., Noguchi, S., Wakabayashi, E., Piluso, G., Belsito, A., Nigro, V., and Ozawa, E. (1997) The fourth component of the sarcoglycan complex. *FEBS Lett.* **403,** 143–148.
14. Moreira, E. S., Vainzof, M, Marie, S. K., Nigro, V., Zatz, M., and Passos-Bueno, M. R. (1998) First missense mutation in the δ-sarcoglycan gene associated with a severe phenotype and frequency of limb-girdle muscular dystrophy type 2F (LGMD2F) among Brazilian sarcoglycanopathies. *J. Med. Genet.* **35,** 951–953.
15. Duggan, D. J., Manchester, D., Stears, K. P., Mathews, D. J., Hart, C., and Hoffman, E. P. (1997) Mutations in the delta-sarcoglycan gene are a rare cause of autosomal recessive limb-girdle muscular dystrophy. *Neurogenetics* **1,** 49–58.
16. Nigro, V., Okazaki, Y., Belsito, A., Piluso, G., Matsuda, Y., Politano, L., et al. (1997) Identification of the Syrian hamster cardiomyopathy gene. *Hum. Mol. Genet.* **6,** 601–608.
17. Nigro, V., Politano, L., Nigro, G., Colonna-Romano, S., Molinari A. M., and Puca, G. A. (1992) Detection of a nonsense mutation in the dystrophin gene by multiple SSCP. *Hum. Mol. Genet.* **1,** 517–520.

16

Molecular Diagnosis of Calpainopathies

Methods Used for Detection of Mutations in CAPN3 Gene Implicated in Limb-Girdle Muscular Dystrophy Type 2A

Isabelle Richard and Jacques Beckmann

1. Introduction

Limb-girdle muscular dystrophy 9LGMD) type 2A (LGMD2A; MIM253600) is an autosomal recessive disorder belonging to the group of progressive MDs. LGMD2A is characterized by symmetrical atrophy of the pelvic, scapular, and trunk muscles, elevated serum creatine kinase and a necrotic–regeneration pattern on muscular biopsies *(1–2)*. The study of these biopsies show that the integrity of the dystrophin-associated complex is preserved in these patients, because immunohistochemical staining for dystrophin, merosin, or the various sarcoglycan (SG) proteins is normal *(2)*. Other than that, there are no specific diagnostic criteria, which explains why, despite having been properly described over a century ago *(3)*, this field has generated much heated controversy, but this clinical entity remained difficult to recognize.

Other autosomic recessive progressive MDs are often also regrouped under the term LGMD2. The latter present an overall similar clinical picture, preferentially involving the proximal musculature, although subtle differences may be recognized by an experienced neurologist *(2)*. Four LGMD2 entities form a subgroup of their own, because they are characterized by a disruption of the SG complex *(4)*. These are each caused by mutations in one of the SG genes *(5–9)*, which were previously referred to as LGMD2C, 2D, 2E, and 2F, and, according to the new genetic nomenclature, are now designated *SGCA*, *SGCB*, *SGCC*, and *SGCD*, respectively. Two additional LGMD2 entities, namely,

From: *Methods in Molecular Medicine, vol. 43: Muscular Dystrophy: Methods and Protocols*
Edited by: K. M. D. Bushby and L. V. B. Anderson © Humana Press Inc., Totowa, NJ

LGMD2B and 2G, present no alterations in the SG complex, and their causative genes are respectively the dysferlin and telethonin genes ***(10–14)***.

The gene responsible for LGMD2A was localized to chromosome 15q15.1-q15.3 ***(12)***, and was subsequently identified by positional cloning ***(16–19)***. It encodes for calpain 3, the skeletal muscle-specific member of the calpain family ***(20)***. This family is composed of ubiquitously expressed and tissue-specific intracellular calpains, cysteine-proteases requiring calcium for their catalytic activities (for a review *see* ref. ***21–23***). To date, 97 distinct LGMD2A mutations have been identified by the authors' group (***19,24–27***; unpublished data): They are distributed uniformly along the length of the *CAPN3* gene, with no obvious mutational hot spots. Most mutations identified thus far represent private variants, although particular mutations were found more than once. The calpain 3 gene (or *CAPN3*) spans a region of about 40 kb ***(19)***. The main calpain 3 isoform expressed in skeletal muscle consists of 24 exons encoding a 3.5-kb transcript. In addition, a recent study demonstrated that this gene is subject to alternative splicing, and may present an alternative promoter (***28–30***).

Because of the lack of suitable specific diagnostic immunological reagents, the definitive identification of LGMD2A still rests almost exclusively on the characterization of the underlying mutation(s) (*see* **Note 1**). This chapter reviews the various detection methods that have been used to uncover *CAPN3* mutations, to demonstrate the role of this gene in the etiology of this disease, and in the molecular diagnosis of patients affected by progressive MDs. This may help other investigators/clinicians to design appropriate screening strategies. Three approaches can be considered, depending on the available materials. Given the large size differences, it is evidently far easier to scan the *CAPN3* cDNA for the presence of mutations or polymorphisms, rather than the corresponding genomic sequence. Thus, the first choice is to scan for mutations on RNA extracted from muscle biopsies; the second one, on RNA extracted from lymphoblastoid cell lines; and, if these fail, or for lack of mRNA preparations, the third one is to screen the different exons (or occasionally introns) at the genomic level, either by indirect methods such as single-strand conformational polymorphism (SSCP) ***(31)*** or heteroduplex analysis (HA) ***(32)***, or directly by DNA sequencing.

2. Materials

2.1. cDNA Preparation

1. RNA-plus solution (Bioprobe Systems, France).
2. 5X reverse transcriptase buffer: 50 m*M* Tris-HCl, pH 8.3, 75 m*M* KCl, and 3 m*M* $MgCl_2$.
3. Random hexamer primers mix 100 μ*M* (pd(N_6); Pharmacia).

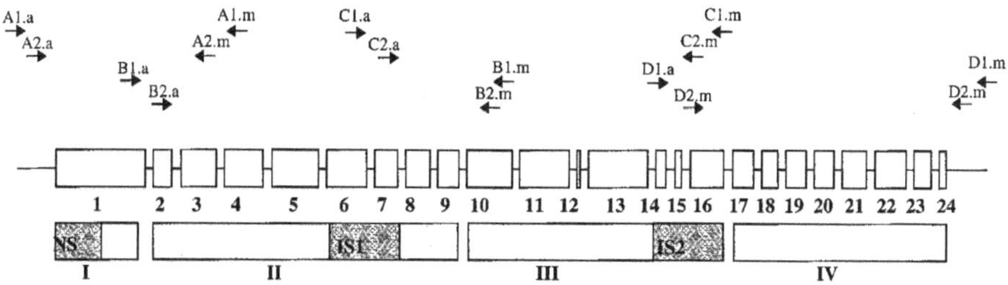

Fig. 1. Position of oligonucleotides used in CDNA analysis.

4. 10 m*M* deoxyribonucleoside triphosphate (dNTP) mix.
5. RNAsin (Promega).
6. Reverse transcriptase.

2.2. Polymerase Chain Reaction

For the position of oligonucleotide (oligo-nt) along the calpain 3 gene, *see* **Fig. 1**.

1. Oligo-nt A1, B1, C1, and D1 for the first polymerase chain reaction (PCR) amplification on cDNA

   A1a CAGCTCGGTTTTTAAGATGG, A1m CGTCCACCCACTCTCCATAG;

   B1a AAGTTCCCCATCCAGTTCGT, B1m GAAGCTTGTCAGACTGCAGA;

   C1a GTCACGCCTACTCTGTCACG, C1m GCTTTTGCTTATCAGGGCTT;

   D1a TTGAAAATACCATCTCCGTG, D1m GGGGTAAAATGGAGGAGGAA.

   (fragment sizes A1 = 674 bp, B1 = 1006 bp, C1 = 912 bp, D1= 869 bp).
2. Oligo-nt A2, B2, C2, and D for the nested PCR amplifications on cDNA

   A2a CTTTCCTTGAAGGTAGCTGTAT A2m AAGATCCCTGCGTAGTTTTCG;

   B2a ATGGAGCCAACAGAACTGAC, B2m GGCCGTGAGGTTGCAGATCT;

   C2a AGGTGGAGTGGAACGGTTCT, C2m GCTCCTTGTTGCTGTTTGCT ;

   D2a CCATCATCTTCGTTTCGGAC, D2m GGGTGAAACTGAAATCCTGA.

   (fragment sizes A2 = 548 bp, B2 = 914 bp, C2 = 760 bp, D2 = 721 bp)
3. 10X PCR buffer: 100 m*M* Tris-HCl, pH 9.0, 500 m*M* KCl, 15 m*M* $MgCl_2$, 0.1% Triton X-100, 0.01% gelatin, 2 m*M* dNTP.
4. *Taq* polymerase.

2.3. Heteroduplex Analysis

1. Hydrolink–MDE gel matrix (Bioprobe Systems).
2. Hydrolink dye.
3. 0.6X Tris-borate–EDTA (TBE).

Table 1
Oligo-nt Used for Genomic Analysis

Amplified region (exon)	Primer sequences (5'-3')	Size (bp)	Annealing temp. (°C)
1	CTTTCCTTGAAGGTAGCTGTAT GAGGTGCTGAGTGAGAGGAC	438	60
2	ACTCCGTCTCAAAAAAATACCT ATTGTCCCTTTACCTCCTGG	239	57
3	TGGAAGTAGGAGAGTGGGCA GGGTAGATGGGTGGGAAGTT	354	58
4	GAGGAATGTGGAGGAAGGAC TTCCTGTGAGTGAGGTCTCG	292	59
5	GGAACTCTGTGACCCCAAAT TCCTCAAACAAAACATTCGC	325	56
6	GTTCCCTACATTCTCCATCG GTTATTTCAACCCAGACCCTT	315	57
7	AATGGGTTCTCTGGTTACTGC AGCACGAAAAGCAAAGATAAA	333	56
8	GTAAGAGATTTGCCCCCCAG TCTGCGGATCATTGGTTTTG	321	58
9	CCTTCCCTTCTTCCTGCTTC CTCTCTTCCCCACCCTTACC	173	56
10	CCTCCTCACCTGCTCCCATA TTTTTCGGCTTAGACCCTCC	251	56
11	TGTGGGGAATAGAAATAAATGG CCAGGAGCTCTGTGGGTCA	355	57
12	GGCTCCTCATCCTCATTCACA GTGGAGGAGGGTGAGTGTGC	312	61
13	TGTGGCAGGACAGGACGTTC TTCAACCTCTGGAGTGGGCC	337	60
14	CACCAGAGCAAACCGTCCAC ACAGCCCAGACTCCCATTCC	230	61
15	TTCTCTTCTCCCTTCACCCT ACACACTTCATGCTCTCTACCC	225	57
16	CCGCCTATTCCTTTCCTCTT GACAAACTCCTGGGAAGCCT	331	56
17	ACCTCTGACCCCTGTGAACC TGTGGATTTGTGTGCTACGC	270	61
18	CATAAATAGCACCGACAGGGA GGGATGGAGAAGAGTGAGGA	258	59
19	TCCTCACTCTTCTCCATCCC ACCCTGTATGTTGCCTTGG	159	57
20–21	GGGGATTTTGCTGTGTGCTG ATTCCTGCTCCCACCGTCTC	333	61

(continued)

Table 1 *(continued)*

Amplified region (exon)	Primer sequences (5'-3')	Size (bp)	Annealing temp. (°C)
22	CACAGAGTGTCCGAGAGGCA GGAGATTATCAGGTGAGATGCC	282	57
22–23	CAGAGTGTCCGAGAGGCAGGG CGTTGACCCCTCCACCTTGA	608	61
24	GGGAAAACATGCACCTTCTT TAGGGGGTAAAATGGAGGAG	375	58

2.4. Single-Strand Conformational Polymorphism

1. 40% Acrylamide–*bis*-acrylamide solution, 37.5:1 (2.6% C).
2. 0.5X TBE.
3. 5% Glycerol.
4. 10% Amonium persulfate.
5. *NNN'N'*-tetramethylethylenediamine.
6. Loading buffer: 0.25% bromophenol blue, 50X formamide.
7. Nylon membrane.
8. 10X reaction buffer: 2 *M*, potassium cacodylate, pH 7.6, 1 m*M* dithiothreoitol, 2 m*M* dNTPs, 10 m*M* $CoCl_3$.
9. Terminal transferase.
10. Gold buffer (ECL) ElectroCChemiluminescence (Amersham).
11. Posthybridization solutions: 3X standard sodium citrate (SSC), 0.1% dosium dodecyl sulfate (SDS); 0.2X SSC; 2X SSC.

2.5. Allele-Specific PCR

1. Primer pairs: For each mutation, two couples are used (*see* **Table 2**): oligo-nt corresponding to the normal allele (1) and mutant allele (2). Nucleotides corresponding to the mutation are underlined.

3. Methods

3.1. cDNA Analysis

The capacity to perform an analysis at the cDNA level presents a particular interest for the calpain gene, considering its relatively large size and exon multiplicity. Thus, whenever possible, i.e., whenever adequate RNA preparations are available, analyzing the cDNA represents the first choice. Besides the size advantages, scanning the cDNA, instead of genomic DNA, also often enables the visualization of splicing defects, but one must have access to an adequate RNA source. The fact the calpain 3 expression was reported to be skeletal-

Table 2
Mutation-Specific Oligo-nt

Mutation	Upper primer 5'–>3'	Lower primer 5'–>3'
550ΔA	(1) TATAGATGACTGCCTGCCAAC (2) TAGATGACTGCCTGCCAC	TTCCTGTGAGTGAGGTCTCG
G222R	(1) CTACGAAGCTCTGAAAGGTG (2) CTACGAAGCTCTGAAAGGTA	GGCTTTCTTCATGATCTTGT
IVS6-1 G–>A	(1) CTCTGGTTACTGCTCTACAA (2) CTCTGGTTACTGCTCTACAG	AGCACGAAAAGCAAAGATAAA
R489W	(1) GCCCTGATGCAGAAGAACC (2) GCCCTGATGCAGAAGAACT	CCAGGAGCTCTGTGGGTCA
R489Q	(1) GCCCTGATGCAGAAGAACCG (2) GCCCTGATGCAGAAGAACCA	CCAGGAGCTCTGTGGGTCA
R572W	(1) AGGGGGAATTCATCCTCCG (2) AGGGGGAATTCATCCTCTG	TTCAACCTCTGGGAGTGGGCC
R572Q	(1) AGGGGGAATTCATCCTCCG (2) AGGGGGAATTCATCCTCCA	TTCAACCTCTGGGAGTGGGCC
S744G	AAGAATGGGGTTGATTTGGAG	(1) GCATTTCGCATCTCGTAGCT (2) GCATTTCGCATCTCGTAGCC
R748Q	AAGAATGGGGTTGATTTGGAGA	(1) TGCGTCGTTGACTGCATTTC (2) TGCGTCGTTGACTGCATTTT
R769Q	AAGAATGGGGTTGATTTGGAGA	(1) ATGTGTTTGTCTGCGTACC (2) ATGTGTTTGTCTGCGTACT
1872C–> T	CACCAGAGCAAACCGTCCAC	(1) CAGGGCTTGTTTTGCCTTTG (2) CAGGGCTTGTTTTGCCTTTA
2069 ΔCA	(1) CAAGGACCTGAAGACACACG (2) CACAAGGACCTGAAGACACG	ACCCTGTATGTTGCCTTGG
2362AG–>TCATCT	(1) CATCTGCTGCTTCGTTAG (2) TGCTGCTTCGTTTCATCT	GGAGATTATCAGGTGAGATGCC

muscle-specific is a considerable impediment, because muscle biopsies are often unavailable or may be of insufficient quality for RNA extraction (e.g., because they were not taken with this purpose in mind). Demonstration of the presence of illegitimate transcripts ***(33)*** of the calpain 3 gene in lymphocytes was therefore of importance ***(19,24)***, because it enabled bypassing the need for muscle biopsies (*see* **Note 2**). Yet, the level of calpain 3 mRNA in lymphoblastoid cells is much lower than in muscle biopsies. Hence, two rounds of PCR are required to visualize the corresponding RNA (using the second-round nested primers).

3.1.2. Total RNA Extraction

This protocol can be used indifferently on lymphoblastoid cells or on muscle biopsies. In the first case, about 10–15 million cells from a lymphoblastoid cell culture are necessary. Cell pellets can be processed immediately or stored at –20°C until use. In the second case, muscle biopsies must first be pulverized either with a mortar, a homogenizor, or, as in the authors' case, with a Fast prep apparatus (Bio 101, La Jolla, CA). Samples must be kept on ice throughout the procedure and handled with RNase-free precautions.

1. Add 1.6 mL RNA-plus solution to the cell pellet or muscle powder, homogenize, and transfer in a 2-mL Eppendorf tube, wash with 200 µL RNA-plus solution.
2. Add 180 µL chloroform; leave 5 min on ice.
3. Centrifuge at 12,000*g* for 15 min at 4°C, transfer the aqueous phase in a 2-mL Eppendorf tube.
4. Add 1 vol isopropanol; leave 15 min on ice.
5. Centrifuge at 13,000*g* for .5 h at 4°C.
6. Wash with 70% ethanol.
7. Centrifuge at 12,000*g* for 15 min at 4°C.
8. Air-dry, and resuspend in 20 µL RNase-free H_2O.
9. Control the quality by gel electrophoresis, and measure of optical density (OD) at 260 nm.

3.1.2. First-strand cDNA Synthesis

Various commercial sources exist to obtain cDNA synthesis kits or required individual reagents. Slight variations in protocols exist.

1. Denature 1 µg RNA (at the concentration of 50 µg/µL) by incubation at 75°C for 3 min.
2. Chill on ice.
3. Add 6 µL 5X reverse transcriptase buffer.
4. Add 1 µL random hexamer primer mix.
5. Add 1.5 µL dNTPs.
6. Add 0.5 µL RNAsin.
7. Add 200 U reverse transcriptase.

8. Incubate at 42°C for 1 h.
9. Stop the reaction by incubation at 75°C for 5 min; chill on ice.

3.1.3. Polymerase Chain Reaction

A first amplification was performed on 1 µL cDNA sample, using one of four sets of primers (A1, B1, C1, D1; *see* **Subheading 2.**) to generate four overlapping DNA fragments spanning the entire *CAPN3* coding sequence. It is also possible to amplify the whole sequence of the calpain gene, using primers located at both ends of the gene. To amplify RNA from lymphoblastoid cells, a second nested PCR is performed. It may be necessary to adapt PCR conditions and amounts of cDNA, depending on the results.

1. Perform four distinct PCR amplifications (40 s at 92°C, 30 s at 60°C, 1 min at 72°C, for a total of 20 cycles), with 1 to 5 µL cDNA as template, using couples A1, B1, C1, and D1.
2. Analyze the PCR amplification products on a 2% agarose gel.
3. For cDNA from lymphoblastoid cells, perform a second round of PCR amplification (40 s at 92°C, 30 s at 60°C, 1 min at 72°C, for 20 cycles) on 1 µL of the first PCR product using the corresponding nested primers (A2, B2, C2, D2).
4. Control on a 2% agarose gel.

3.2. Genomic Analysis

The determination of the calpain 3 genomic organization ***(19)*** allows for exon-specific oligo-nt design, thereby facilitating a systematic mutation screening. Each exon can therefore be amplified by specific intronic primers (**Table 1**). Numerous detection methods can be used to visualize the presence of base changes on PCR products. Those relying on the recognition of electrophoretic mobility alterations are usually simple, easy to implement, and are therefore often used in the process of gene validation. The authors used HA and SSCP.

3.2.1. PCR Amplification

1. To 100 ng genomic DNA, prepared from peripheral blood or lymphoblastoid cell lines, add 5 µL PCR mix, 100 ng of each primer, and 5 U *Taq* polymerase.
2. Bring reaction volume to 50 µL.
3. Add 50 µL oil, in order to prevent evaporation.
4. Denature for 5 min at 94°C.
5. Perform the PCR reaction (92°C 40 s, annealing temperature 30 s, 72°C 30 s, for 30–35 cycles). The annealing temperature correspond to T_m –5°.
6. Run the products on agarose gel, to check the quality of the amplification reaction.

3.2.2. Heteroduplex Analysis

1. To 10 µL PCR product (up to 20 µL), add 3 µL Hydrolink dye.
2. Add 50 µL oil, in order to prevent evaporation.

3. Denature for 5 min at 94°C.
4. Leave in ice for 2 min.
5. Allow to renature at room temperature (RT) for at least 1 h.
6. Run the total amount of product on Hydrolink gel, prepared according to the manufacturer's recommendations. For PCR products around 150 bp, the conditions of migration are an overnight (approx 16 h) run at 400 V.
7. Stain the gel with ethidium bromide.
8. Visualize the products under UV light.

3.2.3. SSCP Analysis

Classic methods were used, except for pattern visualization. To circumvent the use of radioactivity, the samples were transferred onto nylon filters and hybridized according to the ECL protocol (Amersham) with the primers used in the PCR.

3.2.3.1. Electrophoresis

1. To 2.5 µL PCR product, add 5 µL loading buffer.
2. Denature at 95°C for 5 min, and keep on ice until loading.
3. Load 5 µL on a 6–8% acrylamide gel with 5% glycerol, 0.5X TBE.
4. Electrophorese at 8 W for 16 h at RT.
5. Put a nylon membrane onto the gel, and allow to transfer for at least 1 h.

3.2.3.2. Oligo-nt Labeling

1. To 0.12 nmol oligo-nt, add 10 µL reaction buffer and 75 U terminal transferase.
2. Bring reaction volume to 100 µL.
3. Incubate for 2 h at 37°C.
4. Add 4 µL 0.25 *M* EDTA, pH 8.0, to stop the reaction.
5. Separate elongated oligonucleotide from unincorporated nts by gel filtration, using a G25 column.
6. Calculate the extent of elongation after OD measure at 260 nm
7. Combine 200 µg oligo-nt, at the concentration of 10 ng/µL with 20 µL horseradish peroxidase and 20 µL glutaraldehyde.
8. Incubate for 10 min at 37°C, then keep on ice until use.

3.2.3.3. Hybridization

1. Prehybridize at 42°C for 1 h in the hybridization mix.
2. Add the oligo-nt probe at a final concentration of 10 mg/mL.
3. Hybridize at 42°C overnight in Gold buffer.
4. Wash once in 3X SSC–0.1% SDS at 42°C for 15 min.
5. Wash 2× in 0.2X SSC at 42°C for 15 min.
6. Wash once in 2X SSC at RT.
7. Reveal with ECL detection kit, and expose to an X-ray film for the appropriate time.

3.3. Sequencing

Direct sequencing is the definite step giving the nature and precise location of a mutation. It can be used to characterize mutations detected by other methods, but is also a screening method *per se*. Each laboratory has its own protocols for purification of PCR products prior to sequencing, and for the sequencing itself. For the authors, PCR products are purified using microcon devices (Amicon), then subjected to dye–dideoxy sequencing (*see* **Note 3**).

3.4. Mutation-Specific Detection

In several instances, it was useful to develop specific methods that allow rapid, simple detection of a particular mutation with a 100% efficiency (*see* **Note 4**). Direct sequencing can be used, but does not lend itself to parallel screening of a large number of patients. Restriction enzyme changes is applicable in some cases. In the authors' study, allele-specific PCR was developed for mutations that are either recurrently observed or that are specific for selected populations (551ΔA, G222R, IVS6-1G–>A, R489W, R489Q, R572W, R572Q, S744G, R748Q, R769Q, 1872C–>T, 2069ΔCA, and 2362AG–>TCATCT). Oligo-nts were designed in such way that their 3' bases overlap the point of the mutation. For each mutation, alternative sets of oligo-nt are used: one corresponding to the normal allele and the other to the mutated allele (*see* **Subheading 2.5.**).

1. After 5 min denaturation at 96°C, perform a touchdown PCR amplification *(34)* on genomic DNA, using the primers corresponding to the mutation investigated. The touchdown PCR conditions are as follows: 40 s denaturation at 94°C, followed by 30 s annealing steps starting 5°C higher than the annealing temperature, with a decrease of 1°C every two cycles, until the annealing temperature is reached. Twenty additional cycles of amplification, consisting of 40 s at 94°C and 30 s at the annealing temperature, are performed. The buffer conditions were as described above.

   For 551?A, R769Q, R489W, R489Q, 2069 ΔCA, and S744G, use 65 to 60°C.

   For IVS6–1 G–>A and 1872C–>T, use 63 to 58°C.

   For G222R, R572W, R572Q, R748Q, and 2362AG–>TCATCT, use 60 to 55°C.

   To further increase the specificity of some PCR reactions, it is necessary to add a variable concentration of formamide. For G222R, R572Q, R572W, 2069 ΔCA, and S744G, add formamide to a 2% final concentration; for R489W and R489Q to 4%.
2. Monitor the result by electrophoresis on a 2% horizontal agarose gel stained with ethidium bromide.

4. Notes

1. Mutation analysis is a technically demanding and time-consuming procedure. Moreover, to help in differential diagnosis, and considering the genetic heterogeneity of LGMD2 (which has at least eight causative genes, LGMD2A–G), a linkage analysis may be performed when possible, i.e., for informative families, using markers flanking the different LGMD2 chromosomal regions. Identification of linkage allows for the assignment of families to a specific LGMD2 locus. In addition, in the cases of sarcoglycanopathies, antibody-based protein assays exist. This is not the case for LGMD2A. Whenever the SGs are preserved, or in case of high suspicion of a calpainopathy, e.g., based on the specific pattern of muscle involvement, one must validate this hypothesis by a precise molecular diagnosis. At present, this implicates direct search of mutations in the gene. In the future, assessing the state of the protein in muscle biopsies (by Western blot or immunohistochemistry *see* Chapter 22) may become an alternative to mutation screening. Nevertheless, one should be aware that the proteolytic nature of calpain 3 may render this test less obvious than for the SGS, because some missense mutations may lead to a protein increase by affecting its stability.

   A sequencing-based approach may still be required to identify the underlying mutation. As long as the emerging DNA chip technologies or other equivalent methods have not become routine practice, the molecular diagnosis will still rest on conventional DNA sequencing.
2. There are, broadly speaking, different motives to carry a mutation search. Mutation-detection methods are used to incriminate a candidate gene in the etiology of a particular genetic disease. They are also used for the molecular diagnosis of patients and the elucidation of structure/function relationships. In the first and last cases, it is not critical to detect 100% of the defects, but, for diagnostic purposes, a high efficiency is necessary. Hence, the methods used could differ, depending on one's objectives. This laboratory's choice was influenced by the relative ease to implement the various screening technologies, as well as by the characteristics of the *CAPN3* gene. Finally, it was also guided by the nature of the available materials. Not all potentially interesting techniques were explored, e.g., denaturating gradient el electrophoresis ***(35)*** or fluorescent assisted mismatch analysis ***(36)***, for instance, were not tested.

   For the identification of the morbid locus, the authors first used rapid and easy techniques, such as SSCP and HA, since, for this purpose, loss of power, because of their relatively lower efficiencies, was not critical. In addition, the same PCR products could be examined using either of these two methods, and, eventually, for DNA sequencing, too.

   Because of the inherent limitations for mutation detection of the SSCP and HA techniques, the authors chose, in a second step, to sequence directly either the genomic DNA or cDNA derived by RT-PCR on RNA from muscle or from illegitimate transcription products. Results showed that the automated sequencing strategy provides a satisfactory method to identify virtually all mutations in the *CAPN3* gene. cDNA sequencing is attractive, despite the caveat that it can only visualize alterations that are present in the mRNA molecules. Thus, when possible, it should be considered as a method of choice. Illegitimate transcripts do not exactly reflect muscle transcripts. As often observed with illegitimate transcripts (e.g. *see* **ref. *37***), the lymphocyte CAPN3 transcripts present aberrant splicings: a systematic splicing of exon 16 and in half the molecules of exon 6. This observation should be taken into account in a screening process, because it is necessary to complete the analysis by the examination of exons 6 and 16 using a different independent method.

3. In contrast to sequence alterations leading to the creation of a premature stop codon, which are deleterious for the protein function, missense mutations may represent either a causative pathogenic mutation or a neutral polymorphism. Therefore, it is important to obtain other evidences that the observed base change is the cause of the disease. This evidence could be inferred from, among others, the fact that the mutation is located in a region of known function or structure, or in a residue that is conserved in other species, and, thus, is supposed to have a critical role; a drastic change in the nature of the substituted amino acid; the absence of this sequence variant on a large number of normal chromosomes; the observation of a *de novo* mutation; and the modification of particular characteristics or biochemical properties of the protein.
4. It may be useful to discuss the recurrent mutations thus far identified, because this knowledge could be introduced into a general diagnostic procedure. Recurrent mutations can be explained by two distinct mechanisms: a coincidental occurrence resulting from independant mutational event, or the sharing of a common ancestor. The latter can be recognized by the observation of a common core marker haplotype flanking the disease locus, i.e., the sharing of specific marker alleles. In several instances, as outlined hereafter, it was useful to first analyze the families by means of polymorphic markers flanking the *CAPN3* gene. If a previously characterized haplotype was uncovered, this was thus suggestive of the presence of a particular known mutation, which was then subsequently easily identified. This approach is particularly useful when analyzing patients from defined populations, in which high frequency or specific mutations were already detected. In such populations, one should first target the diagnosis to these particular mutations, whether or not the families were haplotyped. This could be performed using rapid assays that require small amounts of genomic DNA and cheap diagnostic methods.

References

1. Fardeau, M., Hillaire, D., Mignard, C., Feingold, N., Mignard, D., de Ubeda, B., et al. (1996) Juvenile limb-girdle muscular dystrophy: clinical, histopathological, and genetic data from a small community living in the Reunion Island. *Brain* **119,** 295–308.
2. Beckmann, J. S. and Fardeau, M. (1998) Limb-girdle muscular dystrophies, in *Neuromuscular disorders: Clinical and Molecular Genetics* (Emery, A. E. H., ed.), Chichester, UK, pp. 123–156.

3. Erb, W. (1884) Ueber die "juvenile form" der progressiven muskelatrophie ihre Beziehungen zur sogenannten pseudohypertrophie der muskeln. *Deutsches Archiv fur Klinische Medizin.* **34,** 467–519.
4. Campbell, K. P. (1995) Three muscular dystrophies: loss of cytoskeleton-extracellular matrix linkage. *Cell* **80,** 675–679.
5. Roberds, S. L., Leturcq, F., Allamand, V., Piccolo, F., Jeanpierre, M., Anderson, R. D., et al. (1994) Missense mutations in the adhalin gene linked to autosomal recessive muscular dystrophy. *Cell* **78,** 625–633.
6. Noguchi, S., McNally, E. M., Ben Othmane, K., Hagiwara, Y., Mizuno, Y., Yoshida, M., et al. (1995) Mutations in the dystrophin-associated protein γ-sarcoglycan in chromosome 13 muscular dystrophy. *Science* **270,** 819–822.
7. Lim, L. E., Duclos, F., Broux, O., Bourg, N., Sunada Y., Allamand, V., et al. (1995) β-Sarcoglycan (43 DAG): characterization and role in limb-girdle muscular dystrophy linked to chromosome 4q12. *Nature Genet.* **11,** 257–265.
8. Bönnemann, C. G., Modi, R., Noguchi, S., Mizuno, Y., Yoshida, M., Gussoni, E., et al. (1995) β-Sarcoglycan (A3b) mutations cause autosomal recessive muscular dystrophy with loss of the sarcoglycan complex. *Nature Genet.* **11,** 266–273.
9. Nigro, V., de Sà Moreira, E., Piluso, G., Vainzof, M., Belsito, A., Politano, L., et al. (1996) Autosomal recessive limb-girdle muscular dystrophy, LGMD2F, is caused by a mutation in the δ-sarcoglycan gene. *Nature Genet.* **14,** 195–198.
10. Bashir, R., Strachan, T., Keers, S., Stephenson, A., Mahjneh, I., Marconi, G., Nashef, L., and Bushby, K. M. D. (1994) A gene for autosomal recessive limb-girdle muscular dystrophy maps to chromosome 2p. *Hum. Mol. Genet.* **3,** 455–457.
11. Bashir, R., Britton, S., Strachan, T., Keers, S., Vafiadaki, E., Lako, M., et al. (1998) A gene related to the *C. elegans* spermatogenesis factor fer-1 is mutated in limb-girdle muscular dystrophy type 2B. *Nat. Genet.* **20,** 37–42.
12. Liu, J., Aoki, M., Illa, I., Wu, C., Fardeau, M., Angelini, C., Serrano, C., et al. (1998) Dysferlin, a novel skeletal muscle gene, is mutated in Miyoshi myopathy and linb-girdle muscular dystrophy. *Nat. Genet.* **24,** 31–36.
13. Moreira, E. S., Wiltshire, T. J., Faulkner, G., Nilforoushan, A., Vainzof, M., et al. (2000) Limb-girdle muscular dystrophy type 2G is caused by mutations in the gene encoding the sarcomeric protein telethonin. *Nat. Genet.* **24,** 163–166.
14. Moreira, E. S., Vainzof, M., Marie, S. K., Sertié, A. L., Zatz, M., and Passos-Bueno, M.-R. (1997) The seventh form of autosomal recessive Limb-girdle muscular dystrophy is mapped to 17q11-12. *Am. J. Hum. Genet.* **61,** 151–156.
15. Beckmann, J. S., Richard, I., Hillaire, D., Broux, O., Antignac, C., Bois, E., Cann, H., et al. (1991) A gene for limb-girdle muscular dystrophy maps to chromosome 15 by linkage analysis. *C. R. Acad. Sci. Paris III* **312,** 141–148.
16. Fougerousse, F., Broux, O., Richard, I., Allamand, V., Pereira de Souza, A., Bourg, N., et al. (1994) Mapping of a chromosome 15 region involved in limb-girdle muscular dystrophy. *Hum. Mol. Genet.* **3,** 285–293.
17. Allamand, V., Broux, O., Richard, I., Fougerousse, F., Chiannilkulchai, N., Bourg, N., et al. (1995) Preferential localization of the limb-girdle muscular dystrophy type 2A gene in the proximal part of a 1 cM 15q15.1-q15.3 interval. *Am. J. Hum. Genet.* **56,** 1417–1430.

18. Chiannilkulchai, N., Pasturaud, P., Richard, I., Auffray, C., and Beckmann, J. S. (1995) A primary expression map of chromosome 15q15 region containing the recessive form of limb-girdle muscular dystrophy (LGMD2A) gene. *Hum. Mol. Genet.* **4,** 717–726.
19. Richard, I., Broux, O., Allamand, V., Fougerousse, F., Chiannilkulchai, N., Bourg, N., et al. (1995) Mutations in the proteolytic enzyme, calpain 3, cause limb-girdle muscular dystrophy type 2A. *Cell* **81,** 27–40.
20. Sorimachi, H., Imajoh-Ohmi, S., Emori, Y., Kawasaki, H., Ohno, S., Minami, Y., and Suzuki, K. (1989) Molecular cloning of a novel mammalian calcium-dependent protease distinct from both m- and mu- type. Specific expression of the mRNA in skeletal muscle. *J. Biol. Chem.* **264,** 20,106–20,111.
21. Croall, D. E. and Demartino, G. N. (1991) Calcium-activated neutral protease (calpain) system: structure, function, and regulation. *Physiol. Rev.* **71,** 813–847.
22. Suzuki, K., Sorimachi, H., Yoshizawa, T., Kinbara, K., and Ishiura, S. 1995. Calpain: novel family members, activation, and physiological function. *Biol. Chem.* **376,** 523–529.
23. Sorimachi, H., Ishiura, S., and Suzuki, K. (1997) Structure and physiological function of calpains. *Biochem. J.* **328,** 721–732.
24. Richard, I. and Beckmann, J. S. (1995) How neutral are synonymous codon mutations? *Nature Genet.* **10,** 259.
25. Richard, I., Brenguier, L., Dinçer, P., Roudaut, C., Bady, B., Burgunder, J.-M., et al. (1997) Multiple Independant molecular etiology for LGMD2A patients from various geographical origins. *Am. J. Hum. Genet.* **60,** 1128–1138.
26. Dinçer, P., Leturcq, F., Richard, I., Piccolo, F., Yalnizoglu, D., de Toma, C., Broux, O., et al. (1997) A biochemical, genetic and clinical survey of autosomal recessive limb-girdle muscular dystrophies in Turkey. *Ann. Neurol.* **42,** 222–229.
27. Richard, I., Roudaut, C., Saenz, A., Pogue, R., et al. (1999) Calpainopathy: A survey of mutations and polymorphisms. *Am. J. Hum. Genet.* **64,** 1524–1540.
28. Fougerousse, F., Durand, M., Suel, L., Pourquié, O., Delezoide, A-L., Roméro, N., Abitbol, M., and Beckmann, J. S. (1998) Expression of genes (CAPN3, SGCA, SGCB, and TTN) involved in progressive muscular dystrophies during early human development. *Genomics* **48,** 145–156.
29. Ma, H., Fukiage, C., Azuma, M., and Shearer, T. R. (1998) Cloning and expression of mRNA for calpain Lp82 from rat lens: splice variant of p94. *Invest. Ophthalmol. Visual Sci.* **39,** 454–461.
30. Herasse, M., Ono, Y., Fougerousse, F., Kimura E., Beley, C., Montarras, D., Pinset, C., et al. (1999) Expression and functional characteristics of Calpain 3 isoforms generated through tissue-specific transcriptional and post-transcriptional events. *Mol. Cell. Biol.* **19,** 4047–4055.
31. Orita, M., Iwahana, H., Kanazawa, H., Hayashi, K., and Sekiya, T. (1989) Detection of polymorphisms of human DNA by gel electrophoresis as single-strand conformation polymorphisms. *Proc. Natl. Acad. Sci. USA* **86,** 2766–2770.
32. Keen, J., Lester, D., Inglehearn, C., Curtis, A., and Bhattacharya, S. (1991) Rapid detection of single base mismatches as heteroduplexes on Hydrolink gels. *Trends Genet.* **7,** 5.

33. Chelly, J., Condorcet, J.-P., Kaplan, J. C., and Kahn, A. (1989) Illegitimate transcription: Transcription of any genes in any cell type. *Proc. Natl. Acad. Sci. USA* **86,** 2617–2621.
34. Don, R. H., Cox, P. T., Wainwright, B. J., Baker, K., and Mattick, J. S. (1991) 'Touchdown' PCR to circumvent spurious priming during gene amplification. *Nucleic Acid Res.* **19,** 4008.
35. Myers, R. M., Maniatis, T., and Lerman, L. S. (1987) Detection and localisation of single base changes by denaturing gradient gel electrophoresis. *Methods Enzymol.* **155,** 501–527.
36. Verpi, E., Biasotto, M., Meo, T., and Tosi, M. (1994). Efficient detection of point mutations on color-coded strands of target DNA. *Proc. Natl. Acad. Sci. USA* **91,** 1873–1877.
37. Roberts, R. G., Bentley, D. R., and Bobrow, M. (1993) Infidelity in the structure of ectopic transcripts: a novel exon in lymphocyte dystrophin transcripts. *Human Mut.* **2,** 293–299.

17

Molecular Investigation of LGMD2B-Haplotype Analysis and Mutation Screening

Rumaisa Bashir, Ruth Harrison, and Robert H. Brown, Jr.

1. Introduction

The limb-girdle muscular dystrophies (LGMDs) are generally characterized by weakness and atrophy of the proximal muscles. In 1994, the authors localized a form of autosomal recessive LGMD (LGMD2B) to chromosome 2p13 *(1)*. Patients with LGMD2B have proximal muscle weakness with onset in the late teens, and highly elevated serum creatine kinase levels: The progression of the disease is generally slow. Muscle CT scanning in some patients indicates involvement of the distal muscles. This finding is relevant, because a distal myopathy, termed "Miyoshi Myopathy" (MM), was also mapped to the same genetic interval as LGMD2B, suggesting allelic heterogeneity *(3)*. MM is characterized by weakness of the distal muscles in the early stages of the disease, and, like LGMD2B, is inherited as autosomal recessive, with onset also in the late teens, and elevated serum creatine kinase levels.

Further evidence that LGMD2B and MM were indeed allelic came from reports *(4,5)* of two large inbred families whose affected members shared the same chromosome 2 haplotypes, yet displayed either the LGMD2B or the MM phenotypes. In the absence of an obvious positional and functional candidate, the authors pursued a positional cloning approach toward identification of the LGMD2B gene. Haplotype analysis of informative LGMD2B families allowed identification of key recombinants that mapped the gene immediately distal to the microsatellite marker, D2S291, which was consistently regarded as the closest marker to the gene.

The authors also identified an expressed sequence tag highly expressed in skeletal muscle and mapping close to D2S291 *(6)*. Sequencing of genomic clones

From: *Methods in Molecular Medicine, vol. 43 : Muscular Dystrophy: Methods and Protocols*
Edited by: K. M. D. Bushby and L. V. B. Anderson

identified exons of this candidate gene, and mutations were found in patients with LGMD2B and MM *(6,7)*. The authors have named this gene "dysferlin," reflecting its role in MD, and its homology to a Caenor-habditis *elegans* protein, FER-1, which is a spermatogenesis factor that has a role in membrane fusion, since, in mutant fer-1 sperm, large membranous vesicles are unable to fuse with the plasma membrane, resulting in sterility *(8)*. Like *fer-1*, dysferlin is a large gene, with an open reading frame of 6 kb arranged across 56 exons spanning more than 150 kb *(9)*. Dysferlin is characterized by a C-terminal anchor and four C2 domains that bind calcium and phospholipid like many other proteins, such as the synaptotagmins *(10)*, which are also involved in membrane fusion. Many mutations have been found in patients with LGMD2B and MM, and these are randomly distributed across the gene, with no apparent hot spots, although several founder mutations, in the Libyan Jews *(6,11)* and the Canadian Aborigines *(12)*, have been reported. A monoclonal antibody, targeted close to the C-terminus, is available, and has confirmed that dysferlin is anchored to the plasma membrane *(13)*, probably facing the cytoplasm. With the availability of specific antibodies and freely available intronic primer sequences to at least 38 exons, estimates of the frequency of dysferlinopathy and genotype–phenotype correlations are now possible.

1.1. Investigative Strategies for Identifying Dysferlinopathy.

Because of the heterogeneity of LGMD, any muscle samples positive for dystrophin, the sarcoglycans, and caveolin-3 are all potential candidates for involvement of dysferlin. The authors believe that an integrated clinical, protein-based (*see* Chapter 19), and genetic approach will be the most efficient approach towards identifying patients with dysferlinopathy. This integrated approach will sometimes be limited, because muscle samples and DNA from family members may not be available for immunofluorescence and haplotype analysis, but, where possible, the protein and genetic analysis should be performed, and will be very useful in directing mutation screening, especially since the dysferlin gene is so big and is not expressed in lymphoblastoid cells, thus requiring genomic DNA for mutation screening.

1.1.1. Microsatellite Analysis

There are many markers mapping to the LGMD2B/MM locus that can be used to generate haplotypes for diagnosis (**Table 1**). The markers that are most useful are marked with an asterisk, but, if these are uninformative, the additional markers shown in the table should be analyzed. The authors have identified a single polymerase chain reaction (PCR) program that is effective for the amplification of all of the markers listed, and have analyzed them radioactively by kinase-labeling the forward primer for the PCR reaction. PCR reac-

Table 1
Microsatellites Mapping to LGMD2B Region

Marker	Primer sequences (5'-3')	Product size (bp)
104-SAT	AGGAATGAGATTAATCCGTGTG GGGAAAATTCTATGAGT	156
Cy172-H32	CCTCTCTTCTGCTGTCTTCAG TGTGTCTGGTTCACCTTCGTG	199
D2S2443	GAGAGGGCAAGACTTGGAAG ATGGAAGAGCGTTCTAAAACA	250
D2S292	GCATGATGAACCCCACTG TGTGATGGAACCAAATTCAA	190
D2S327	GCTGTCCCAGATACAGGACT TGGGCACACAGTGTTTTG	129
D2S291	TGGCCCCAAGTTGGATTT CCCCCTAGCCATCCTAGACG	184
D2S1394	GGCATCTTTATCCTTAGCCC CGGGGTCTGCATTACAGTAT	156
D2S2110	AAGGGTAGTATGTCACTCCATT GCTTACCATATGATCAGGGG	200
D2S2111	CAGGAATGCTAGTGCATACACTC ACCCTCATGCTGGTCGTAAT	216

tions are performed independently, and the polyacrylamide gel electrophoresis (PAGE) is multiplexed, so that up to three different markers can be resolved on the same gel, as long as their products differ by 20–25 bp. However, many laboratories are now using the ABI automated sequencer for multiplex genotyping using fluorescently tagged primers, and, if this resource is available, it will speed the genotype analysis considerably, and also has the added advantage of not using radiation.

1.1.2. Multiplex SSCP and HA

The authors use single-strand conformation polymorphism (SSCP) analysis and heteroduplex analysis (HA) for mutation screening, because these techniques are simple, quick, and relatively cheap, and do not require elaborate equipment. Intronic primer sequences to 38 exons of dysferlin are presented in **Table 2**, together with additional information on their location in the cDNA, and optimal amplification conditions. Following PCR, SSCP and HA are performed simultaneously on the same gel, followed by silver staining. Any bands consistently migrating differentially are subcloned for sequencing.

Table 2
Amplification of Dysferlin Exons for SSCP/HA

Exon	Sequence (5'-3') Forward	Reverse	Annealing temp. (°C)
1	GACCCACAAGCGGCGCCTCGG	GACCCCGGCGAGGGTGGTCGG	53
2	TGTCTCTCCATTCTCCCTTTTGTG	AGGACACTGCTGAGAAGGCACCTC	53
3	AGTGCCCTGGTGGCACGAAGG	CCTACCTGCACCTTCAAGCCATGG	56
4	CAGAAGAGCCAGGGTGCCTTAGG	CCTTGGACCTTAACCTGGCAGAGG	53
5	CGAGGCCAGCGCACCAACCTG	ACTGCCGGCCATTCTTGCTGGG	56
6	CCAGGCCTCATTAGGGCCCTC	CTGAAGAGGAGCCTGGGGTCAG	56
7	CTGAGATTTCTGACTCTTGGGGTG	AAGGTTCTGCCCTCATGCCCCATG	53
8	CTGGCCTGAGGGATCAGCAGG	GTGCATACATACAGCCCACGGAG	53
9	GAGCTATTGGGTTGGCCGTGTGGG	ACCAACACGGAGAAGTGAGAACTG	56
10	CCACACTTTATTTAACGCTTTGGCGG	CAGAACCAAAATGCAAGGATACGG	53
11	CTTCTGATTCTGGGATCACCAAAGG	GGACCGTAAGGAAGACCCAGGG	53
12	CCTGTGCTCAGGAGCGCATGAAGG	GCAGACCTCCCACCCAAGGGCG	53
13	GAGACAGATGGGGGACAGTCAGGG	CCTCCCGAGAGAACCCTCCTG	53
14	GGGAGCCCAGAGTCCCCATGG	GGGCCTCCTTGGGTTTGCTGG	53
15	GCCTCCCCAGCATCCTGCCGG	TCACTGAGCCGAATGAAACTGAGG	53
16	TGTGGCCTGAGTTCCTTTCCTGTG	GGTCAAAGGGCAGAACGAAGAGGG	56
17	CCCGTCCTTCTCCCAGCCATG	CTCCCCTGGTTGTCCCCAAGG	53
18	CGACCCCTCTGATTGCCACTTGTG	GGCATCCTGCCCTTGCCAGGG	53
19	TCTGTCTCCCCTGCTCCTTG	CTTCCCTGCCCCGACGCCCAG	53
20	GCTCCTCCCGTGACCCTCTGG	GGGTCCCAGCCAGGAGCACTG	56
21	CAGCGCTCAGGCCCGTCTCTC	TGCATAGGCATGTGCAGCTTTGGG	53
22	CATGCACCCTCTGCCCTGTGG	AGTTGAGCCAGGAGAGGTGGG	60
23	CATCAGGCGCATTCCATCTGTCCG	AGCAGGAGAGCAGAAGAAGAAAGG	56
24	GTGTGTCACCATCCCCACCCCG	CAAGAGATGGGAGAAAGGCCTTATG	56
25	CTGGGACATCCGGATCCTGAAGG	TCCAGGTAGTGGGAGGCAGAGG	56

26	TCCCACTACCTGGAGCTGCCTTGG	GGCTCTCCCCAGCCCTCCCTG	56
27	CAGAGCAGCAGAGACTCTGACCAG	TAGACCCCACCTGCCCCTGAG	56
28	TCCTCTCATTGCTTGCCTGTTCGG	TTGAGAGCTTGCCGGGGATGG	56
29	AAGTGCCAAGCAATGAGTGACCGG	CTCACTCCCACCCACCACCTG	56
30	CCCACCGGCCTCTGAGTCTGC	ACCCTACCCAAGCCAGGACAAGTG	53
31	GAATCTGCCATAACCAGCTTCGTG	TATCACCCCATAGAGGCCTCGAAG	56
32	CAGCCACTCACTCTGGCACCTCTG	AGCCCACAGTCTCTGACTCTCCTG	56
33	ACATCTCTCAGGGTCCCTGCTGTG	CCTGTGAGGGGACGAGGCAGG	56
34	GCCCTGGGTAAGGGATGCTGATTC	CCTGCCTGGGCCTCCTGGATC	56
35	GAGGGTGATGGGGGCCTTAGG	GCAATCAGTTTGAAGAAGGAAAGG	56
36	CCCCTCTCACCATCTCCTGATGTG	GGCTTCACCTTCCCTCTACCTCGG	60
37	CACCTTTGTCTCCATTCTACCTGC	CTCCCAGCCCCCACGCCCAGG	56
38	CTGAGCCACTCTCCTCATTCTGTG	TGGAAGGGGACAGTAGGGAGG	60
39	GGCCAGTGCGTTCTTCCTCCTC	TCCCTGACCTGCCCATCATCTC	56
40	GCCCCTGTCAGGCCTGGATGG	TGACCCAGGCCTCCCTGGAGG	56
41	CTGAAATGGTCTCTTTCTTTCTAC	CACACCGACTGTCAGACTGAAGAG	50
42	TTGTCCCCTCCTCTAATCCCCATG	GGGTTAGGGACGTCTTCGAGG	60
43	CAGCCAAACCATATCAACAATG	CTGGGGAGGTGAGGGCTCTAG	56
44	GAAGTGTTTTGTCTCCTCCTC	ACTAGACTGTGGGTTATCCTGT	56
45	GGGTGCCCTGTGTTGGCTGAC	GCAGGCAGCCAGCCCCCATC	56
46	CTCGTCTATGTCTTGTGCTTGCTC	CACCATGGTTTGGGGTCATGTGG	60
47	TCTCGCTTCCCCAGCTCCTGC	TCTGGAGTTCGAGGACTCTGGG	56
48	AGAAGGGTGGGGAGAGAACGG	CAGCTCAGAGCCTGTGGCTGG	56
49	AAGGCCTTCCCATCCTTTGGTAGG	ACAACCCAGAGGGAGCACGGG	60
50	GTTGACGATGTATATACTGTGTTGG	GCTGGCACCACAGGGAATCGG	56
51	GCCTCTCTCTAACTTTGCTTCCTTG	AGCCCCCATGTGCAGAATGGG	56
52	GGCTACAGGCTGGCAGTGATCGAG	TTCCCCCATGCCCTCCACTGG	56
53	AGCCTTCGTGCCCCTAACCAAGTG	CTGTGGGCATTGGGGCTCAGG	56
54	GGATGCCCAGTTGACTCCGGG	CCCCACCACAGTGTCGTCAGG	56
55	GCCCCAGTGGGATCACCATG	ATGCTGGAGGGGACCCCACGG	56

1.1.3. Sequencing of Subcloned PCR Products

Any samples showing mobility shifts by SSCP and HA are further analyzed by sequencing, to characterize any sequence changes. The authors prefer to subclone the PCR products and sequence both strands using vector primers rather than direct sequencing. DNA from at least five independent clones is sequenced following the ABI automated DNA sequencer guidelines. The authors use the Bigdye [HG1] dye terminator or the dye primer sequencing kits, although there are many other kits and manual sequencing methods that can also be used.

2. Materials

2.1. Nonradioactive PCR

1. Sterile 0.5-mL and 1.5-mL microcentrifuge tubes (Sarstedt) or thermowell 96 well PCR plates (Greiner, Solingen, Germany; or Costar, Cambridge, MA).
2. 5-mL sterile bijous or tubes.
3. Sterile 2–5 µL, 200 µL, and 1 mL pipet tips.
4. Molecular-biology grade water (BDH, London) filter-sterilize or autoclave.
5. Template DNA: approx 100 ng/µL.
6. 10X *Taq* polymerase buffer (Promega): 100 m*M* Tris-HCl, pH 9.0, 500 m*M* KCl, 15 m*M* $MgCl_2$. The buffer is available with and without $MgCl_2$, to allow calibration. The authors prefer to use the buffer with $MgCl_2$ f.c. 1.5 m*M*.
7. Deoxyribonucleoside triphosphate (dNTP) mix (Boehringer Mannheim): Stocks are 100 m*M*. Pipet 100 µL each of the dNTPs into a sterile 5-mL container, and dilute 50-fold, i.e., add 4.6 mL sterile molecular biology water, to give a working solution of 2 m*M*. Store at –20°C as 1-mL aliquots.
8. Primers: See Table 1 for microsatellite primers, and Table 2 for the SSCP/HA primers for mutation screening. The authors usually synthesize 50 n*M* primers requesting standard purity. The primers are resuspended in 1 mL molecular-biology-grade H_2O, to a concentration of 100 µ*M*, to yield stocks that are stored at –20°C. When necessary, the stocks are diluted 10-fold, to give 10 µ*M* working solutions, which are also stored at –20°C. Forward and reverse primers are used at equal concentration, with a final concentration in the PCR reaction of 0.25–0.5 µ*M*.
9. Taq DNA polymerase (Promega): usual concentration is 5 µ/µL. Other sources for the enzyme include Pharmacia, Boehringer Mannheim, and Perkin-Elmer (Norwalk, CT). Store at –20°C.
10. Mineral oil (Sigma).
11. Electrophoresis buffer, 10X Tris-acetate–EDTA (TAE): (0.4 *M* Tris-acetate; 0.01 *M* EDTA). Weigh 48.4 g Trizma base (Sigma) in 900 mL molecular-grade water containing 20 mL 0.5 *M* EDTA. Adjust the pH to 8.2 using 12 mL glacial acetic acid, and adjust the volume to 1 L. Note that EDTA is insoluble in water, until the pH is adjusted to 8.0 with 5 *M* NaOH. For electrophoresis, 10X TAE is diluted 10 fold, to yield a working solution of 1X TAE.

12. Agarose: SeaKem LE from FMC Bioproducts (Rockland, ME), or any other molecular-biology-grade.
13. Ethidium bromide (EtBr) (2 μg/mL).
14. Loading buffer (6X concentrated solution): 0.25% bromophenol blue, 0.25% xylene cyanol, and 40% (w/v) sucrose or 30% glycerol (all from Sigma), made up to volume with molecular biology water and stored at 4°C. Working concentrate is 1X.
15. 1 kb and 100 bp DNA size marker (Promega): Dilute with the accompanying loading buffer, to give a working solution of 1 μg/20 μL, and use 10–20 μL.
16. Equipment: automated thermocycler (Hybaid Omnigene, Tedington, UK; or Perkin-Elmer Cetus), electrophoresis tanks (Pharmacia GNA100 [100-mL capacity] or GNA200 [200-mL capacity]) with 14-well or 22-well combs, power supply (Pharmacia; Bio-Rad, Hercules, CA), UV transilluminator, visor, gloves, and face mask.

2.2. Radioactive PCR

Microsatellites are analyzed by radioactive PCR, which involves three steps: kinase, or end-labeling, of the forward PCR primer; radioactive PCR; and separation of the fragments on large denaturing polyacrylamide gels (PAGs). Radioactive PCR needs **items 1–10** described in **Subheading 2.1.**, and, in addition the following:

1. Redivue [γ-32P] deoxyadenosine triphosphate (dATP) at 10 mCi/mL (Amersham, ICN). Can store up to a month at 4°C.
2. T4 polynucleotide kinase (New England Biolabs, Beverly, MA; Promega, and so on) at a concentration of 10 U/μL. Store at –20°C.
3. T4 kinase buffer (10X): 700 m*M* Tris-HCl, pH 7.6, 50 m*M* dithrothreitol, 100 m*M* $MgCl_2$. This is usually supplied with the enzyme and the f.c. is 1X.
4. Sequagel concentrate (National Diagnostics).
5. *N,N,N',N'*,-tetramethylethylenediamine (TEMED) (Sigma).
6. 25% Ammonium persulphate (APS) (Sigma).
7. 10X Tris-borate–EDTA TBE electrophoresis buffer, 1 *M* Tris-borate, 0.02 *M* EDTA. Dissolve 108 g Trisma base (Sigma) and 55 g boric acid (Sigma) in 850 mL molecular-biology-grade water, add 40 mL 0.5 *M* EDTA (pH 8.0), and adjust volume to 1 L. Dilute 10-fold, to make working solution.
8. Stop buffer: 10 m*M* EDTA, 0.05% bromophenol blue, 0.05% xylene cyanol, and 98% v/v formamide (Sigma, BDH). Store at room temperature.
9. Pyroneg or any laboratory detergent for washing the plates and the spacers.
10. Repelcote (VS) (BDH).
11. 10% methanol/10% acetic acid (v/v) fixing solution. The authors only fix the gels after PAGE if there is not a quick exposure (>50 count on gel, and within a few hours).
12. 95% ethanol.
13. N-Dex nitrile gloves (Best Manufacturing).

14. Kodak Biomax X-ray film.
15. Saran Wrap or cling film.
16. 3MM blotting paper (Whatman).
17. Equipment: sequencing apparatus (gels, combs, and tank) (Bio-Rad), Geiger counter, gel dryer, incubator, hot block, cassettes, and trays.

2.3. Single-Strand Conformational Polymorphism/HA

Need **items 1–10** described in **Subheading 2.1.**, and **items 5–9** and **12–14** in **Subheading 2.2.** In addition, the following:

1. MDE gel solution (Flowgen). This is mutation-detection enhancement Hydrolink acrylamide.
2. 10% APS.
3. Plastic pipets.
4. Gell Saver II Fine Pipette tips (Laboratory Sales).
5. Potean II xi system (Bio-Rad) or Hoefer Sturdier Vertical Gel Electrophoresis Units (Pharmacia Biotech).

2.4. Subcloning and Sequencing

1. 90-mm Petri dishes.
2. pGEM-T Easy Vector Systems (Promega).
3. PCR amplified DNA to be sequenced (1–2 µL of a 20 µL reaction).
4. JM109 high-efficiency competent cells (Promega).
5. 0.1 *M* isopropylthio-β-D-galactoside (IPTG) stock solution (Sigma, Boehringer Mannheim): Dissolve 1.2 g in 50 mL water and filter-sterilize. Store frozen.
6. *N,N'*-dimethyl-formamide (BDH, Sigma).
7. 50 mg/mL (X-Gal) (Sigma, Boehringer Mannheim): Dissolve 100 mg 5-bromo-4-chloro-3-indolyl-β-D-galactoside in 2 mL dimethylformamide. Cover the tube in aluminum foil, and store at –20°C.
8. LB medium: Dissolve 10 g tryptone, 5 g yeast extract (Oxoid, Basingstoke, UK; Difco E Molesley, Surrey, UK) and 5 g NaCl in 950 mL sterile water, adjust the pH to 7.0, bring to 1 L with water, and autoclave. Store at room temperature.
9. 50 mg/mL Ampicillin (Sigma): Dissolve 1 g in 20 mL water and filter-sterilize. Store as 5-mL aliquots at –20°C.
10. LB agar with ampicillin–IPTG–X-Gal: Add 15 g agar (Oxoid, Difco) to the bottle before adding 1 L LB medium. Autoclave, cool to 50°C, and add 200 µL ampicillin, 5 mL IPTG, and 1.6 mL X-Gal. Mix gently, and pour plates. After the plates have set, store them at 4°C, covered in foil.
11. Glass spreader for plating cells.
12. 95% ethanol.
13. Sterile loops.
14. QIAprep Spin Miniprep Kit (Qiagen).
15. ABI Bigdye Dye Terminator Cycle Sequencing Kits (Perkin-Elmer): Kits for 24, 100, 1000, and 5000 reactions are available. The authors normally buy the 100 reactions.

16. Equipment: 37°C incubator with and without a shaking platform, Mistral centrifuge, microcentrifuge, Perkin-Elmer DNA thermocycler, ABI Sequencer 373/377.

3. Methods

3.1 Radioactive PCR

1. Thaw the forward microsatellite primer, 10X T4 polynucleotide kinase buffer, and store on ice, along with the T4 polynucleotide kinase.
2. Set up the kinase-labeling reaction as described:

   Example

	1 sample (μL)	10 samples (μL)
Forward primer (10 μ*M*)	0.2	2 (f.c. 2 pmols)
T4 poly-nt kinase buffer (10X)	3.0	3 (f.c. 1X)
[γ^{32}P] dATP (10 mCi/mL)	1.0	1 (10 μCi)
T4 poly-nt kinase (10 U/μL)	1.0	1 (10 U)
Sterile H_2O	23.8	23.8
Total volume	30	30

   We use approx 0.5 μCi/sample, but always to the nearest μL. Therefore if 30 samples are to be amplified we will use 30 μCi of radiation and the reactions are always performed in a total volume of 30 μL.
3. Incubate the labeling reaction at 37°C for 45 min.
4. While the forward primer is labeling, make the PCR master mix. Thaw the reverse primer, dNTPs, *Taq* polymerase buffer, and patient DNA.
5. Make the PCR master mix, minus the DNA, as below:

   Example

	10 samples (μL)
Reverse primer (10 μ*M*)	2 (f.c. 2 pmols)
dNTPs (2 m*M*)	10 (f.c. 0.2 m*M*)
10X Taq polymerase buffer (10X)	10 (f.c. 1X)
Kinase-labeled mix	30
Taq polymerase (5 U/μL)	1 (0.5 U)
Sterile H_2O	37
DNA	10 (50–100 ng)
Total volume	100

   Always make more mix than needed, e.g., if 15 samples are to be amplified, make enough mix for 20 samples.
6. Aliquot 9 μL PCR mix into appropriately labeled PCR tubes or wells, if using the thermowell plates for PCR.
7. Add 1 μL DNA into each tube or well, and mix the contents by pipeting.

8. Overlay with a drop or 50 μL mineral oil, and transfer the tubes or the plate to the DNA thermocycler.
9. Program the machine according to the manufacturer's instructions, using the following PCR program: denaturation at 94°C for 4 min for 1 cycle, followed by denaturation at 94°C for 30 s, annealing at 55°C for 1 min, and extension at 72°C for 1 min, for 30 cycles. Evening PCR runs should have an extra soaking step of 4°C after the run is complete.

3.2. Polyacrylamide Gel Electrophoresis

3.2.1. Casting the Gel

1. Wash both the front and the back plate and the spacers with Pyroneg or other laboratory detergent, and dry.
2. Wash the front and the back plate with 95% ethanol, and air-dry.
3. Silanize the back plate (the one with the buffer tank), using Repelcote.
4. Assemble the plates and clamp.
5. Make 6% denaturing gel mix as described below:

Small gel (21 × 50; maximum 34 samples)		Big gel (38 × 50; maximum 68 samples)
66 mL	8 *M* Urea	132 mL
24 mL	Sequagel	48 mL
10 mL	10X TBE	20 mL

Mix well.

6. Place two strips of 3MM paper into the casting tray, to form the wick for the plug.
7. Place the assembled gel plates into the casting tray, and use the screws in the casting tray to fit the gel firmly.
8. Make the plug by mixing 25 mL (small gel) or 50 mL (big gel) of the gel mixture from above with 150 or 300 μL 25% ammonium sulphate and 150 and 300 μL TEMED, respectively.
9. Mix, and pour the plug immediately into the casting tray, to set.
10. After 5 min, check that the gel in the plug has solidified, using a pair of tweezers.
11. Pour some water into the buffer chamber in the back plate, so that the electrode is covered (this protects the electrode from any polymerized acrylamide).
12. When the plug is ready, pour the gel by adding 300 or 600 μL 25% APS and 30 and 60 μL TEMED to 75 mL (small gel) or 150 mL (big gel) of the gel mixture from above, respectively.
13. Mix, and pour the mixture into a plastic squeezy bottle.
14. Lift the gel assembly with the casting tray, at an angle, toward you, and start pouring the gel in a constant flow rate, but without any air bubbles (bubbles in the gel will distort the movement of the DNA).
15. Insert the appropriate comb, so that the edge of the wells is visible when looking at the apparatus from the top.

16. Pour some of the gel mixture on top of the comb, and allow the gel to set for a minimum of 1 h.
17. When the gel has set, remove the gel assembly from the casting tray, and discard any loose acrylamide from the bottom of the apparatus.
18. Place the gel assembly into the electrophoresis setup, and prepare the samples for loading.

3.2.2. Gel Loading and Electrophoresis

1. Prepare 2 L (big gel) or 1 L (small gel) of 1X TBE buffer, and warm in a microwave oven to 50°C.
2. Pour into the buffer chamber of the back plate and into the buffer tank.
3. Add 7 μL stop solution to the amplified DNA samples, and denature at 95°C for 3 min.
4. Remove the comb and wash the wells with 1X TBE buffer from the back chamber, using a plastic pipet to remove urea from the wells.
5. Load 3–4 μL of the samples, if using 0.75-mm-thickness well combs, and 1–2 μL for 0.4-mm-thickness well combs.
6. Electrophorese at 100 W, constant power for a large gel, and at 50 W, constant power for a small gel, for up to 3 h. The dye fronts of the dark blue bromophenol blue (26-bp–6% gel) and the light blue of xylene cyanol (120-bp–6% gel) in the stop mix are a good indicator of the fragment size, and the authors usually stop the electrophoresis when the light blue dye front is 15 cm from the bottom of the gel, for DNA fragments of 150–230 bp.
7. If you are multiplexing the PAGE, load the shorter amplified DNA fragments first, as described in step 5 above, and electrophorese at the conditions described above for 40 min, then stop the run, and load the larger DNA fragments. Electrophorese using the conditions described above, making sure that the shorter fragments have not migrated from the bottom of the gel.
8. After electrophoresis, remove the gel assembly from the tank, and pour the now-radioactive buffer carefully from the back chamber of the back plate down the sink.
9. Separate the gel plates, using your thumbs or a wedge.
10. The gel should remain attached to the front plate; monitor the gel, using a Geiger counter to assess the success of the amplification, using the dye fronts as an indicator for the position of the amplified fragments.
11. If the gel counts are less than 50, fix the gel on the front plate with 10% methanol/10% acetic acid solution for 5–10 min. Pour the fixer back in the bottle for reuse.
12. Place 3MM Whatman paper onto the gel, and ensure contact by pressing on the paper gently.
13. Lift the 3MM paper with the gel stuck to it, and cover with Clingfilm. Using a pen, mark the orientation of the samples on the gel.
14. Place on a gel dryer, with a sheet of 3MM paper below and above the gel, and dry at 70°C for 2–3 h.

15. When dry, place the gel in a cassette, and expose. Exposure times will vary, depending on the number of counts on the gel; for >50 counts, 3–6 h, and for less than 50 counts, an overnight exposure is usually necessary.

3.3. Nonradioactive or Cold PCR

1. Thaw the following components of the PCR reaction mix: forward and reverse primers, 10X *Taq* DNA polymerase buffer, dNTP mix, and template DNA, and pulse briefly in a microcentrifuge. Store on ice, along with the enzyme.
2. Make a PCR master mix without the DNA as described below:

   Example

	1 sample (µL)	10 samples (µL)
Forward primer (10 µ*M*)	1.3	13 (f.c. 0.25 µ*M*)
Reverse primer (10 µ*M*)	1.3	13 (f.c. 0.25 µ*M*)
dNTPs (2 m*M*)	2.5	25 (f.c. 200 µ*M*)
Buffer (10X)	2.5	25 (f.c. 1X)
Taq polymerase (5 U/µL)	0.1	1 (f.c. 0.5 U)
Sterile H_2O	16.3	163
DNA	1.0	10 (f.c. 50–100 ng)
Total volume	25	250

   Again, as for the radioactive PCR, always make more mix than for the actual number of samples. Also, always set up the appropriate controls, a –ve control 1 µL water, instead of DNA and a +ve control, which is a DNA sample known to give the required product.
3. Aliquot 24 µL PCR master mix into appropriately labeled PCR tubes or wells, if using microtiter plates.
4. Add 1.0 µL DNA sample to each tube or well, except the –ve control, to which 1 µL H_2O should be added.
5. Overlay with a drop or 50 µL mineral oil, and, if using tubes, microcentrifuge briefly to mix the contents.
6. Place the tubes or the plate into the thermocycler and program the machine according the manufacturer's instructions, using the following guidelines: denaturation at 94°C for 4 min for 1 cycle, followed by denaturation at 94°C for 30 s, annealing at 45–60°C (*see* **Table 1** for the annealing temperature for the exons) for 1 min, extension at 72°C for 1 min for 30 cycles, followed by a final extension step at 72°C for 10 min. If the program is running on the overnight slot, then an additional step of 4°C "on hold" should be added.
7. Prepare a 2% agarose gel in 1X TAE buffer, and add a drop of EtBr (2 µg/mL), and pour 100 mL (small gel) or 200 mL (big gel), depending on the number of samples to be analyzed.
8. To 5 µL amplified DNA, add 1 µL loading buffer and 5 µL water.
9. Mix, and load DNA into wells, including 10 µL of the 100-bp size ladder.

10. Electrophorese in 1X TAE buffer at 80 V for 2 h, and soak the gel in dH_2O, to remove unbound EtBr, and visualize under UV light.
11. If a clear single fragment of the expected is seen in the samples only, and not in the –ve control, the samples are ready for SSCP/HA.

3.4. Single-Strand Conformational Polymorphism/HA

3.4.1. Preparation of MDE Hydrolink Gel and Sample Loading

1. Clean the glass plates and the spacers with Pyroneg, rinse in 95% ethanol, and assemble the vertical gel apparatus according the manufacturer's instructions.
2. For 24 × 14 cm standard gels, 50 mL gel mix will be adequate: To 25 mL MDE Hydrolink acrylamide, add 3 mL 10X TBE buffer, 5 mL 50% glycerol, 300 μL 10% APS, and 75 μL TEMED. Mix by inverting the Falcon tube gently, and pour the gel, using a plastic pipet. Insert the comb, and allow to polymerize for 1 h.
3. To 7 μL PCR product, add 7 μL denaturing loading buffer, then denature the samples at 94°C for 5 min, and immediately place on ice.
4. Remove the combs from the polymerized gels, and wash the wells thoroughly with 0.6X TBE buffer.
5. Load the wells using the fine tips, and attach the plates to the gel-running apparatus according to the manufacturer's instructions and electrophorese at 140 V for 1 h, followed by 300 V overnight (or 18 h). If possible, cool the gel apparatus during electrophoresis by cold-water circulation through rubber tubing, or, alternatively, the samples can be electrophoresed in the cold room.
6. Following electrophoresis, dismantle the apparatus, and, using a wedge or your thumbs, pry apart the gel plates. The gel should remain attached on one plate.

3.5. Subcloning PCR Products for Sequencing

1. Amplify DNA samples from affected carrier(s) and controls, showing mobility shifts by SSCP/HA analysis, and electrophorese 5 μL of the reaction on 2% agarose gels, to assess specificity and concentration.
2. If the samples have amplified and a single band is present of the expected size, ligate 2 μL fresh DNA sample (do not freeze) into the pGEM T-Easy Vector, following the manufacturer's instructions.
3. Following ligation, transform the ligated insert into JM109-competent cells, according to the manufacturer's instructions.
4. Dry the required number of LB + ampicillin–IPTG–X-Gal plates in a 50°C oven, by removing the lids and placing the plate and the lid upside down on a tray for 10 min.
5. Plate 2× 50 μL transformation mixture onto LB–ampicillin–IPTG–X-Gal plates, using a glass spreader that has been sterilized by flaming, after soaking in 95% ethanol. Cover the plates with aluminium foil, and allow to dry at room temperature for 10 min.
6. Incubate the plates, agar-side-up, overnight at 37°C.
7. Pick five white single colonies (those without any satellite colonies), and innoculate 5 mL LB broth containing 100 μg/mL ampicillin. Grow overnight at 37°C.

8. Harvest the cells by centrifugation at 3000*g* for 10 min, and extract DNA, using the Qiaprep Spin Miniprep kit.
9. Analyze 5 μL extracted DNA on a 1% agarose gel with a 1 kb-size-ladder, to assess concentration.
10. Sequence 0.5–1 μg cloned DNA, using the ABI BigDye dye terminator cycle sequencing kit, and purify the products according to the manufacturer's instructions.
11. Prepare the PCR products for ABI 373/377 Sequencer.

4. Notes

1. If PCR contamination is a common problem, use a separate area for setting up PCR reactions with a dedicated set of pipets and presterilized self-sealing tips, such as the Aerosol Resistant Tips (Molecular Bio Products).
2. Aliquoting buffers and reagents for PCR also avoids contamination.
3. If you have problems amplifying the DNA, start by using fresh aliquots of all reagents and DNA. If the problem still persists, reduce the annealing temperatures by a few degrees. If this also fails, try different concentrations of Mg^{2+}. Normally, the *Taq* buffers with magnesium have 1.5 m*M* (f.c.) Mg^{2+} ions. Try using 1.8, 2, and 2.5 m*M*, annealing at the recommended temperature. If all else fails, redesign the primers.
4. **CAUTION:** EtBr is a powerful carcinogen, and should be handled with extreme care; gloves should be worn at all times.
5. The authors use the liquid concentrates of acrylamide and *bis*-acrylamide to reduce exposure to these neurotoxins, and also always wear nitrile gloves, rather than latex for protection.
6. **CAUTION:** Take care when handling TEMED: It is corrosive and flammable, and inhalation can be fatal.
7. A precipitate may form when concentrated solutions of TBE (10X) are stored for long periods, and any batches that develop a precipitate should be discarded.
8. **CAUTION:** Formamide and *N,N'*-dimethyl-formamide are both very toxic, and should be stored and dispensed in the fume hood.
9. Repelcote (BDH) has replaced dimethylchlorosilane, and is less toxic, so it can be handled on the bench, and is also ozone friendly.
10. The glass spreader is made by holding a glass pipet in a flame, until the end collapses to form a spreader. Sterilize by soaking in ethanol, and flaming.
11. The authors usually store ethanol for sterilization in a wide glass sealable container. Always store after use in a metal solvent container, and, when in use, keep away from the flames.

Acknowledgments

This work is supported by the Muscular Dystrophy Campaign, the Medical Research Council (UK), Action Research.

References

1. Bashir, R., et al. (1994) A gene for autosomal recessive limb-girdle muscular dystrophy maps to chromosome 2p. *Hum. Mol. Genet.* **3,** 455–457.
2. Mahjneh, I., et al. (1996) The phenotype of chromosome 2p-linked muscular dystrophy. *Neuromusc. Disord.* **6,** 483–490.
3. Bejeoui, K., et al. (1995) Linkage of Miyoshi myopathy (distal autosomal recessive muscular dystrophy) locus to chromosome 2p12-14. *Neurol*ogy **45,** 768–772.
4. Weiler, T., et al. (1996) Limb-girdle muscular dystrophy and Miyoshi Myopathy in an Aboriginal Canadian kindred map to LGMD2B and segregate with the same haplotype. *Am. J. Hum. Genet.* **59,** 872–878.
5. Illarioshkin, S. N., et al. (1997) Refined genetic location of the chromosome 2p-linked progressive muscular dystrophy gene. *Genomics* **42,** 345–348.
6. Bashir, R., et al. (1998) A gene related to the *Caenorh-abditis elegans* spermatogenesis factor *fer-1* is mutated in limb-girdle muscular dystrophy type 2B. *Nature Genet.* **20,** 37–42.
7. Liu, J., et al. (1998) Dysferlin, a novel skeletal muscle gene is mutated in Miyoshi myopathy and limb-girdle muscular dystrophy. *Nature Genet.* **20,** 31–36.
8. Achanzar, W. E., et al. (1997) A nematode gene required for sperm vesicle fusion. *J. Cell Sci.* **110,** 1073–1081.
9. Aoki, M., et al. (2000) Genomic organization and novel mutations in the dysferlin gene in Miyoshi myopathy and limb-girdle dystrophy Type 2B. *Neurol*ogy **53,** 1119–1122.
10. Rizo, J. and Sudhof, T. (1998) C2–domains, structure and function of a universal Ca^{2+} binding domain. *J. Biol. Chem.* **273,** 15,882–15,897.
11. Argov, Z., et al (2000) Cluster of dysferlin related muscular dystrophy in Libyan Jews-clinical and genetic features. *Brain* **123,** 1229–1237.
12. Weiler, T., et al. (1999) Identical mutations in patients with limb-girdle muscular dystrophy type 2B or Miyoshi myopathy suggests a role for modifier gene(s). *Hum. Mol. Genet.* **8,** 871–878.
13. Anderson, L. V. B., et al. (1999) Dysferlin is a plasma membrane protein and is expressed early in human development. *Hum. Mol. Genet.* **8,** 855–862.

18

Molecular Analysis of Facioscapulohumeral Muscular Dystrophy (FSHD1)

Silvère M. van der Maarel, Egbert Bakker, and Rune R. Frants

1. Introduction

Although facioscapulohumeral muscular dystrophy (FSHD) is genetically heterogeneous, in 97% of cases the disease is associated with a submicroscopic rearrangement on 4q35 (FSHD1). This rearrangement is the result of deletions of an integral number of tandemly arrayed 3.3-kb repeat units *(1,2)*. The repeat number in the normal population varies between 12 and 100 copies, but FSHD1 patients consistently show one allele with 12 copies or less. Because the entire repeat array resides on a single *Eco*RI fragment, the rearrangement can be demonstrated by an *Eco*RI digestion, followed by hybridization with the probe, p13E-11, recognizing a sequence of this restriction fragment proximal to the repeat units themselves (**Fig. 1**; *1*). Southern analysis has been complicated by the presence of a highly homologous repeat array of similar size on chromosome (chr) 10 *(3)*. In most cases, chr-10-derived repeat units can be discriminated from chr-4-derived units by a chr-10-specific *Bln*I restriction site within each repeat unit (**Fig. 1**; *4*). In 20% of the population, an exchange between chr-10- and chr-4 derived repeat units has been observed, complicating FSHD1 diagnosis in approx 1% of cases *(5)*. Because of these complex rearrangements, and because of the size of the repeat array (*Eco*RI fragments ranging from 7 to 300 kb), the authors strongly encourage use of pulsed-field gel electrophoresis (PFGE) for the molecular analysis of FSHD1, which will enable visualization of all 4q35 and 10q26 alleles.

By combining PFGE with frequent cutting-restriction enzymes, such as *Eco*RI (the repeat arrays reside on an *Eco*RI restriction fragment) and *Bln*I (to

From: *Methods in Molecular Medicine, vol. 43: Muscular Dystrophy: Methods and Protocols*
Edited by: K. M. D. Bushby and L. V. B. Anderson © Humana Press Inc., Totowa, NJ

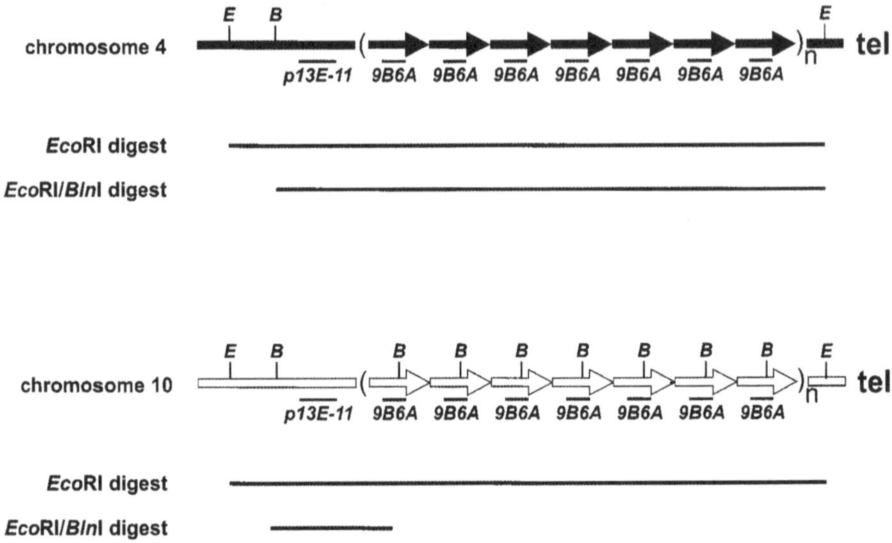

Fig. 1. Schematic representation of the chr-4 and chr-10 subtelomeric repeat arrays involved in FSHD. Filled arrow represents the chr-4 repeat unit; open arrows, chr-10-derived repeat units. The number of arrows may vary. *Eco*RI and *Bln*I restriction sites are indicated with an E and B, respectively. The probes, p13E-11 and 9B6A, are drawn at the probe-recognition site. A line beneath the chrs represents the resulting fragments after *Eco*RI and *Eco*RI/*Bln*I digestion, respectively.

discriminate between chr-4- and chr-10-derived repeat units), salt-extracted liquid DNA can be applied for this analysis, which circumvents the time-consuming procedure of immobilizing cells in agarose plugs, but requires careful handling of the liquid DNA. Therefore, in this laboratory, much emphasis has been placed on DNA extraction (adapted from ref. *6*) and handling during the entire procedure.

The PFGE apparatus at the authors' disposal is a homemade device. Therefore, the running conditions for PFGE analysis employed will not be directly applicable in other cases, and it is inappropriate to extensively describe the running conditions for this gel system. Protocol here is limited to the definition of the parameters of importance for proper size separation.

The probe, p13E-11 (D4S104F), used for analysis, is a single-copy fragment from a region proximal to the repeat array *(1)*. This probe only recognizes the chr 4 and chr 10 repeat arrays and a 9.5-kb Y-allele, but not the other homologous repeat arrays dispersed over the genome. To visualize the repeat unit itself, the authors often rehybridize the blot with probe 9B6A (D4Z4), which recognizes 320 bp of the repeat unit proper

(1). This hybridization may be very helpful in case of inconsistent results after hybridization with p13E-11.

In most laboratories, normal Southern blot analysis is performed for molecular FSHD1 diagnosis. However, because of the size of the normal repeat arrays (35–300 kb), this technique fails to recognize all four alleles. With accumulating evidence for dynamic recurrent subtelomeric rearrangements on chr 4 and chr 10 *(5,7)*, it is of importance to be able to identify all four alleles. Therefore, the protocol described is written for PFGE. However, the protocol can also be applied for conventional Southern blot analysis.

2. Materials

2.1. DNA Isolation

1. Erythrocyte lysis buffer: 155 m*M* NH_4Cl, 10 m*M* $KHCO_3$, 1 m*M* Na_2-EDTA, pH 7.4.
2. Nucleus lysis buffer: 10 m*M* Tris-HCl, pH 8.2, 2 m*M* Na_2-EDTA, 400 m*M* NaCl.
3. 20% Sodium dodecyl sulphate (SDS).
4. Pronase (20 mg/mL).
5. 6 *M* NaCl (saturated).
6. 96% Ethanol.
7. 70% Ethanol.
8. Tris-EDTA (TE): 10 m*M* Tris-HCl (pH 8.0), 1 m*M* Na_2-EDTA. Autoclaved.

2.2. Restriction Enzyme Digestion

1. *Eco*RI.
2. *Bln*I.
3. Restriction buffer: 5 m*M* Tris-HCl (pH 7.5), 1 m*M* $MgCl_2$, 10 m*M* NaCl, supplemented with 3.3 m*M* spermidine.
4. 6X loading buffer: 0.25% bromophenol blue, 0.25% xylene cyanol, 15% Ficoll (400) in H_2O.

2.3. Gel Electrophoresis

1. 1% PFGE-grade agarose in 0.5X Tris-borate–EDTA (TBE) (PFGE) or 1% agarose (Agarose MP, Boehringer) in 1X TBE (conventional gel electrophoresis).
2. 0.5X TBE: 45 m*M* Tris-borate, 1 m*M* Na_2-EDTA (pH 8.0).
3. 1X TBE: 90 m*M* Tris-borate, 2 m*M* Na_2-EDTA (pH 8.0).

2.4. Southern Blotting

1. Alkaline blotting solution: 0.4 *M* NaOH, 1.6 *M* NaCl (fresh).
2. Neutralization solution: 0.2 *M* Tris-HCl (pH 8.0), 2X standard sodium citrate (SSC) (1.75% NaCl, 0.88% Na-citrate), 3MM paper (Whatman).
3. Blotting membrane: Hybond N^+ (Amersham).
4. Paper towels.

2.5. Probe Hybridization

1. Hybridization solution: 0.125 *M* Na_2PO_4, pH 7.2, 0.25 *M* NaCl, 1 m*M* EDTA, 7% SDS, and 10% polyethylene glycol-6000, supplemented with 10 µg/mL denatured salmon sperm DNA.
2. Hybridization probes: The probe routinely used for FSHD1 analysis is p13E-11 *(1)*. For refined analysis, the probe, 9B6A, can be used *(1)*. The DNA is radioactively labeled using the Megaprime labeling kit (Amersham).

2.6. Hybridization Analysis

1. Washing solution: 2X SSC (1.75% NaCl, 0.88% Na-citrate), 0.1% SDS.
2. Phosphorimager.

3. Methods

3.1. DNA Isolation

Mostly, fresh EDTA blood is collected for analysis. The blood is left overnight at room temperature (RT) prior to DNA isolation. The protocol used for DNA isolation from blood is adapted from Miller et al. *(6)*.

1. Transfer 20 mL blood to a 50-mL tube, and add Erythrocyte lysis buffer, mix the tube thoroughly, and place the tube on ice for 15 min.
2. Centrifuge at 900*g* for 10 min, discard the supernatant, and resuspend the pellet in 25 mL erythrocyte lysis buffer, and place the tube on ice for 15 min.
3. Centrifuge at 900*g* for 10 min, discard the supernatant, and wash the pellet carefully with 2 mL erythrocyte lysis buffer, to remove the remaining erythrocytes.
4. Add 3 mL nucleus lysis buffer, and resuspend the pellet by pipeting.
5. Add 100 µL pronase (20 mg/mL) and 150 µL 20% SDS; mix gently.
6. Incubate overnight at RT.
7. Transfer the suspension to a 10 mL tube containing 1 mL 6 *M* NaCl.
8. Shake thoroughly for 20 s.
9. Centrifuge 15 min at 2800*g*.
10. Decant the clear supernatant to a 50-mL tube, add 2 vol 96% ethanol, and mix gently.
11. Remove the DNA using a Pasteur pipet, and wash the DNA in 70% ethanol.
12. Dissolve the DNA in 500 µL TE at 65°C for 10 min and overnight at RT.
13. Measure the DNA concentration at OD_{260}.
14. Store the DNA at 4°C.

3.2. Restriction Enzyme Digestion

Digest 5 µg genomic DNA in 30 µL restriction buffer, supplemented with 3.3 m*M* spermidine and either 20 U *Eco*RI, or 20 U *Eco*RI and 20 U *Bln*I, respectively. Incubate the DNA for at least 6 h at 37°C. Add 6 µL DNA loading buffer prior to loading on gel.

3.3. Pulsed-Field Gel Electrophoresis

The PFGE system is developed by the department, and therefore the running conditions cannot be copied. The conditions the authors apply may serve as a guideline for individual setup. Conditions have been optimized for separation in the range of 10–200 kb within 20 h at 18°C. DNA is separated on a 1% agarose (PFGE-graded) gel in 0.5X TBE at 8.5 V/cm, in four identical cycles. During these cycles, switch time is linearly increased from 1 to 20 s, including a 2% pause interval of the forward switch.

3.4. Conventional Gel Electrophoresis

Most laboratories use a conventional gel electrophoresis for FSHD analysis with the probe p13E-11. To properly estimate the size of the *Eco*RI fragment, up to 30–35 kb, the authors suggest running 36-h electrophoresis at 35 V in 1X TBE. Electrophoresis is done on a 0.5–0.7% agarose (Agarose MP, Boehringer) gel.

3.4.1. Southern Blotting

To transfer the high-mol-wt DNA fragments efficiently to the blotting membrane, the authors nick the DNA prior to blotting. Although several blotting membranes are available, the best results have been when using Hybond N^+ membrane (Amersham).

1. Remove the gel from the PFGE apparatus, and stain the DNA for 20 min in 0.5X TBE, supplemented with 2 µg/mL ethidium bromide, under gentle shaking. Photograph the gel over UV transilluminator.
2. Nick the DNA by a UV-crosslinker (Stratagene) at 180,000 J/cm^3.
3. Denature the gel 2× 20 min in alkaline blotting solution, with gentle shaking.
4. Simultaneously, prewet the Hybond N^+ membrane 10 min in water, and subsequently 15 min in alkaline blotting solution.
5. Transfer the DNA to the Hybond N^+ membrane overnight, using the alkaline blotting solution and capillary action.
6. After Southern transfer, neutralize the blot 5 min in neutralization solution, and air-dry.
7. Bind the DNA to the membrane by a UV-crosslinker (Stratagene) at 180,000 J/cm^3.

3.4.2. Probe Hybridization

1. Prehybridize the membrane for at least 30 min at 65°C in hybridization solution, in the smallest hybridization volume possible (i.e., 10–30 mL).
2. Label 10 ng p13E-11 DNA by the random nonamer priming method (Multiprime Kit, Amersham) with [α-^{32}P]dCTP to a specific activity of >1 × 10^7 cpm/µg.
3. Separate the radiolabeled DNA from the unincorporated [α-^{32}P]dCTP molecules through a Sephadex G50 column.

4. Denature the probe for 10 min at 95°C, prior to hybridization.
5. Add the denatured probe to the prehybridization solution, and incubate overnight at 65°C.
6. Wash the membranes with washing solution (set at 65°C) 3× for 5 min.
7. Expose the blot to a phosphorimager screen or an X-ray film.
8. Prior to reprobing membranes, the old probe is stripped from the membrane with boiling 0.1% SDS/0.1X SSC. Membranes are reprobed successfully in this laboratory up to 2×.

3.4.3. Hybridization Analysis

The authors use a phosphorimager to analyze hybridization results. However, exposure to X-ray films is also possible, but, because of the greater sensitivity of phosphorimager screens, longer exposure times are necessary for X-ray films. Usually, blots are exposed 18–48 h to phosphorimager screens.

3.5. Notes to Interpret the Results

The interpretation of the result obviously depends on the quality of the Southern blot obtained. Since the use of liquid DNA for the analysis of such large fragments is tricky, the authors cannot overstate the quality of the DNA preparation. Moreover, it takes experience to recognize false hybridization results caused by partial digestions or running artifacts of the PFGE. Because of the complexity of the rearrangement, and the presence of multiple highly homologous repeat structures in the genome, correct interpretation may also be complicated. The analysis is performed for both familial cases, as well as sporadic cases.

The probe p13E-11 recognizes the *Eco*RI fragment on which the repeat locus resides. It does not recognize the repeat unit itself, but a unique sequence adjacent to it. Also, this probe recognizes highly homologous chr-10 repeat array and a Y-chr-specific fragment of 9.5 kb. The latter fragment can be used as a control for the hybridization quality. In contrast to the chr-4 repeat unit, the chr-10 repeat unit contains a *Bln*I site, which can be used to discriminate between both chr. After digestion with *Eco*RI, four alleles will be identified, two from chr 4 and two from chr 10. After *Eco*RI and *Bln*I digestion, however, the chr-10 alleles will be fragmented in 3.3-kb units; the chr-4 alleles will remain, apart from a *Bln*I site 3 kb distal to the proximal *Eco*RI site, undigested (Fig. 1). In 10% of individuals, a fragment smaller than 38 kb is present on chr 10q. These can be easily discriminated from the chr-4 FSHD, causing arrays by the *Eco*RI/*Bln*I double digest. However, in some cases, an exchange between the chromosome 4 and the chr-10 repeat units has been observed, and a small 10-like allele on chr 4 also causes FSHD1 (1% of FSHD cases). A typical example of a familial diagnosis is shown in **Fig. 2**; on overview of the possi-

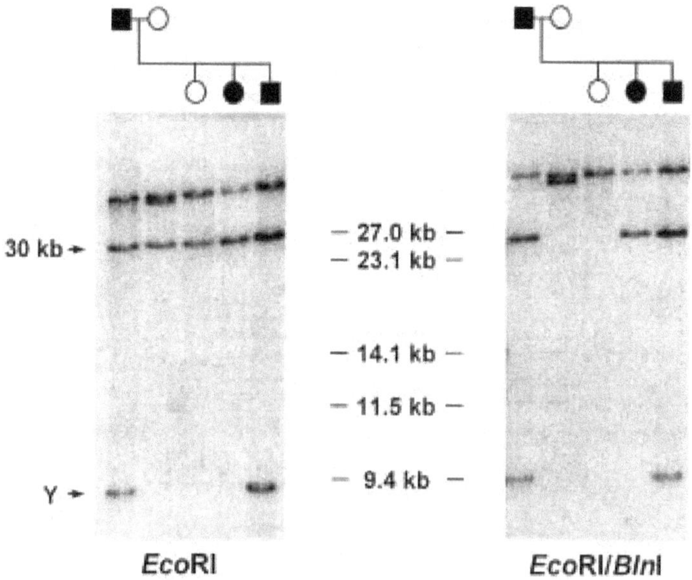

Fig. 2. Typical example of the molecular diagnosis of a FSHD kindred. Filled boxes and circles are affected individuals, open boxes and circles healthy individuals. After *Eco*RI digestion, the affected and unaffected individuals show a 30-kb repeat fragment, which remains undigested after digestion with *Eco*RI and *Bln*I in the affected individuals, and is therefore the pathogenic chr-4 allele. However, the repeat arrays of similar size in the unaffected individuals disappear after *Bln*I digestion, and therefore reside on chr 10. Note the presence of the 9.5-kb Y-allele hybridizing in all male individuals.

bilities is given in **Fig. 3A,B**. **Table 1** can be used as a quick reference for FSHD1 diagnosis.

There is an overall correlation between the size of the deletion (i.e., the size of the remaining repeat array) and the age of first onset *(8)*. The specificity of this test is >99%; the sensitivity is >95%; in <1% of the patients, a chr-10-repeat array smaller than 38 kb may reside on chr 4, and, in 2–3% of the FSHD families, locus heterogeneity is observed *(9)*.

4. Notes

1. EDTA-blood should be left overnight at room temperature prior to DNA isolation. Never chill the EDTA-blood. The size of the *Eco*RI fragments requires careful handling of the genomic DNA. We have optimized our DNA isolation protocol for high molecular weight DNA. For pipetting, we recommend large bore pipet tips.
2. The use of PFGE electrophoresis for this analysis, requires an optimal blotting procedure. In the past, we have obtained variable results with different blotting

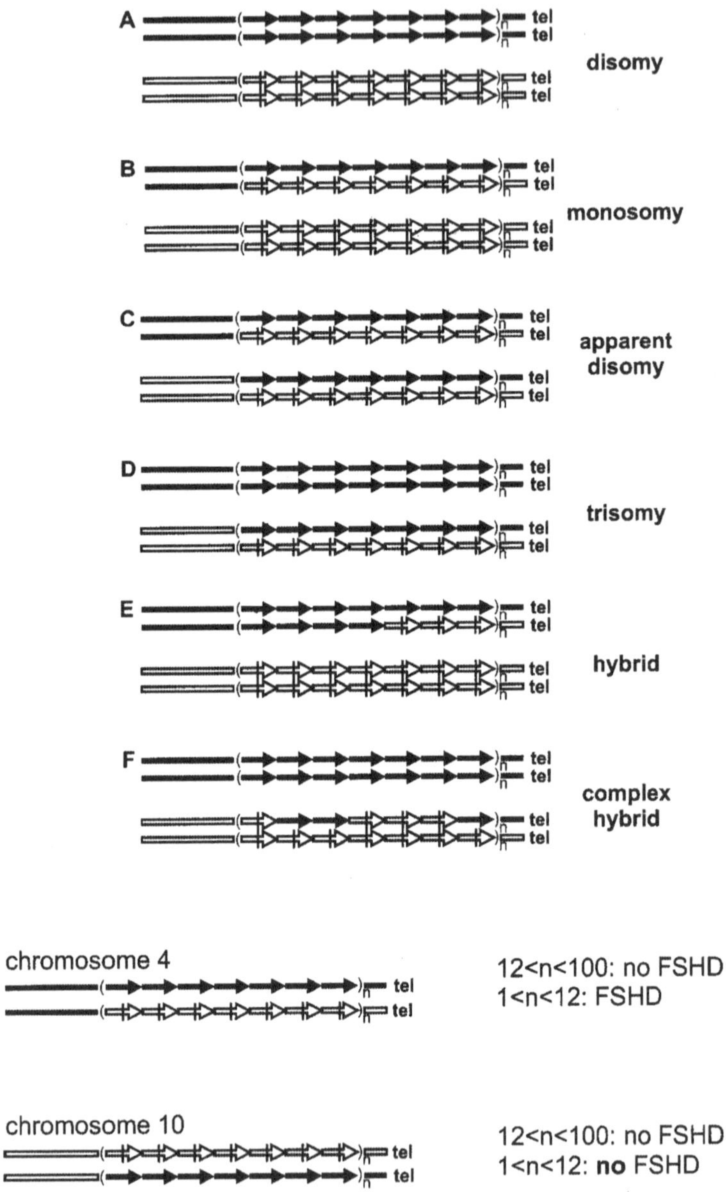

Fig. 3. **(A)** Schematic representation of the (sub)telomeres of the chrs 4q and 10q. Chromosome-10 sequences are represented by open bars and open arrows, with vertical lines representing the *Bln*I site; chr-4 sequences are filled. The 3.3 kb repeat unit is shown by an arrow. The repeat array can vary between 1 and 100 copies per allele, as indicated by the parentheses. The repeats derived from chr 10 (open arrows) can be

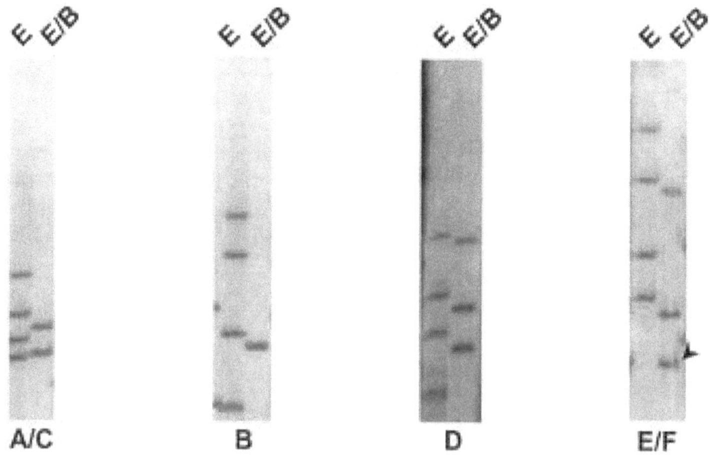

discriminated from those derived from chr 4 (filled arrows) by a *Bln*I digest. This restriction will fragment the chr-10 repeats in 3.3 kb units; chr-4 repeats remain undigested. Normally, two *Bln*I-resistant and two *Bln*I-sensitive alleles will be identified **(A)**. Occasionally, only one repeat will remain undigested **(B)**, suggestive of a chr-10-like repeat array on chr 4 (monosomy). The apparent disomy **(C)**, in which a 4-like repeat array resides on chr 10 and a 10-like repeat array on chr 4, cannot be recognized by this technique. Also, three chr-4-like arrays resistant for *Bln*I restriction have been encountered **(D)**. Here, a 4-like repeat resides on chr 10 (trisomy). Finally, the repeat arrays may consist of clusters of both chr-4- and chr-10-derived repeat units **(E, F)**. This will yield unexpected fragments after hybridization with p13E-11 or 9B6A. Note that FSHD is only associated with a repeat array smaller than 12 units on chr 4, irrespective of the structure (i.e., chr-4 repeat units or chr-10 repeat units) of this array. **(B)** Examples of Southern blots of *Eco*RI and *Eco*RI/*Bln*I digested DNA from control individuals after hybridization with p13E-11. After *Eco*RI digest, four alleles will be identified, two from chr 4 and two from chr 10. Double digestion with *Eco*RI and *Bln*I will fragment the chr-10 repeat arrays; chr-4 repeat arrays will remain undigested, apart from one *Bln*I site 3 Kb distal to the proximal *Eco*RI site. The first figure shows a normal karyotype (or an apparent disomy: **A/C**). The second figure shows an individual carrying one 4-like repeat array (monosomy: **B**); three arrays are sensitive for *Bln*I digestion, and thus consist of 10-like repeat units. The third figure shows three repeat arrays resistant to *Bln*I, which consist of chr-4-like repeat units (trisomy: **D**). The last figure shows a complex repeat array. Here, two chr-4 repeat arrays and two chr-10 repeat arrays are detected. However, a unexpected p13E-11 fragment is also visible (arrow). This fragment must be derived from one of the chr-10 repeat arrays. Thus, this chr-10 subtelomere consists of a cluster of 4-like repeat units, followed by a cluster of 10-like repeat units, which are digested by *Bln*I **(E/F)**.

Table 1
Overview of Possibilities Obtained after Hybridization with p13E-11

Size *Eco*RI fragment	Size *Eco*RI/*Bln*I fragment	Diagnosis	Remarks
<38 kb	3 kb smaller	FSHD1 (>99%)	Chr 4: FSHD1 confirmed
>38 kb	Fragmented in 3.3-kb units	No FSHD1 (<5%)[a]	Chr 10: FSHD1 unlikely
<38 kb	Fragmented in 3.3-kb units	FSHD1 unlikely (<10%)[b]	(Sub)telomeric exchange between chrs 4 and 10 possible
>38 kb	3 kb smaller	FSHD1 unlikely (<5%)	Exclude chr 4 by linkage analysis or haplotype analysis with D4S139 and D4S163

[a]Some FSHD families have been described who are not linked to 4q35.

[b]This fragment probably resides on chr 10. In 10% of the population, however, an exchange between chr-10 repeat units and chr-4 repeat units have been observed. In this situation, additional PFGE experiments and haplotyping are required to determine the diagnosis. Also, repeat arrays may be partially digested by *Bln*I. In this case, the array consists of clusters of both chr-4, as well as chr-10 repeat units *(7)*. Again, additional experiments are required.

papers, and with different batches of the same blotting paper. Currently, prior to large scale usage, we test different batches of blotting paper with previously tested DNA. Batches with satisfactory results, are reserved for this purpose only.

3. As an internal control, we always run a previously tested DNA sample on the new gel. This sample contains four different sized *Eco*RI fragments ranging from 50 to 200 kb and allows us to assess the quality of the entire procedure.
4. We always run a male sample on the gel. This will allow a quality control at the 9.5 kb Y chromosome fragment.
5. Recently we obtained evidence for deletions of p13E-11 *(7)*. As long as the repeat array remains >38 kb, these deletions are non-pathogenic. The incidence of these deletions in the population is unknown. However, these results emphasize again the use of PFGE for FSHD diagnosis since this procedure allows the identification of all 4 alleles. Employing PFGE, we demonstrated the presence of a short repeat array in a patient carrying a deletion of p13E-11 on the same chromosome. The repeat was visualized with the probe 9B6A.
6. To obtain sharper fragments in the 40–70 kb range, a double digestion with *Eco*RI and *Hin*dIII can be used instead of *Eco*RI alone. *Hin*dIII has, like *Eco*RI, no restriction sites in the repeat array. An *Eco*RI/*Hin*dIII double digest will reduce the average fragment size thereby enhancing the resolution in the 40–70 kb range.
7. For conventional gel electrophoresis, we recommend to run at least 36 h at 35 V in 1X TBE. Optimization of the electrophoresis in the range of 2.5–50 kb will allow a quality control of the *Eco*RI/*Bln*I digest. After hybridization with p13E-11, a 2.6 kb *Eco*RI/*Bln*I fragment should be detected.

8. As size markers we use (DNA digested with *Hin*dIII and a ladder of (concatamers. The ladder can easily be generated by adding 1 mL of 1% low melt agarose (SeaPlaque GTG agarose, FMC) in TE to 1 mL (DNA in TE (20 µg/mL) at 50°C. Gently mix and aliquot by pipetting 40 µL in agarose plug molds. After solidifying at 4°C, incubate the plugs 3.5 h at 37°C and subsequently overnight at room temperature in 10 mL 1% sarcosyl (N-lauroylsarcosine, Sigma)/0.5 *M* EDTA supplemented with 125 µL (20 mg/mL) pronase. Wash the plugs 4 times 2 h in TE and store them in 0.5 *M* EDTA at 4°C.
9. As discussed in **Subheading 3.5.** and shown in **Fig. 3**, sometimes we observe chromosome 4-type repeat arrays on chromosome 10, and, vice versa, chromosome 10-type repeat arrays on chromosome 4. However, only a short repeat array on chromosome 4, irrespective of the repeat type, is associated with FSHD1. Therefore, with inconsistent results, always define the chromosomal origin of the short repeat array by linkage analysis (D4S163, D4S139, D10S555, and D10S590).

References

1. Wijmenga, C., Hewitt, J. E., Sandkuijl, L. A., Clark, L. N., Wright, T. J., Dauwerse, H. G., et al. (1992) Chromosome 4q DNA rearrangements associated with facioscapulohumeral muscular dystrophy. *Nat. Genet.* **2,** 26–30.
2. van Deutekom, J. C., Wijmenga, C., van Tienhoven, E. A., Gruter, A. M., Hewitt, J. E., Padberg, G. W., et al. (1993) FSHD associated DNA rearrangements are due to deletions of integral copies of a 3.2 kb tandemly repeated unit. *Hum. Mol. Genet.* **2,** 2037–2042.
3. Bakker, E., Wijmenga, C., Vossen, R. H. A. M., Padberg, G. W., Hewitt, J. E., van der Wielen, M., Rasmussen, K., and Frants, R. R. (1995) The FSHD linked locus D4F104S1 (P13E 11) on 4q35 has a homologue on 10qter. *Muscle Nerve* (Suppl) S39–S44.
4. Deidda, G., Cacurri, S., Piazzo, N., and Felicetti, L. (1996) Direct detection of 4q35 rearrangements implicated in facioscapulohumeral muscular dystrophy (FSHD). *J. Med. Genet.* **33,** 361–365.
5. van Deutekom, J. C., Bakker, E., Lemmers, R. J., van der Wielen, M. J., Bik, E., Hofker, M. H., Padberg, G. W., and Frants, R. R. (1996) Evidence for subtelomeric exchange of 3.3 kb tandemly repeated units between chromosomes 4q35 and 10q26: implications for genetic counselling and etiology of FSHD1. *Hum. Mol. Genet.* **5,** 1997–2003.
6. Miller, S. A., Dykes, D. D., and Polesky, H. F. (1988) A simple salting out procedure for extracting DNA from human nucleated cells. *Nucleic. Acids. Res.* **16,** 1215.
7. Lemmers R. J. L. F., van der Maarel S. M., van Deutekom J. C. T., van der Wielen, M. J. R., Deidda, G., Dauwerse, H. G., Hewitt, J., Hofker, M., Bakker, E., Padberg, G. W., and Frants, R. R. Inter- and intrachromosomal subtelomeric rearrangements on 4q35: implications for facioscapulohumeral muscular dystrophy (FSHD) aetiology and diagnosis. *Hum. Mol. Genet.* **7,** 1207–1214.

8. Lunt, P. W., Jardine, P. E., Koch, M. C., Maynard, J., Osborn, M., Williams, M., Harper, P. S., and Upadhyaya, M. (1995) Correlation between fragment size at D4F104S1 and age at onset or at wheelchair use, with a possible generational effect, accounts for much phenotypic variation in 4q35-facioscapulohumeral muscular dystrophy (FSHD). *Hum. Mol. Genet.* **4,** 951–958.
9. Bakker, E., van der Wielen, M. J., Voorhoeve, E., Ippel, P. F., Padberg, G. W., Frants, R. R., and Wijmenga, C. (1996) Diagnostic, predictive, and prenatal testing for facioscapulohumeral muscular dystrophy: diagnostic approach for sporadic and familial cases. *J. Med. Genet.* **33,** 29–35.

III

Protein Analysis in the Muscular Dystrophies

19

Analysis of Protein Expression in Muscular Dystrophies

Louise V. B. Anderson

1. Introduction

The preceding chapters have dealt with the detection of gene mutations and the following chapters deal with protein analysis. This chapter links the two by describing the effect that different types of mutations have on protein synthesis, and how this may be used in the investigation of muscular dystrophy (MD). Analysis at the DNA level can be performed with a simple blood sample, but analysis at the protein level requires a sample of the tissue expressing the target protein. Although proteins such as emerin may be detected in a skin biopsy, most of the diagnostic proteins are only expressed in muscle. The taking of a skeletal muscle biopsy for histological analysis has been part of the routine for a diagnostic work-up for many years, and the practice of storing such samples in an archive was of great importance when diagnostic protein analysis first started in the MDs, with the identification of the Duchenne/Becker gene product, dystrophin. Now that there is an increasing range of gene products to analyze, the taking of a muscle biopsy is an invaluable asset to the diagnostic protocol ***(1)***, and analysis of protein expression is established as an essential link between the underlying genotype and the manifestations of clinical severity.

2. Gene Mutations and Protein Synthesis

Figure 1 outlines the stages in the synthesis of a protein: DNA is transcribed into pre-mRNA inside the nucleus. Pre-mRNA is processed to mature mRNA by excision of the intronic sequences and ligation of the exons. The mRNA is exported from the nucleus, attached to ribosomes, and the nucleotide coding sequences are translated into the string of amino acids that form proteins. Codons are the triplets of nucleotides that code for all the different aas. In

From: *Methods in Molecular Medicine, vol. 43: Muscular Dystrophy: Methods and Protocols*
Edited by: K. M. D. Bushby and L. V. B. Anderson © Humana Press Inc., Totowa, NJ

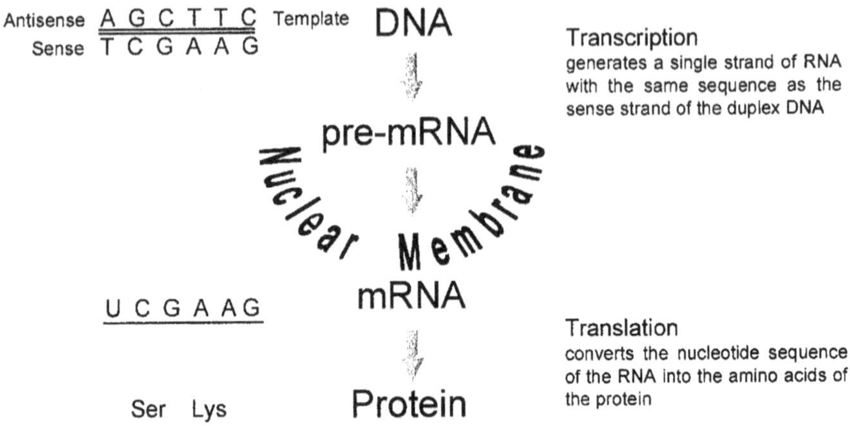

Fig. 1. Stages in the synthesis of a protein.

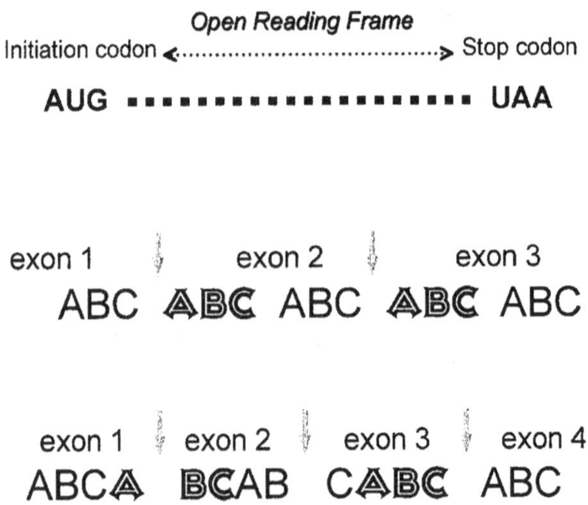

Fig. 2. Codons and the boundaries between exons.

addition, certain triplets code for initiation (AUG) and stop signals (UAA, UGA, UAG), and the sequence between the two is the open reading frame (ORF). Codons may need to span the boundaries between exons, so it is critically important to get the exon-splicing correct (**Fig. 2**). Defective splicing is a common type of frame-shifting mutation (*see* **Table 1**). DNA deletions are

Table 1
Types of Gene Mutation

Premature termination:
Nonsense
Point mutation in which one base is exchanged for another.
Stop codon replaces a codon for an amino acid.
Frame-shifting deletion/insertion/duplication
Codons altered → wrong amino acids and/or stop codon.
Splice site mutation
Point mutation occurs, which alters splicing of introns and exons.
Exon not included, reading frame is disrupted → wrong amino acids and/or stop codon.
Normal termination
Missense
Point mutation causes an incorrect amino acids to be substituted.
Resultant changes in charge or shape may alter functional sites.
In-frame deletion/duplication
Codons maintained → whole amino acids removed/repeated.
Splice-site mutation
Point mutation occurs, which alters splicing of introns and exons.
Exons not included, reading frame is maintained, but functional sites may be altered.

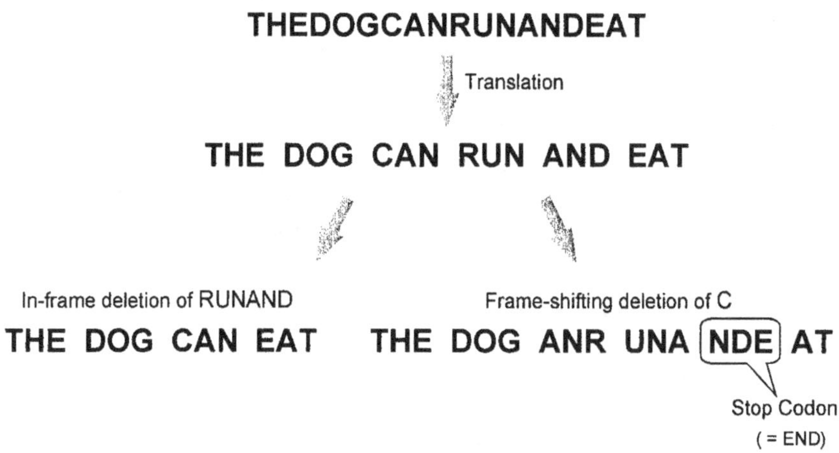

Fig. 3. Demonstration of the effect of in-frame and frame-shifting deletions.

also common, and these may maintain or disrupt the ORF. **Figure 3** demonstrates the effect that these two types of deletion might have on protein synthesis. In the in-frame deletion, a protein is synthesized to the end (the words make sense), but it is smaller than expected, and is missing a functional unit (part of the information is missing): This corresponds to a smaller semi-functional protein. With the frame-shifting deletion, protein synthesis is started (the first words make sense), but, after the deletion, the template is scrambled, and a few incorrect aas are made before a premature stop codon is generated (a variant of "end"). In practice, the very short peptides that are synthesized up to the premature stop codon are flagged by the cell as inappropriate, and are rapidly removed.

3. Analysis of Protein Expression

Protein analysis may achieve the following objectives:

1. Aid accurate diagnosis
   a. Indicate type of inheritance (e.g., X-linked, dominant) = improve genetic counseling.
   b. Indicate where to start the search for gene mutations = improve efficiency of mutation analysis.
2. Aid prognosis, in some instances
   a. Indicate type of mutation = demonstrate disruption or maintenance of protein synthesis.
   b. Indicate improvement in animal models of gene therapy = demonstrate restoration of missing proteins.
3. Aid location of functionally important regions in a protein via its mutations:
   a. Missense mutations in association with a pathological phenotype = improve understanding of the protein's role in normal muscle.
   b. In-frame deletions with a mild clinical phenotype = regions that may be less essential (has been used to guide minigene approaches to gene therapy).

How effective the analysis is at achieving these different objectives varies with the protein under consideration. Defective expression of dystrophin or emerin indicates an X-linked condition, and this has a major impact on the counseling of family members. In cases in which the differential diagnosis was Becker muscular dystrophy (MD) or a form of autosomal recessive limb-girdle muscular dystrophy (LGMD), the impact on any daughters is considerable.

Sometimes, the presenting clinical symptoms are nonspecific, and the choice for differential diagnosis is between several different forms of MD. This would mean a huge amount of work if every one of the possible genes had to be screened for mutations, but protein analysis has developed into a very effective way of guiding the search *(2)*. Such analysis does have limitations in the sarcoglycanopathies, because this group of proteins has very close interactions, and a mutation in one member protein may cause an absence of protein expression for all four *(3,4)*. Nevertheless, it now appears that, particularly for γ-sarcoglycanopathy, the absence of labeling for one member of the complex may be accompanied by a mere reduction in the others *(5,6)*. In these cases, the protein with the most severely altered expression has proved to be the one with the mutated gene, indicating that protein analysis may be useful even in these dystrophies.

Analysis of dystrophin protein expression has proven to be very useful for prognosis. The pattern of muscle involvement in Duchenne MD and BMD is very characteristic, but the intellectual problems associated with the Xp21-linked dystrophies can sometimes result in a young boy appearing to be more physically affected than he really is when he presents for the first time in a clinic. Protein analysis with antibodies to different regions of the dystrophin molecule, including the C-terminus, can show what type of mutation (frame-shifting or in-frame) is present in the boy, and hence whether he is likely to have Duchenne-like or Becker-like disease severity (**Fig. 3**). Early mutation analysis involved Southern blotting of the whole gene, but the current use of multiplex PCR analysis, targeted to the mutation hot spots in the dystrophin gene, means that the exact extent of a deletion may not be delineated. Thus, protein analysis can be used to predict the effect of a mutation on the ORF. The situation is more complicated in the autosomal recessive dystrophies, but, as a general rule, a total lack of protein expression is frequently associated with homozygous null mutations (**Table 1**) and more severe clinical phenotypes.

Protein expression may also provide an explanation as to why, in particular genes, missense mutations result in a pathological pheneotype. Whether a protein has a structural, enzymatic, or regulatory role in normal muscle physiology, there will be certain regions or aa sequences that are critical for the normal function of that protein. A reduction in protein expression accompanying a homozygous missense mutation suggests that the modified protein may be unstable and unable to fulfill its normal function. For example, the homozygous Arg91 → Pro missense mutations in β-sarcoglycanopathy are associated with protein absence, presumably because of the inability of the modified molecules to be incorporated into the muscle membrane correctly *(4)*. Thus, incorrect localization leads to rapid clearance of the redundant molecules. Equally, sites on a protein that are not important may be indicated by correct localization of an abundant protein in the presence of in-frame deletions and mild clinical phenotypes *(7)*. This approach has been used to generate minigenes for gene therapy *(8)*.

It is important to note that there are exceptions to every rule. Underlying gene mutations may be modified at the somatic level, resulting in an alteration of the expected phenotype (e.g., boys with frame-shifting deletions in the dystrophin gene may synthesize enough dystrophin in their muscle to produce an intermediate *[9]* or even Becker phenotype *[10]*). Likewise, the literature on every MD contains reports of variation in clinical phenotype among patients with identical mutations. Other factors (environmental, nutritional, hormonal, age-related, unknown) may modify the phenotype, or even the underlying genotype (as in myotonic dystrophy).

References

1. Anderson, J. R. (1997) Recommendations for the biopsy procedure and assessment of skeletal muscle biopsies. *Virchows Arch. Int. J. Pathol.* **431,** 227–233.
2. Anderson, L. V. B. (1996) Optimised protein diagnosis in the autosomal recessive limb-girdle muscular dystrophies. *Neuromusc. Disord.* **6,** 443–446.
3. Nigro, V., de Sá Moreira, E., Piluso, G., Vainzof, M., Belsito, A., Politano, L., et al. (1996) Autosomal recessive limb-girdle muscular dystrophy, LGMD2F, is caused by a mutation in the δ-sarcoglycan gene. *Nature Genet.* **14,** 195–198.
4. Bönnemann, C. G., Passos-Bueno, M. R., McNally, E. M., Vainzof, M., de Sá Moreira, E., Marie, S. K., et al. (1996) Genomic screening for β-sarcoglycan gene mutations: Missense mutations may cause severe limb-girdle muscular dystrophy type 2E (LGMD 2E). *Hum. Mol. Genet.* **5,** 1953–1961.
5. Sewry, C., Taylor, J., Anderson, L. V. B., Ozawa, E., Pogue, R., Piccolo, F., et al. (1996) Abnormalities in α-, β- and γ-sarcoglycan in patients with limb-girdle muscular dystrophy. *Neuromusc. Disord.* **6,** 467–474.
6. Vainzof, M., Passos-Bueno, M. R., Canovas, M., de Sá Moreira, E., Pavanello, R. C. M., Marie, S. K., et al. (1996) The sarcoglycan complex in the six autosomal recessive limb-girdle muscular dystrophies. *Hum. Mol. Genet.* **5,** 1963–1969.
7. England, S., Nicholson, L. V. B., Johnson, M. A., Forrest, S. M., Love, D. R., Zubrzycka-Gaarn, E. E., et al. (1990) Very mild muscular dystrophy associated with the deletion of 46% of dystrophin. *Nature* **343,** 180–182.
8. Vincent, N., Ragot, T., Gilgenkrantz, H., Couton, D., Chafey, P., Grégoire, A., et al. (1993) Long-term correction of mouse dystrophic degeneration by adenovirus-mediated transfer of a minidystrophin gene. *Nature Genet.* **5,** 130–134.
9. Nicholson, L. V. B., Johnson, M. A., Bushby, K. M. D., Gardner-Medwin, D., Curtis, A., Ginjaar, H. B., et al. (1993) Integrated study of 100 patients with Xp21 muscular dystrophy using clinical, genetic, immunochemical, and histopathological data. Part 2: Correlations within individual patients. *J. Med. Genet.* **30,** 737–744.
10. Malhotra, S. B., Hart, K. A., Klamut, H. J., Thomas, N. S. T., Bodrug, S. E., Burghes, A. H. M., et al. (1988) Frame-shift deletions in patients with Duchenne and Becker muscular dystrophy. *Science* **242,** 755–759.

20

Immunological Reagents and Amplification Systems

Caroline A. Sewry and Qui Lu

1. Introduction

Immunohistochemistry/immunocytochemistry (ICC) and allied techniques are used to visualize and localize specific tissue components. The principle of ICC is the binding of an antibody (Ab) to a specific antigen. Allied techniques include the labeling of glycoproteins with lectins, the labeling of receptors with ligands such as toxins, and the labeling of nucleic acids by *in situ* hybridization. These methods are based on similar principles of specific affinity, and similar methods of detection and amplification have been developed.

Although histochemical procedures still continue to be of major importance in the assessment of muscle biopsies, these are now complemented by ICC and the specificity that it provides. ICC has made a major contribution to the differentiation of the various muscular dystrophies (MDs), and has led to the identification of genes responsible for, as well as playing a major role in defining the clinical spectrum of some disorders. It is now an essential diagnostic tool for the identification of primary defects.

Monoclonal and polyclonal Abs are available to a wide number of muscle proteins, many of which are commercially available. With advances in knowledge of isoforms of many proteins, however, the specificity of some Abs produced several years ago now must be reassessed. It is essential to fully characterize any Ab to meet the specific requirements of the investigation, particularly if the commercial source is unknown, or the specificity has not been fully evaluated.

This chapter concentrates on practical applications of ICC relevant to the field of MDs. Aspects of the technique considered in this chapter are specimen preparation, detection, amplification, visualization options, the most important Abs for studies in the field, the need for controls, and problems that may arise.

From: *Methods in Molecular Medicine, vol. 43: Muscular Dystrophy: Methods and Protocols*
Edited by: K. M. D. Bushby and L. V. B. Anderson © Humana Press Inc., Totowa, NJ

2. Specimen Preparation

2.1. Tissues

Most ICC studies relevant to the diagnosis of MDs are performed on muscle biopsies. In some situations, however, when a protein of interest is known to be expressed in another tissue, other less-invasive sampling techniques may be useful. For example, in congenital muscular dystrophy (CMD) and Emery-Dreifuss muscular dystrophy (EDMD), the expression of laminin α_2 and emerin, respectively, can be assessed in a skin biopsy ***(1,2,3)***. Emerin can also be assessed in buccal smears ***(4)***. Also, ICC studies of chorionic villus samples are a useful prenatal diagnostic test for cases of CMD with an absence of laminin α_2 ***(5,6)***.

2.2. Tissue Preparation

All samples should be less than 5 mm in diameter and rapidly frozen in isopentane cooled in liquid nitrogen ***(7)***. Once frozen, tissue blocks can be stored indefinitely at –80°C, or in liquid nitrogen. Not only is tissue architecture better in frozen material than in fixed material, but many antigens are only recognized, or accessible, in unfixed tissue. Some Abs, however, may only work on fixed material, in which case, frozen sections can be postfixed with a variety of fixatives (*see* **Subheading 2.4.**). If only formalin-fixed, wax-embedded material is available, and various antigen-retrieval techniques using pretreatment of sections with enzymes and/or microwaving can be tried. Abs to some relevant muscle proteins can be localized following these retrieval techniques, but they have not been extensively investigated, and must be evaluated along with control samples, and the established pattern in frozen sections. The use of frozen sections is preferred.

2.3. Sectioning and Section Collection

Cryostat sections of muscle (5–7 μm) should be cut at about –23°C. They can be collected onto glass cover slips or slides (*see* **Note 1**). Sections should be air-dried for about 20 min before use, or before storage at –20 or –80°C for long-term storage. For storage, slides are wrapped back-to-back in Clingfilm and sealed in foil; cover slips are placed in racks, and wrapped in foil. If only a few sections from a package are required, the remainder should not be allowed to thaw. Before immunolabeling sections should be warmed and dried at room temperature (RT).

2.4. Fixation of Sections

Many of the Abs used for diagnostic assessment of muscle do not require fixation (*see* **Note 2**). If necessary, acetone or methanol are the most frequently used fixatives. 1% formaldehyde or paraformaldehyde is also often used. The use of these fixatives, or permeabilization with Triton X-100 (0.05–0.2%), saponin (0.05–0.1%) or Tween-20 (0.05–2%), are often necessary for localization of intercellular antigens in cultured muscle cells. If fixation is required, the optimal conditions of time and concentration, and the most suitable fixative, must be experimentally determined.

2.5. Immunolabeling and Washing

Dry sections must be placed in a moist atmosphere for labeling, to prevent evaporation of the small volumes of reagents. This can be done in a Petri dish containing damp filter paper, or in commercially available staining trays. The use of a hydrophobic PAP pen (Agar Aids), to draw around each section, is a convenient way to reduce the volume of reagents used, and to prevent them spreading. Cover slips or slides can be placed in racks and washed collectively in a dish, or they can be rinsed individually. Three rinses of buffer for 3–5 min each are generally used, or, in the case of individual cover slips, 10-s dip-washes are adequate.

2.6. Blocking Agents

Nonspecific background labeling, which reduces the signal-to-noise ratio, may present problems in human muscle. Additives to the buffer, such as bovine serum albumin (0.1%) or detergents (0.2% Triton X), or normal serum from the same species as the secondary Ab (usually neat-10% is adequate), can be used to block nonspecific binding of secondary Abs. Some tissue may contain endogenous enzymes, such as peroxidase or alkaline phosphatase. These need to be blocked with hydrogen peroxide (1%) or levimisole (1 m*M*), respectively. Endogenous biotin can be blocked by applying unconjugated avidin followed by biotin. This is (commercially available as a kit) (*see* **Note 3**).

2.7. Antigen Retrieval

If only fixed material is available, some Abs of interest to the MDs can be applied after protease and/or microwave treatment of the section (e.g., laminins and emerin). The mechanism(s) by which these work is not fully understood, but it is thought to be achieved by breaking the crosslinking bonds formed by fixatives, or by denaturation of proteins and/or exposure of epitopes. Many different methods have been developed, including protease digestion with trypsin or pronase, microwaving, pressure-cooking, or autoclaving. The best method and optimal conditions for each Ab must be experimentally determined.

2.8. Primary Abs

A wide variety of primary Abs to muscle proteins are now commercially available, particularly those that detect primary defects in MDs (*see* **Note 4**).

Table 1 summarizes the most important Abs for the diagnosis of MDs, and the source and dilutions the authors have used with the standard methods shown below. The table shows Abs used to detect both primary and relevant secondary defects, and some that are important as controls. Several companies now sell relevant primary Abs, and details can be found on the Internet, or in directories such as that sold by Lippscott. Dilution of primary Ab should always be assessed by titration in each laboratory, and is dependent on such factors as supplier, poly- or monoclonal Ab, secondary Ab, and time and temperature of incubation. Incubation times can vary from 30 to 60 min at RT, to overnight at 4°C, depending on the Ab and the level of acceptable background (*see* **Note 5**). Incubation at 4°C overnight may allow greater dilution of Ab, with increased signal intensity. With an incubation time of 30 min at RT, with the primary and secondary AB, followed by a fluorescent conjugate, it is possible to complete the immunolabeling in less than 2 h, and several proteins can be assessed on a batch of biopsies within a day.

2.9. Detection Systems

Following the application of primary Abs, most techniques now utilize an indirect detection method with a secondary Ab against the immunoglobulin G (IgGs) of the species in which the primary was raised. The secondary Ab may be conjugated to either an enzyme or a fluorochrome. A three-step system is now also commonly used, in which a biotinylated secondary Ab is followed by streptavidin labeled with a marker of choice. This technique has the advantage of enhancing the signal, through the multiple labeling of the biotinylated secondary Ab by labeled streptavidin molecules. A preformed adin–biotin complex (ABC) can also be applied, instead of labeled streptavidin *(8)*. Peroxidase–anti-peroxidase also provides enhancement, but is now less frequently used. Recently, several methods have been developed to give greater enhancement, such as a tryamide amplification system (e.g., Life Science, St. Petersburg, FL). This uses peroxidase to catalyze the deposition of biotin or fluorophore-labeled tryamide onto the section close to the antigen–Ab binding site. The deposited biotin is then visualized by streptavidin conjugated to an enzyme or fluorochrome.

The choice of label to visualize the Ab is often a matter of personal preference but it is also governed by the type of microscope available, the need for a permanent preparation, and the of amount and localization pattern of antigen. Enzyme labels, such as peroxidase or alkaline phosphatase, provide permanent results and a good overview of tissue morphology, particularly if counterstained. Fluorescent labels, on the other hand, produce an image of sharp contrast against a dark background, making it easier to distinguish areas of low expression. With improvements in aqueous mountants, the rate of photobleaching has been reduced, and fluorescent signals can be retained for several

Table 1
Antibodies Used for Studies of Muscular Dystrophies and Their Suppliers

Antigen	Supplier and code	Dilution	Application
Dystrophin N-terminal	Novocastra NCL-Dys 3	1:20	Absent in DMD Reduced, uneven in BMD Mosaic in manifesting carrier occasionally reduced in sarcoglycanopathies
Dystrophin rod domain	Novocastra NCL-Dys 1	Neat	As above
Dystrophin C-terminal	Novocastra NCL-Dys 2	1:20	As above
Dystrophin rod domain	Sigma D-8168 MANDYS8	1:400	As above
Dystrophin C-terminal	Sigma D-8403 MANDRA1	1:100	As above
β-Spectrin	Novocastra NCL-SPEC1	1:20	Control for dystrophin Reduced on regenerating fibers
α-Sarcoglycan	Novocastra NCL a-SARC	1:50	Reduced or absent in some LGMD
β-Sarcoglycan	Novocastra NCL b-SARC	1:50	Reduced or absent in some LGMD
γ-Sarcoglycan	Novocastra NCL g-SARC	1:30	Reduced or absent in some LGMD
δ-Sarcoglycan	Novocastra NCL-d-SARC	1:25	Reduced or absent in some LGMD
β-Dystroglycan	Novocastra NCL-b-DG	1:5	Reduced in DMD and BMD
Emerin	Novocastra NCL-emerin	1:20	Absent nuclear labeling in EDMM
Laminin α_2 (80 kDa)	Chemicon MAB 1922	1:4000	Absent or reduced in some CMDs
Laminin α_2 (300 kDa)	Alexis 4H8	1:2	Absent or reduced in some CMDs
Laminin α_2	Novocastra NCL-merosin	1:50	Absent or reduced in some CMDs
Laminin α_5	Chemicon MAB1924	1:4000	High on regenerating fibers Overexpressed if laminin α_2 reduced
Laminin β1	Chemicon MAB 1928 MAB 1921	1:4000 1:2000	Reduced in some dystrophies

(continued)

Table 1 *(continued)*

Antigen	Supplier and code	Dilution	Application
Laminin γ1	Chemicon MAB 1914	1:4000	Control for laminins
	MAB 1920	1:2000	
Utrophin	Novocastra NCL- DRP2	1:2	High on regenerating fibers Overexpressed in DMD and BMD
Fetal myosin	Novocastra NCL-MHCn	1:20	High in regenerating fibres (various stages)
Fast myosin	Novocastra NCL-MHCf	1:10	Fast/type 2 fibers
Slow myosin	Novocastra NCL-MHCs	1:20	Slow/type 1 fibers
Slow myosin[a]	Chemicon MAB 1628	1:5	slow fibers
HLA class I ABC (W6/32 clone)	Several companies	1:50	Regenerating fibers Overexpressed in inflammatory myopathies

[a]Same clone also available from Sigma.

NB, other Abs to some of these proteins are also available (e.g., from Alexis, Transduction Laboratories, Gibco); DMD, Duchenne muscular dystrophy; BMD, Becker muscular dystrophy; LGMD, limb-girdle muscular dystrophy; EDMD, Emery-Dreifuss muscular dystrophy; CMD, congenital muscular dystrophy.

weeks or months, depending on the Ab and its localization. Several fluorescent counterstains are also now available. Fluorescent methods are usually time-saving, and avoid the use of hazardous substances such as diaminobenzamine (DAB). Also, double or multiple labeling is easier, using two fluorochromes, than with enzyme conjugates, and, with image-capturing facilities, the geographical relationship of different antigens can be precisely determined.

2.9.1. Fluorescent Labels

The most commonly used fluorochromes are fluorescin, rhodamine, Texas Red, AMCA, Cy3, and Cy5. The choice is often of personal preference but factors such as cost, intensity, filters fitted to the microscope, and fading also need to be considered (*see* **Note 6**). For multiple labeling, it is also important to use fluorochromes that do not have overlapping wave lengths. Labels such as the Cy range give a particularly high signal, and their popularity is increasing. Development and improvements in a technique have obvious advantages, but the pathological assessment of muscle often requires comparisons of intensity, and new baselines may have to be established if methods are changed.

2.9.2. Enzyme Labels

Peroxidase detected with DAB has traditionally been the most-used enzyme label. This produces a brown end product, which is stable for long periods at RT. Additional contrast and enhancement of the DAB end product can be achieved using nickel or silver to produce a black product. Other colors, such as red, with aminoethyl carbazole, or blue, with 4-chloro-1-naptholol, can also be obtained with different substrates. A common alternative to peroxidase is alkaline phosphatase, which, with the appropriate substrate, can be visualized as a red end product. β-galactosidase is useful for double-labeling, and provides good contrast against the brown from peroxidase or red from alkaline phosphatase. Amplification systems with peroxidase are discussed in **Subheading 2.9.**

2.10. Counterstaining and Mounting

Counterstains provide an overall impression of the morphology of the tissue, and can be nuclear or cytoplasmic. They are not essential, and their use is often one of individual choice. In sections expected to show no labeling of nuclei, such as in EDMD, nuclear counterstains should be avoided. The choice of counterstain is dependent on the color of the end product, or the fluorochrome. Hematoxylin or methyl green are common nuclear counterstains used after peroxidase. For immunofluorescence, (DAPI) (1 μg/mL; blue under UV), ethidium bromide (1 μg/mL; red), Hoersch dye (10 μg/mL; blue under UV), or Evans blue can be used. Mountants containing a counterstain are also commercially available (e.g., with DAPI: Vector Labs).

The choice of mountant is dependent on the use of fluorescent or enzyme markers. Fluorescent markers require aqueous mountants, and several commercial ones are now available that reduce fading (*see* **Note 7**). Storage of slides in the dark at 4°C may also help to prevent fading. It is important to avoid bubbles in the mountant, and to use only a small drop per section. For enzyme markers dehydration in alcohol, clearing and mounting in synthetic resins (e.g., DPX) can be used.

3. Methods

3.1. Slide Coating

3.1.1. Slide Coating: A

1. 1 mg/mL poly-L-lysine.
2. Spread about 10 μL over a slide with the end of another slide.
3. Drying will be almost instantaneous.
4. Batches of slides can be prepared at least a week in advance.

3.1.2. Slide Coating: B

1. Dip slides 2% 3-aminopropyltriethoxysilane in acetone, 10 s.
2. Rinse briefly in acetone.
3. Rinse in distilled water.
4. Air-dry.

3.2. Buffer

This buffer is used for all dilutions and washing.

1. 0.1 *M* phosphate-buffered saline (PBS), pH 7.2 (e.g., 8 g/L NaCl, 2 g/L KCl, 1.44 g/L $Na_2HPO_4{\cdot}2H_2O$, 0.2 g/L KH_2PO_4) (*see* **Note 8**).
   or
2. Commercial PBS tablets (Sigma = 0.01 *M*, Oxoid [Basingstoke, UK] = 0.2 *M*).

3.3. Immunoperoxidase Labeling with a Three-Step Biotin/Streptavidin Method

1. Air-dry sections on the bench for 15 min. Place slides or cover slips in a moist atmosphere (e.g., Petri dish with damp filter paper; slides or cover slips are placed flat, and drops of each reagent placed on top).
2. Optional: Cover each section with methonal or acetone for 10 min (RT, unless specified by supplier); drain, and air-dry.
3. Circle each section with hydrophobic PAP pen (Agar Aids).
4. Soak with PBS for 10 min.
5. Incubate with 1% hydrogen peroxide in PBS at RT for 20 min.
6. Rinse with PBS.
7. Incubate with 5% normal serum of the same species which the secondary AB was raised, for 20 min (approx 20–25 µL, to cover each section); drain, but do not wash.
8. Incubate (approx 20–25 µL) with diluted primary Ab at RT for 1 h.
9. Wash with PBS for 5 min, 3×.
10. Incubate with diluted biotinylated secondary Ab (e.g., Amersham 1:100 or 1:200) at RT for 1 h.
11. Wash with PBS for 5 min, 3×.
12. Incubate with diluted streptavidin-peroxidase at RT for 1 h (e.g., Dako 1:200).
13. Wash slides with PBS for 5 min, 3×.
14. Prepare DAB solution (1 mg/mL DAB in PBS; just before use, add 0.1% H_2O_2). **Caution:** *See* **Note 9**.
15. Incubate in DAB–peroxide solution (enough to cover whole section) at RT for 4 min.
16. Rinse with distilled water.
17. Counterstain with hematoxylin, 30–60 s.
18. Rinse thoroughly with tap water, and soak for 5–10 min.
19. Dehydrate through graded alcohols, 70, 90, 100%; clear in two changes of xylene. Leave in xylene until ready to mount.
20. Cover each section with a drop of DPX mounting medium, and cover with a cover slip (*see* **Note 10**).

3.4 Immunofluorescence Labeling Using a Three-Step Biotin/Streptavidin Method

1. Air-dry unfixed cryostat sections, place flat in a moist atmosphere, such as a Petri dish, with damp filter paper. Optional methanol or acetone fixation for 10 min, followed by air-drying, as above.
2. Circle each section with a hydrophobic PAP pen (Agar Aids).
3. Incubate with primary Ab (approx 20–25 µL, to cover each section), diluted in PBS, RT, 30 min.
4. Rinse in PBS: Dip-wash each slide or cover slip 10 s, 3×; or place in racks, and wash in dishes for 5 min, 3×.
5. Incubate with secondary biotinylated Ab from appropriate species (e.g., Amersham 1:200) at RT for 30 min.
6. Rinse in PBS as in **step 4**.
7. Incubate with streptavidin–Texas Red diluted in PBS (e.g. Amersham 1:200) at RT, 15 min.
8. Rinse in PBS as in **step 4**.
9. Mount in Hydromount (Merck). Carefully blot the slides with filter paper and slight pressure, to ensure even distribution of the mountant (*see* Note 10).

4. Controls

Controls for ICC are essential, and a single biopsy should not be labeled in isolation. Controls should include both sample and Ab controls (**Fig. 1**). To ensure that working procedures and reagents are correct at least one sample known to be positive should be included. In practice, a group of biopsies should be labeled, and these should not all have the same provisional diagnosis (e.g., if Duchenne muscular dystrophy (DMD) is suspected, a sample in which dystrophin expression will be normal should be labeled in parallel). Concurrent labeling of several biopsies with several Abs controls for problems with reagents, and each Ab and sample will act as a control for the others. It is also good practice to include one section from each sample that is only incubated with the working buffer, instead of primary Ab, followed by the same detection system. This controls for the specificity of the primary Ab. With immunofluorescence specific labeling can be distinguished from autofluoresence by changing the excitation/emission filter. Autofluorescence (i.e., fluorescence is apparent at all wavelengths) is commonly associated with large blood vessels. Lipofuscin, which is often perinuclear, is also autofluorescent.

It is also important to check the quality and preservation of tissue samples. Abs to β-spectrin give a good indication of the preservation of the plasma membrane, and should always be used when assessing the plasma membrane proteins. Necrotic fibers usually lose their plasma membrane and appear negative with all Abs to plasmalemma proteins (**Fig. 2**). A similar effect often occurs in postmortem material. There is therefore a danger of false-negative results if

Insert Fig. 1 A-F Here

Fig. 1. A biopsy from a case of Duchenne muscular dystrophy (DMD) (**A**, **B**, **C**) and a control (**D**, **E**, **F**), immunolabeled with Abs to β-spectrin (**A, D**), C-terminal dystrophin (**B**, **E**) and α-sarcoglycan (**C**, **F**). Note the normal uniform sarcolemmal labeling in the control, but absence of dystrophin, presence of β-spectin, and a secondary reduction of α-sarcoglycan in the case of DMD. Bar = 50 μm.

Insert Fig. 2 A & B Here

Fig. 2. Sections from a case of CMD immunolabeled with Abs against β-spectrin (**A**) and fetal myosin (**B**), showing reduced labeling of a group of regenerating fibers that also express fetal myosin. Note also the number of other fibers of varying size that also express fetal myosin. Bar = 50 μm.

Insert Fig. 3 A & B Here

Fig. 3. Sections from a case of limb-girdle muscular dystrophy immunolabeled with Abs to β-spectrin (**A**) and C-terminal dystrophin (**B**), showing loss of dystrophin caused by loss of membrane integrity. β-Spectrin is an essential control for assessing sarcolemmal proteins. Bar = 50 μm.

the tissue is of poor quality. Low expression of β-spectrin and C-terminal dystrophin can also occur on regenerating fibers, and, if these are abundant, it may give a false impression of a mosaic pattern (**Fig. 3**). The preservation of the basal lamina should also be checked, particularly if a defect in the laminin α_2-chain is suspected, because necrotic fibers may lose their basal lamina. Although the basal lamina is often well-preserved when the plasma membrane is lost, occasionally, some plasma membrane may be retained in the absence of basal lamina. A good control for laminin α_2 labeling is laminin γ_1.

ICC assessment of dystrophic muscle should also take into account the presence of regenerating fibers. β-spectrin expression is low on regenerating fibers, but other proteins, such as utrophin, MHC-class I antigens, and laminin α_5, are highly expressed in immature fibers. It is therefore necessary to compare serial areas with an Ab to fetal myosin, to identify immature/regenerating fibers. Assessment of human skeletal muscle should always take into account this developmental regulation of proteins. Those relevant to the diagnosis of the MDs are mentioned here, but the expression of several other proteins is known to differ in fetal, neonatal, and adult in human muscle. If the developmental expression of a new Ab is not known, this should be experimentally tested before interpreting pathological samples.

The assessment of immunolabeling relies on the presence, absence, or reduced intensity of the visual marker. If only one Ab to a protein is used, it should be remembered that a negative result will be obtained if the Ab recognizes a portion that corresponds to a deleted a region. Protein resulting from an in-frame mutation may then be missed. For this reason, more than one Ab to a protein is helpful. For example, it is essential to use a panel of Abs to dystrophin that correspond to N-terminal, rod, or C-terminal domains, to avoid false interpretations. Abs to more than one fragment of laminin α_2 are also commercially available (*see* **Table 1**).

5. Trouble Shooting

5.1. Sections Come Off the Slides

The most common causes are poor tissue or section quality. This may be caused by poor initial freezing or subsequent handling, resulting in bad freezing artifact, or repeated thawing and freezing of stored sections. If only a few sections are required from a package stored in the freezer, the remainder must not be allowed to thaw. Samples containing much fat and connective tissue, or very necrotic tissue, may also cause adhesion problems. Coated or Superfrost slides may help in these situations (*see* **Note1**). Sections should be well dried before use, and should not be too thick (less than 10 µm), or adhesion may be a problem. Similarly, sections of uneven thickness, or wrinkled, may be less adhesive.

5.2. High Background

Endogenous immunoperoxidase, alkaline phosphatase, or biotin can be blocked (*see* **Subheading 2.6.**). Sections should not be allowed to dry out during the immunostaining procedure, because this also causes nonspecific binding of Abs, resulting in high background. Some polyclonal primary Abs may produce high background, which may be reduced by blocking the sections with a high percentage (up to 50%) of normal serum of the species in which the secondary Ab was raised. Short incubation times and a maximum dilution of the primary Ab may also reduce background.

5.3. Weak or No Signal

Because a reduced label, rather than the absence of a label, is common in the MDs, either as a primary or secondary pathological feature (**Fig. 1**), it is important that the appropriate controls are carried out to interpret a weak signal. First, the positive control should be checked (e.g., cases labeled in parallel). If this shows a similar result, all Abs and solutions should be tested, and the date when Abs were first used checked. Abs do not give consistent results indefinitely; suppliers advice for storage should be followed, if given. Azide (0.1%) should be added if storage is at 4°C (most commercial Abs contain azide), but azide should not be used in buffers, because it inhibits enzyme activity. Freezing may preserve an Ab for long lengths of time, but repeated freeze–thaw should be avoided. It is therefore advisable, and convenient to freeze aliquots of suitable volume for use, but very small volumes (less than 5 µL) or high dilutions should be avoided. If the result of the control is good, the preservation of the testing tissue should be checked morphologically, and with other Abs (*see* **Subheading 4.**). Optimizing dilutions and incubation times, incubating at 4°C, or choosing a more powerful amplification system may improve a weak signal.

5.4. Uneven Labeling

Poor tissue preservation, poor sections, sections drying out, bubbles over the section during labeling, or bubbles in the mountant are common causes of uneven results. Sections should be completely dry before applying the primary Ab, and all labeling should be carried out in a moist chamber. Bubbles over the section must be avoided and enough antibody used.

6. Notes

1. Frozen sections adhere well to cover slips, and no adhesive coating is required. Slides, however, should either be the Superfrost or Superfrost Plus type, which are designed for good adhesion. If sections do not adhere well, slides may be coated with poly-L-lysine or 3-aminopropyltriethoxysilane (Sigma). The extra cost of Superfrost slides is offset by convenience. Similarly, coated slides are also available commercially (e.g., Merck; Ray Lamb).
2. Although acetone or methanol, may be used for studies of muscle sections, in the authors' experience, this is of no advantage for human muscle.
3. In the authors' experience, nonspecific background labeling of human muscle is not a problem, if fluorescent labels are used. Furthermore, with the exception of blocking endogenous peroxidase, the authors have found that there is rarely an advantage in using blocking agents for ICC of human muscle. Good washing and optimal dilution of the Abs are more critical factors.
4. High background will be experienced when mouse monoclonal Abs are used on sections of mouse tissues (e.g., in mouse models of human MDs). This results from the binding of the secondary Ab (e.g., conjugated rabbit antimouse Igs) to endogenous mouse Igs in the tissue. Use primary Abs from a different species to the tissue being examined, if at all possible (commercial kits for mouse or mouse tissues are now available).
5. The authors have found that at RT 30 min is adequate for most Abs.
6. The authors have found Texas Red useful, because using labels in the red region reduces some of the autofluorescence in muscle, such as that associated with blood vessels. Texas Red also fades less quickly than some fluorochromes.
7. Hydromount (Merck) gives good results with Texas Red. The mountant dries to hold the cover slip in place, and fluorescence last for several weeks or months.
8. Other recipes and molarities are also suitable, but the pH should be in the range of 7.2–7.4.
9. **Caution:** DAB is potentially carcinogenic, and a face-mask should be used when weighing the powder. To avoid frequent weighing of the powder, 1-mL aliquots of

DAB in PBS can be frozen, and thawed when required. DAB is also commercially available as tablets (e.g., Sigma) or liquid (e.g., Chemicon, El Segundo, CA).

10. Sections must not be allowed to dry out at any stage, and bubbles must be avoided. Some buffer will remain on the sections after washing, but this should be kept to a minimum, to avoid alterations to the dilution of the next Ab. The volume of secondary and tertiary layers required will vary with the amount of buffer left on the section. The PAP pen circle helps to minimize the spread of these layers after washing.

References

1. Sewry, C. A., Philpot, J., Sorokin, L., Wilson, L. A., Naom I., Goodwin F., et al. (1996) Diagnosis of merosin (laminin α_2)-deficient congenital muscular dystrophy by skin biopsy. *Lancet* **347,** 582–584.
2. Sewry, C. A., D'Alessandro, M., Wilson, L. A., Sorokin, L. M., Naom, I., Bruno, S., Dubowitz, V., and Muntoni, F. (1997) Expression of laminin chains in skin in merosin-deficient congenital muscular dystrophy. *Neuropediatrics* **28,** 217–222.
3. Manilal, S., Sewry, C. A., thi Man N., Muntoni, F., and Morris, G. E. (1997) Diagnosis of X-linked Emery-Dreifuss muscular dystrophy by protein analysis of leukocytes and skin. *Neuromusc. Disord.* **7,** 63–66.
4. Sabatelli, P., Squarzoni, S., Petrini, S., Capanni, C., Ognibene, A. Cartegni, L., et al. (1998) Oral exfoliate cytology for the non-invasive diagnosis in X-linked Emery-Dreifuss muscular dystrophy patients and carriers. *Neuromusc. Disord.* **8,** 67–71.
5. Muntoni, F., Sewry, C., Wilson, L., Angelini, C., Trevisan, C. P., Brambati, B., and Dubowitz, V. (1995). Prenatal diagnosis in congenital muscular dystrophy. *Lancet* **345,** 591.
6. Naom, I., Sewry, C., D'Alessandro, M., Topaloglu, H., Ferlini, A., Dubowitz, V., and Muntoni, F. (1997) Prenatal diagnosis of merosin deficient congenital muscular dystrophy: the role of linkage and immunocytochemical analysis. *Neuromusc. Disord.* **7,** 176–179.
7. Dubowitz, V. (1985) *Muscle Biopsy: A Practical Approach.* Bailliere Tindall, London.
8. Hsu, S.-M., Raine, L., and Fanger, H. (1981) Use of avidin-biotin-peroxidase complex (ABC) in immunoperoxidase techniques. *J. Histochem. Cytochem.* **29,** 577–580.

21

Immunocytochemical Analysis

Margaret A. Johnson

1. Introduction

The inadequacy of conventional histological and histochemical examination for many aspects of the differential diagnosis of the muscular dystrophies (MDs) is well recognized. However, as specific antibodies (Abs) have become available to the proteins and glycoproteins that are causally involved in the MDs, the immunocytochemistry (ICC) applications of these probes have developed in parallel with advances in immunoblotting techniques, and have revolutionized diagnostic practice over the past decade. One of the attractions of ICC is that it is a rapid and relatively simple technique, requiring no specialized equipment in addition to that already found in most histopathology laboratories. Its main strength is that it provides unique information on the precise localization of tissue proteins, which is unobtainable by any other means. However, ICC has its limitations, as well as advantages. Although it is well suited for comparative assessment, such as variability of protein expression within muscle fiber populations, it is of limited value when absolute quantitation is required. Because of this, the ideal approach is to use both ICC and immunoblotting in parallel, because the two techniques are complementary.

The preceding chapter, on the immunological reagents, detection procedures, and amplification systems currently available, has set out the wide variety of immunofluorescence and immunoenzyme techniques that can be used. The choice of detection system employed will be influenced by context of usage, since the requirements and priorities of routine diagnostic protocols may differ from those of specific research applications. There is a tendency for routine laboratories to favor immunoperoxidase techniques, because these give durable permanent preparations that can be easily stored. They are also more amenable to counterstaining procedures, which help to delineate general tissue

From: *Methods in Molecular Medicine, vol. 43: Muscular Dystrophy: Methods and Protocols*
Edited by: K. M. D. Bushby and L. V. B. Anderson © Humana Press Inc., Totowa, NJ

morphology. On the other hand, exponents of immunofluorescence techniques will stress their extra rapidity and convenience, since no development of label reaction product is necessary. Most diagnostic laboratories tend to keep to one basic detection procedure to maximize reproducibility of results and comparability within series of patients who may be investigated over a considerable time span. The formulation of ICC protocols for routine diagnostic use will continue to evolve as greater numbers of specific probes become available. The investigations described in this chapter utilize Abs to dystrophin, utrophin, emerin, sarcoglycans (SGs), dystroglycans, laminins, lamin A/C, caveolin-3, dysferlin, telethanin, and β-spectrin. The constitution of protocols will also vary according to the precise questions of differential diagnosis that are being addressed. Suggestions and recommendations for the content of Ab panels used in diagnostic screening are given at the end of this chapter.

2. Materials and Methods

2.1. Sections

An important prerequisite of satisfactory immunolabeling of tissue sections is good tissue preparation. Skeletal muscle and cardiac muscle need to be frozen in isopentane at –150°C to avoid ice-crystal artifact. Other tissues that may be investigated, such as skin and placenta, may be frozen directly in liquid nitrogen. Frozen sections should be cut at a thickness of about 6 μm (*see* **Note 1**) and mounted on slides coated with 0.5% gelatin–0.5% chrome alum, to ensure good adhesion. For most antigens investigated in the diagnosis of the MDs, a standard drying time of 1 h is appropriate, after which the sections may be wrapped in Clingfilm, and stored at –40 to –80°C until used (up to several months, if necessary). Before use, allow stored sections to equilibrate to room temperature (RT) before unwrapping, to avoid condensation, then air-dry for a further hour.

2.2. Immunoperoxidase Labeling

1. Apply primary Ab, diluted appropriately in phosphate-buffered saline (PBS: 12.5 m*M* phosphate) pH 7.3 containing 1% bovine serum albumin (BSA); 1 h at RT.
2. Wash 3× in PBS; total time 30 min.
3. Apply secondary Ab (e.g., peroxidase-conjugated rabbit antimouse immunoglobulin G, if using mouse monoclonal primary Ab) appropriately diluted in PBS/BSA; 1 h at R.T.
4. Wash 3× in PBS; total time 30 min.
5. Develop peroxidase label reaction product using 1.5 m*M* 3,3'-diaminobenzidine hydrochloride (DAB) as chromogen and 0.01% hydrogen peroxide as substrate, in 0.1 *M* phosphate pH 7.3; 10 min at R.T.
6. Discard incubation medium into dilute hypochlorite, to polymerize DAB before disposal.

7. Wash sections well in tap water, rinse in dH_2O.
8. Counterstain nuclei with hematoxylin (optional); dehydrate, clear, and mount.

The use of duplicate sections for each Ab used is recommended as a precaution in case of accidental damage to sections, and also to act as a control for the consistency of labeling.

3. Results: Investigation of Specific Dystrophies

3.1. Xp21-Linked Disorders (Dystrophinopathies)

The spectrum of Xp21-linked MD encompasses patients whose biopsies show no detectable dystrophin, and also those in whom dystrophin expression appears indistinguishable from normal on ICC labeling. Between these two extremes there is a great diversity of patterns of dystrophin expression, differing both in labeling intensity and in cellular distribution. It is important to use Abs directed against several sites in the dystrophin molecule, because false-negative results may occur if a particular deletion has removed the epitope recognized by the antidystrophin Ab used. A panel of Abs directed against N-terminus, rod domain, and C-terminus is in common usage, and allows some assessment to be made of the integrity of separate molecular domains.

3.1.1. Duchenne Muscular Dystrophy

Experience in individual diagnostic laboratories may differ somewhat, but on average about 40% of biopsies from Duchenne muscular dystrophy (DMD) patients will be found to show no detectable dystrophin on tissue sections (**Fig. 1A,B**). Thus, over one half of DMD biopsies will be expected to show some evidence of dystrophin expression, sometimes confined to a small proportion of the muscle fiber population (**Fig. 1C,D**), and sometimes widespread at low labeling intensity. When assessing DMD biopsies, it is therefore useful to use some form of grading system, such as the one outlined in **Table 1** *(1)*.

The ability to detect very low levels of any antigen will depend on the sensitivity of the labeling system (*see* Chapter 20), and also on the absence of unwanted nonspecific binding of Abs, which would otherwise detract from the totally negative or clean appearance of control sections. The detection of a small percentage of labeled fibers in an otherwise negative biopsy will obviously depend on the size of the biopsy sample. The current trend away from open biopsy procedures, in favor of needle or conchotome biopsies, may result in failure to detect isolated fibers or small clusters of fibers, that express some dystrophin.

The status of the sporadic, strongly dystrophin-positive fibers in some DMD biopsies has been the subject of some debate, but it can be demonstrated that the dystrophin in these fibers has an intact C-terminus *(2)*. The usual out-of-frame

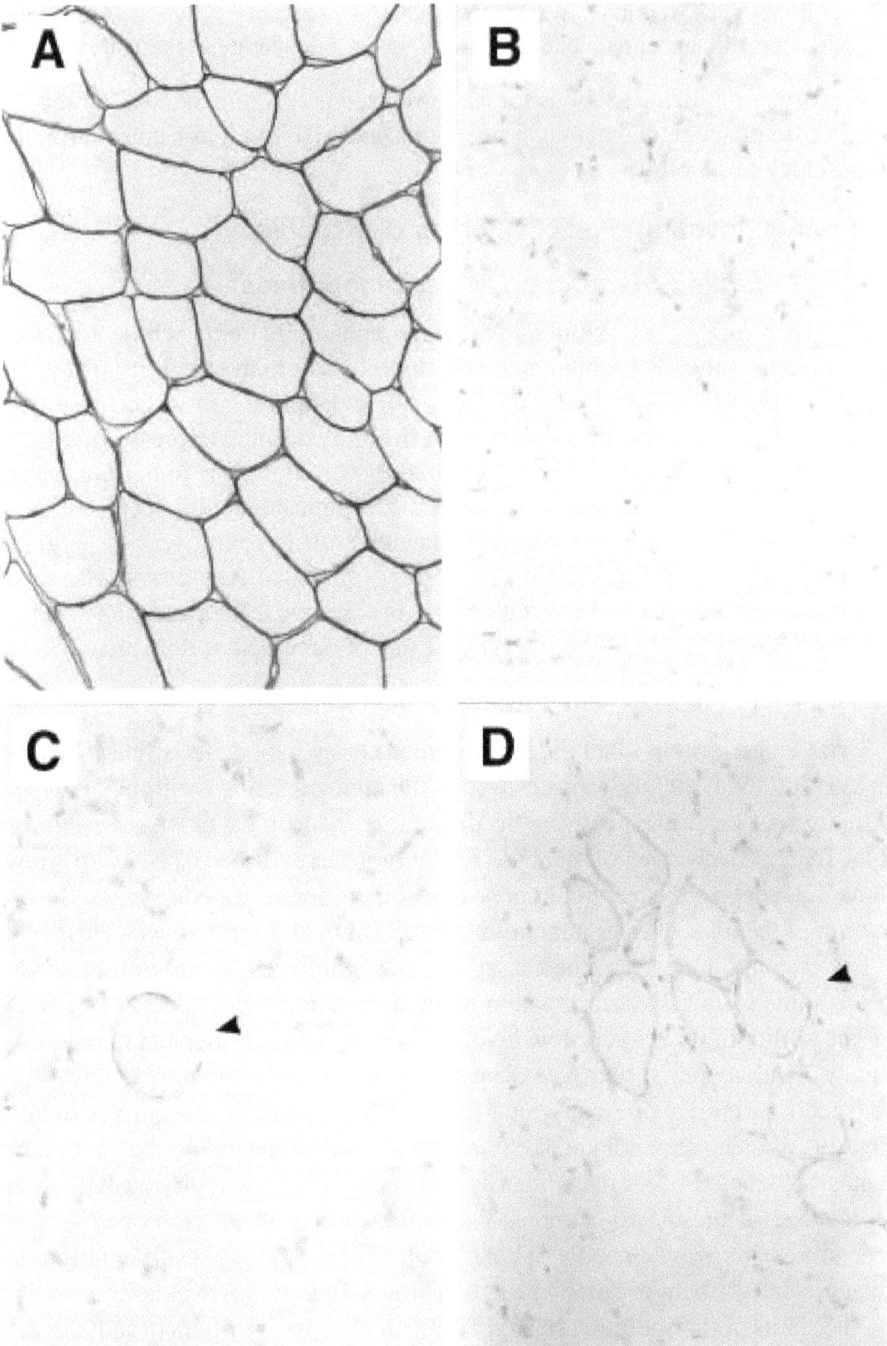

Table 1
Grading System for Dystrophin Labeling

Grade	Dystrophin Labeling On Sections
1	No labeling on any muscle fibers.
2	Faint labeling on occasional fibers; majority of fibers negative.
3	Clear labeling on occasional fibers, generally less than 1%.
4	Low intensity labeling on up to 50% fibers (± occasional more strongly labeled fibers).
5	Low-intensity labeling on almost all fibers.
6	Variable intensity labeling (variation between and/or within fibers).
7	Moderately and uniformly decreased labeling.
8	Near-normal labeling intensity.

Grades 1–5 are relevant to DMD biopsies, and grades 5–8 to Becker MD biopsies.

deletions that occur in DMD would not allow dystrophin synthesis up to the C-terminus, but evidence has been documented for restoration of the open reading frame in these occasional dystrophin-positive fibers *(3)*. It has been shown that a variety of secondary somatic mutations may take place within one affected individual, each extending the deletion in such a way as to bring it back into frame *(4,5)*. The distribution of widely scattered single dystrophin-positive fibers is consistent with this interpretation. Small clusters of dystrophin-positive fibers (**Fig. 1D**) normally show identical profiles, when reacted with panels of antidystrophin Abs, and are thought to derive from clones of myoblasts bearing the same secondary mutation. Although dystrophin-positive fibers are commonly referred to, if these fibers are studied by serial sectioning or in longitudinal sections, it is found that the length of dystrophin-positive fiber segments is often less than 1 mm *(6)*. Monitoring the influx of calcium and albumin in serial sections showed that these indicators of membrane damage were present in the dystrophin-negative rather than dystrophin-positive fiber segments *(7)*. The overall incidence of dystrophin-positive fibers (or fiber segments) is rarely greater than 1% of total cross-sectional area.

Fig. 1. *(opposite page)* **(A)** Biopsy from control patient aged 29 yr, showing normal dystrophin immunolabeling. **(B)** DMD: biopsy from patient aged 4 yr, showing total absence of immunolabeling. **(C)** DMD: biopsy from patient aged 5 yr, illustrating an isolated dystrophin-positive muscle fiber. **(D)** DMD: biopsy from patient aged 7 yr, showing a cluster of dystrophin-positive fibers. Dystrophin (rod domain)/immunoperoxidase ×200.

The presence of widespread, faint, or low-intensity labeling in tissue sections (grades 4 or 5) correlates with milder phenotype when DMD populations are analyzed *(1,6,8)*, but this may not be a meaningful indicator in individual patients. In a subset of patients defined as intermediate DMD/Becker muscular dystrophy (BMD) with loss of independent walking between 12 and 16 yr, 100% biopsies showed unequivocal dystrophin labeling, compared with 65% biopsies from DMD patients who lost independent ambulation between 9 and 12 yr, and about 50% DMD biopsies from patients confined to wheelchairs before 9 yr *(1)*. It would appear that the presence of dystrophin, even an abnormally shortened molecule, can confer extra survival potential on individual muscle fibers, and autopsy samples of DMD muscle may show higher proportions of dystrophin-positive fibers than biopsy samples taken years earlier from the same patient.

Utrophin, the chromosome (chr) 6-encoded dystrophin homolog, is expressed in normal adult skeletal muscle at the neuromuscular junction only, and not at extrajunctional plasma membranes. However, in DMD biopsies, it is seen to be strongly upregulated in almost all fibers. Occasional exceptions are the sporadic dystrophin-positive fibers. There is thus a roughly reciprocal relationship between dystrophin and utrophin expression *(9)*, although a precise complementary relationship is uncommon, possibly because many dystrophin-negative fiber segments are restricted in extent. Utrophin is strongly expressed in regenerating fibers, whatever their origin (i.e., in inflammatory myopathies and in non-Xp21-linked disorders, as well as in DMD and BMD), since it is developmentally regulated, and this phenomenon should not be misinterpreted as upregulation caused by dystrophin deficiency *(10)*.

Dystrophin is linked via a complex of transmembrane dystroglycan and SG proteins to the outside of the muscle fiber. As a result of this direct association, levels of the dystrophin-associated glycoproteins are generally severely decreased in situations in which dystrophin is absent *(11,12)*, but the extent of the decrease varies from biopsy to biopsy.

3.1.2. Becker Muscular Dystrophy

The extremely low levels of dystrophin labeling seen in DMD biopsies enable diagnosis to be made on ICC evidence alone. However, this is often not possible with BMD. In this milder phenotype, dystrophin expression varies from low intensity labeling on all or almost all fibers (grade 5) to near-normal labeling (grade 8) (*see* **Table 1**) indistinguishable by ICC alone from that seen in normal muscle, or more relevantly, from that seen in nonXp21-linked MDs *(13)*.

In BMD, the most commonly observed abnormality of dystrophin immunolabeling in tissue sections is that of excessive variability in labeling intensity (*see* **Note 2**), which is present in about 80% of BMD biopsies. Intrafiber variation (variation in labeling intensity within individual fibers) can consist of a gradation of high- and low-intensity labeling around the fiber periphery, or may include areas that are dystrophin-negative (**Fig. 2A**). At its most dramatic, interfiber variation (variation between fibers) can consist of all gradations of labeling intensity, from negative to supranormal (**Fig. 2B**). The latter is found mostly in hyaline fibers, and is probably associated with overcontraction. Implicit in the concept of variable labeling, whether interfiber or intrafiber, is that there must be some local decrease in intensity, even if this is only moderate. However, variability in labeling intensity can occur in conjunction with an overall decrease, which may be mild, moderate, or severe (**Fig. 2C**).

In BMD biopsies, a moderate decrease in labeling intensity, without any excessive variability, is encountered much less frequently (grade 7 on the dystrophin-labeling scale). The final category (grade 8) covers the small percentage of BMD biopsies in which labeling intensity cannot be distinguished from normal (**Fig. 2D**). Biopsies from this group are generally also mildly affected, from a histopathological viewpoint, often with only a mild fiber size variability and few other abnormalities.

At the ICC level, it is easy to detect the difference between 0% dystrophin and 10% dystrophin, but difficult, if not impossible, to discriminate between 90 and 100%. This is one of the chief reasons why immunoblotting and its associated quantitative analysis should be employed in parallel with ICC investigations. If a small proportion of BMD biopsies cannot be distinguished from non-Xp21-linked disorders on ICC criteria, it also follows, as an inconvenient but important corollary, that non-Xp21-linked disorders cannot be definitively identified as such, without immunoblotting to demonstrate the presence of dystrophin of normal size and abundance. Utrophin labeling can sometimes provide useful corroborative evidence when attempting to discriminate between normal dystrophin labeling and dystrophin that is marginally decreased. The expression of utrophin and dystrophin is broadly reciprocal, and increased utrophin expression may be easier to detect than minimally decreased dystrophin expression.

When panels of dystrophin Abs are used on BMD biopsies, the patterns of labeling abnormality seen in tissue sections show some correlation with dystrophin size as estimated by immunoblotting. In a recent study of almost 60 BMD patients, a panel of Abs, to N-terminus, C-terminus, to three separate locations within the rod domain, and to the cysteine-rich domain, was used ***(14)***. About one-half the biopsies showed excessively variable labeling with all Abs used. In this subset, immunoblotting showed normal or slightly decreased dystrophin size in all but two patients who showed a slightly larger than normal protein. The other subset showed ICC abnormalities that were mostly associated with one major domain, sometimes with variable abnormalities in an

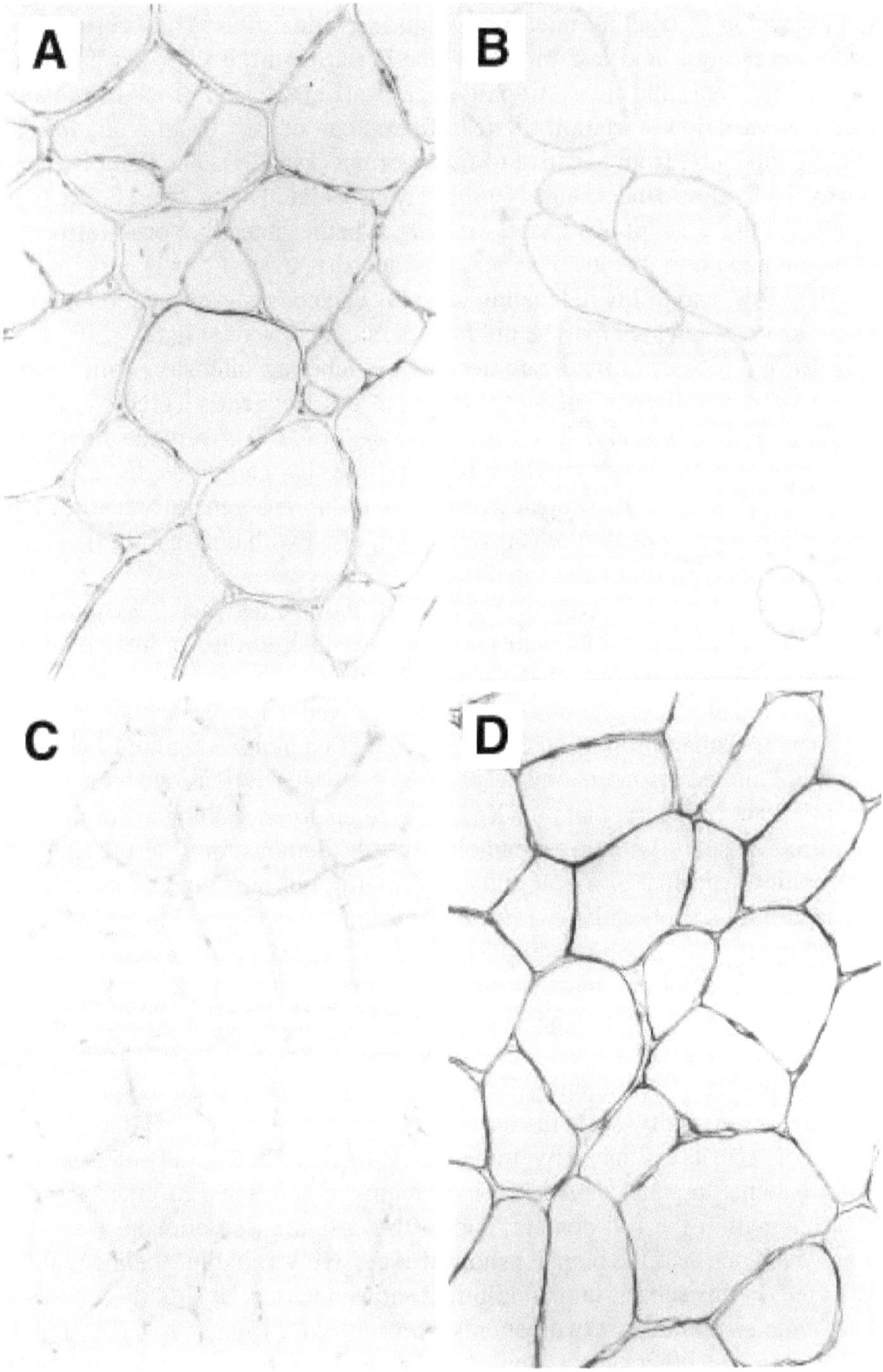
A
B
C
D

adjacent domain. Immunoblotting of these biopsies generally showed more severe size decreases. This group also included all the patients who showed either a uniform moderate decrease in ICC labeling or labeling that was indistinguishable from normal. These made up about 8 and 5%, respectively, of all BMD biopsies assessed. The second group was clinically milder, suggesting that the larger-scale deletions associated with loss of N-terminus or rod domain segments could result in dystrophin molecules, which were more functional than those of normal or near-normal size, but with a patchy distribution at the plasma membrane.

An extreme example of clinically mild BMD was seen in a patient in whose muscle almost 50% of the dystrophin molecule was missing, because of a large-scale deletion of the rod domain, but which showed virtually normal N- and C-terminus labeling ***(15)***. A patient with a huge duplication, resulting in a dystrophin molecule of 600 kDa, was also a mild BMD phenotype, and showed near-normal labeling on tissue sections, although there was some variation from fascicle to fascicle ***(16)***. Individuals with BMD who present clinically as quadriceps myopathy, although mildly affected, show variability in dystrophin labeling, which is often at least as severe as that seen in BMD patients with more generalized muscle involvement ***(17)***. This seems to apply both to the affected quadriceps muscles and to minimally affected muscles, such as biceps brachii ***(18)***.

3.1.3. Carriers of Xp21-Linked Disorders

Many women who are carriers of DMD or BMD show no abnormalities of dystrophin labeling in muscle sections. If one assumes that random X-inactivation ***(19)*** results in approx 50% normal nuclei and 50% nuclei in which the abnormal dystrophin gene is expressed, then muscle syncitia may contain a random and equal mixture of nuclei that can direct the synthesis of normal dystrophin and nuclei that cannot. Under these circumstances, dystrophin immunolabeling appears indistinguishable from normal, presumably because of complementation across normal and abnormal nuclear domains.

In other individuals, the process of X-inactivation may not be truly random, leading to an excess of myoblast clones with the defective X chr, and, later, in myogenesis, to the presence of dystrophin-deficient muscle fibers or fiber segments (*see* Chapter 10). The mosaic appearance of dystrophin-positive and

---

Fig 2. *(opposite page)* **(A)** BMD: biopsy from patient aged 17 yr, showing intrafiber variation in labeling intensity. **(B)** BMD: patient aged 18 yr, illustrating interfiber variation in labeling intensity. **(C)** BMD: patient aged 22 yr, showing severe uniform decrease in labeling intensity. **(D)** BMD: patient aged 30 yr, whose biopsy shows near-normal labeling intensity. Dystrophin (rod domain)/immunoperoxidase ×200.

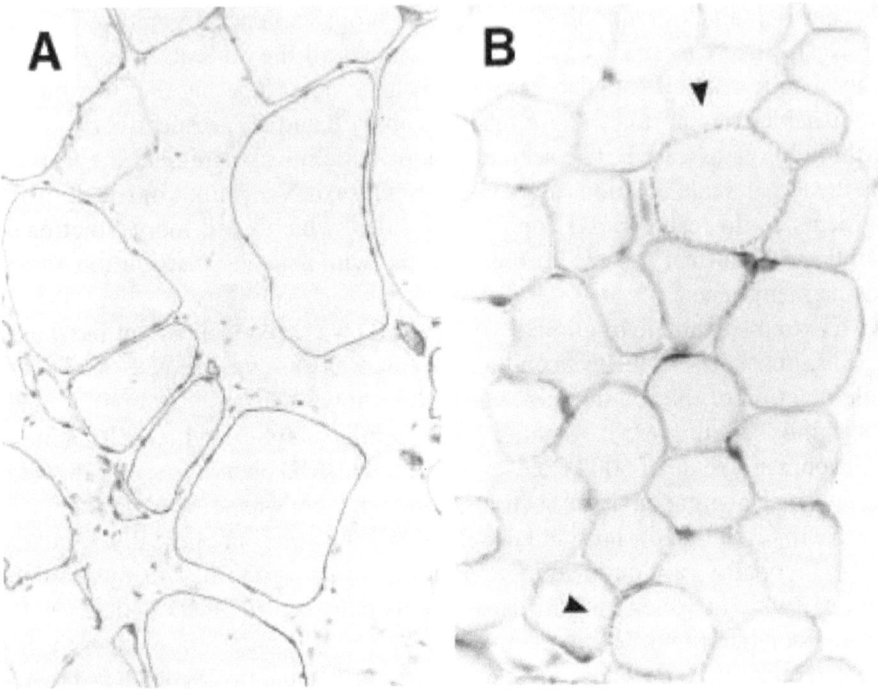

Fig 3. (A) DMD carrier: patient aged 23 yr, showing a mosaic of dystrophin-positive and dystrophin-negative muscle fibers (×200). **(B)** BMD carrier: patient aged 4 yr, illustrating variable decrease in dystrophin labeling with an occasional beaded labeling pattern (×400). Dystrophin (rod domain)/immunoperoxidase.

dystrophin-deficient fibers is, as one would expect, much more prevalent in manifesting carriers (**Fig. 3A**) than in nonmanifesting carriers. In the latter group, up to about 5% dystrophin-deficient fibers have been reported, although 0–2% is more common ***(20)***. In manifesting carriers, the proportion may be as high as 70% or as low as 2%, but considerable intrasample variation may be seen, if large biopsies are examined. It must therefore be recognized that proportions of dystrophin-negative or deficient fibers estimated from small samples may not be truly representative, and, if muscle biopsy is undertaken with the particular aim of investigating Xp21 carrier status, it is obvious that small samples should be avoided (*see also* **Note 3**).

Manifesting carriers of BMD are rarer than manifesting carriers of DMD, even allowing for the greater incidence of the latter. Obviously, one reason for this is that the phenotype would be expected to be mild and possibly misdiagnosed. BMD carriers who do manifest muscle weakness and degeneration often do so late in life (fourth decade onwards). It is not unknown to find mild histological abnormalities, but severe dystrophin abnormalities, with over 25% dystrophin-negative fibers *(21)*. Since all daughters of BMD patients are obligate carriers, the increased efficiency of ascertainment of BMD means that more potentially manifesting females will be monitored from an early age. One 4-yr-old girl, the daughter of a patient with clinically typical BMD, showed more severe dystrophin abnormalities by ICC labeling than did her father, though she herself was as yet mildly affected. Her pattern of dystrophin labeling was characterized by a high proportion of negative fibers, and also scattered fibers showing a regular "dotted line" of discontinuous labeling, not present in biopsies from either her father or affected uncle (Fig. 3B). Further ICC investigation showed that β-spectrin labeling in serial sections showed a similar "dotted-line" pattern in this BMD carrier, a finding suggestive of a more generalized membrane defect. It was speculated that the co-existence of two molecular species of dystrophin might lead to faulty targeting and location of other membrane-associated proteins *(22)*.

In addition to the investigation of manifesting and nonmanifesting carriers from known DMD and BMD families, the ICC detection of dystrophin abnormalities has proved to be particularly valuable in the detection of Xp21 carrier status in female patients with myopathy, but with no informative family history *(23)*. Many such patients have previously been misdiagnosed, on clinical and/or histopathological grounds, as affected by other forms of MD or by nonhereditable disorders (*see* **Note 4**).

3.2. Emery-Dreifuss Muscular Dystrophy

X-linked Emery-Dreifuss muscular dystrophy (EDMD1) is caused by mutations in the *STA* gene (chr Xq28), which encodes a 34-kDa protein known as emerin *(24)*. This protein is expressed in many tissues, and, unlike many of the molecules that are causally associated with human MDs, emerin is not located at the muscle fiber surface. It is associated with the nuclear membrane, and may have a hydrophobic C-terminus within the inner nuclear membrane, with the rest of the molecule extending into the nucleoplasm *(25,26)*. Its function is currently unknown.

Emerin can be labeled by immunofluorescence or immunoenzyme methods in tissue sections, without recourse to any of the additional permeabilization procedures that are often necessary for demonstrating antigens within membrane-bound organelles, such as lysosomes and mitochondria (**Fig. 4A,B**). If immunoperoxidase or other immunoenzyme methods are used, it is preferable not to add a nuclear counterstain, which may obscure the immunolabeling, unless very lightly applied. A good alternative method for making sure that all nuclei are labeled is to use phase-contrast microscopy. This is particularly valuable in the examination of biopsies from possible carriers in whom a variable proportion of muscle nuclei may be emerin-negative.

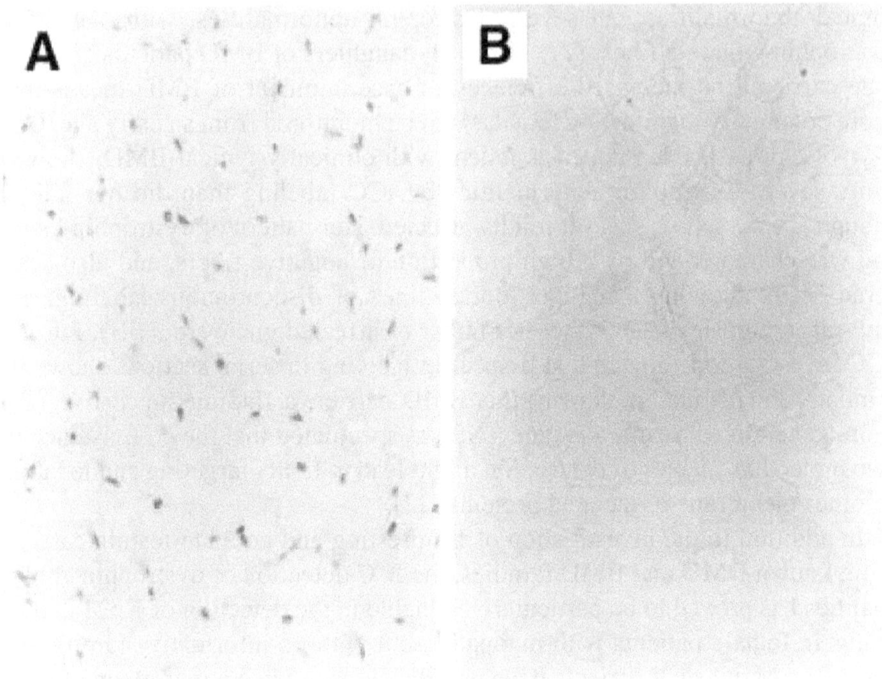

Fig 4. (A) Control patient aged 9 yr, showing normal labeling for emerin localized at the nuclear membranes in muscle tissue. **(B)** EDMD: patient aged 13 yr, whose muscle biopsy shows complete absence of emerin immunolabeling. Emerin/immunoperoxidase ×200.

EDMD1 patients and carriers may also be investigated using skin biopsy, which is a less-invasive procedure than muscle biopsy. In both skin and muscle, 100% of nuclei are emerin-negative in EDMD1 patients (*see* **Note 5**); as yet, no laboratories have reported any instances of residual emerin labeling, or, by analogy with dystrophin in DMD, of any revertant emerin. The proportion of nuclei that are emerin-positive in carriers may be as low as 10% in skin biopsies *(27)*. Whereas leucocytes may be used in immunoblotting of emerin, ICC studies have been hampered by the need to fix and permeabilize leucocytes before labeling, and by the fact that emerin epitopes appear to be adversely affected by many commonly used fixatives. EDMD2 is an autosomal dominant disorder, encoded on chr1 and associated with defective lamin A/C; like emerin this protein is located in the inner nuclear lamina and shows a characteristic perinuclear labeling pattern. It is likely that EDMD2 is allelic with LGMD1B (*see* **Subheading 3.3.8.**).

3.3 Sarcoglycanopathies and Limb-girdle Muscular Dystrophies

In recent years, the clinicopathological classification of limb girdle muscular dystrophies (LGMD), both juvenile and of later onset, has been superceded by a classification based on genetic and protein analysis. The disorders formerly classed as severe childhood autosomal recessive MD were described as having Duchenne-like severity, whose autosomal mode of transmission was most readily detected in large families with consanguinity and/or multiple affected members of both sexes *(28,29)*. Both from a clinical standpoint and in terms of histopathology, this type of childhood MD seemed profoundly different from most adult-onset LGMDs. However, identification of the same SG defects, both in these severe childhood disorders and in milder adult myopathies *(30–32)*, has compelled the classification to be modified.

The starting point for SG analysis is usually the finding of normal dystrophin immunolabeling in tissue sections, and confirmation of this result by immunoblotting *(33)*. This preliminary step serves to differentiate young sarcoglycanopathy patients from DMD or early BMD, and adult LGMD patients from adult BMD (*see* **Note 4**). Manifesting carriers of DMD/BMD also figure in this stage of differential diagnosis. SG analysis by ICC and immunoblotting is particularly important, because most mutations identified in LGMD patients are small, so that any technique that indicates the probable site of the gene defect, thus saving time involved in DNA analysis, is of great practical value (***34***; *see* **Note 6**).

There are currently five proteins that are classified as belonging to the SG group (α-, β-, γ-, δ-, and ε-SG), and pathological mutations causing forms of MD have been found in the first four (*see* Chapters 13, 14, and 15). None has yet been identified in the ε-*SG* gene *(35)*. The proteins appear to function as a group, and the absence of one member of the complex generally affects all the other members of the complex *(36)*. However, labeling for one member protein may appear more severely reduced than the others, indicating that the primary gene defect lies in the gene for this protein, and the reduction in the other proteins is a secondary phenomenon *(32,37)*. When one SG is clearly more radically affected than the rest, immunolabeling may give useful information about the best place to begin DNA analysis. However, in many biopsies, no one particular SG is predominantly affected. All may be absent or decreased to a roughly equivalent extent. Where there is generalized absence of detectable SGs, the clinical phenotype is generally severe. More moderate decreases in all four SGs is usually associated with a milder clinical phenotype and survival beyond the third decade.

3.3.1. α-Sarcoglycanopathy (LGMD2D)

The first SG defect to be identified in the context of childhood LGMD patients was that involving α-SG (initially called “adhalin”), a 50-kDa glycoprotein

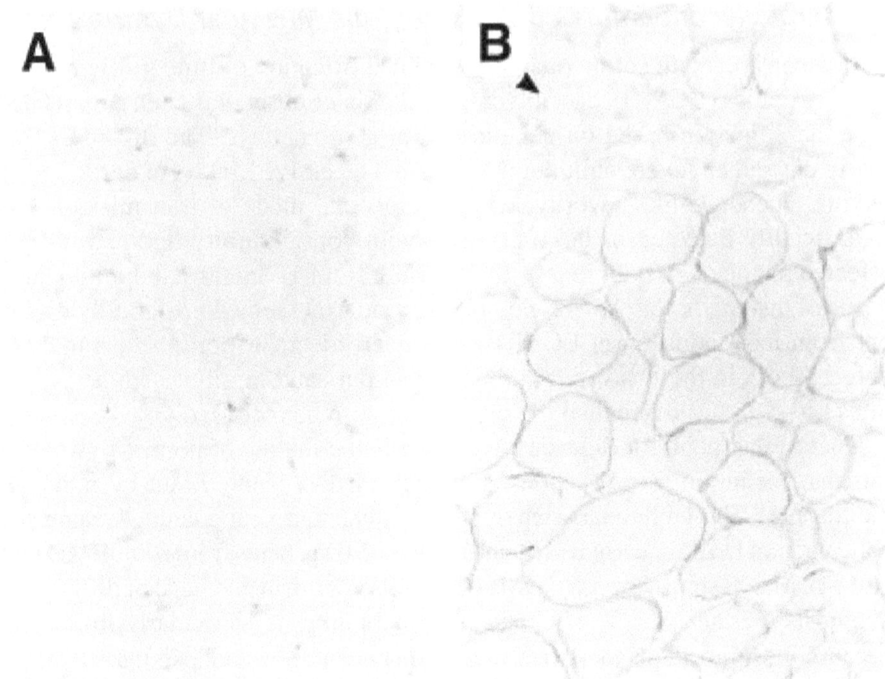

Fig 5. **(A)** LGMD2D: patient aged 6y showing total absence of α-SG (adhalin) immunolabeling. α-SG/Immunoperoxidase ×200. **(B)** Serial section to A, showing near-normal dystrophin labeling, except in clusters of regenerating fibers where it is of lower intensity. Dystrophin (C-terminus)/immunoperoxidase ×200.

occupying a transmembrane location at the sarcolemma ***(12)***. In many juvenile patients with α-SG defects, the molecule appears to be totally absent from the sarcolemma (**Fig. 5**), frequently accompanied by variable decreases in labeling for the other SGs. However, where the observed decrease in α-SG labeling is partial, not total, it is possible that missense mutations may have occurred, often leading to less severe phenotypes ***(38,39)***. The missense mutation, R284C, is particularly associated with residual protein expression and a milder clinical phenotype ***(40)***. It has been estimated that only about 5% of juvenile non Xp21-linked MDs are caused by primary mutations in the α-SG gene ***(41)***, reduced levels of the protein often being associated with primary defects in other genes (*see* **Note 7**).

3.3.2. β-Sarcoglycanopathy (LGMD2E)

Mutations in the β-SG gene pose a particular problem in SG analysis, because they are generally associated with the loss, not only of the 43-kDa β-SG pro-

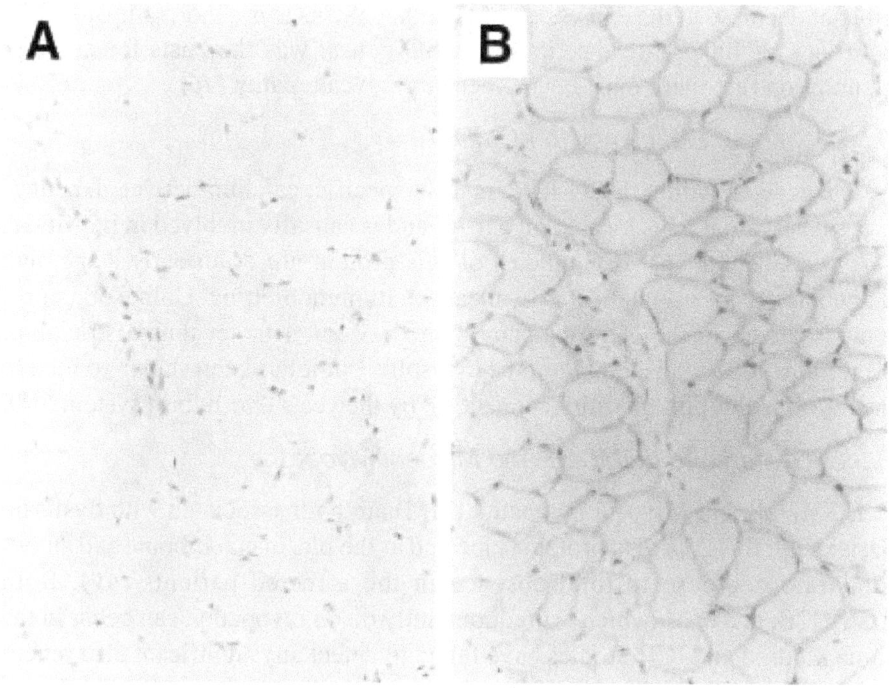

Fig 6. (**A**) LGMD2C: patient aged 7 yr, showing total absence of γ-SG labeling. γ-SG/immunoperoxidase ×200. (**B**) Serial section to 6, showing α-sarcoglycan (adhalin) labeling, which is only moderately decreased. α-SG/immunoperoxidase ×200.

tein, but of the whole SG complex *(36,42)*. Missense mutations in this gene may be associated with severe phenotypes *(39,43)*.

3.3.3. γ-Sarcoglycanopathy (LGMD2C)

Many patients with severe childhood autosomal recessive MD prove to have a primary defect in the gene for the 35-kDa γ-SG protein. This form of sarcoglycanopathy is particularly prevalent in North Africa *(44)*, but is also common in Europe, and elsewhere. It is of particular note that the absence/severe reduction of γ-SG labeling on sections may be accompanied by a mere decrease in the expression of the other SGs *(37)*. This has certainly been the author's experience in Newcastle (*see* **Fig. 6A,B**).

3.3.4. δ-Sarcoglycanopathy (LGMD2F)

Mutations in the gene for the 35-kDa δ-SG protein are uncommon *(45)*. As well as the absence or severe decrease in δ-SG, LGMD2F patients show a significant decrease in the expression of the other sSGs. This abnormality, together with lack of linkage to the first three SG genes, was the basis for an early assumption that there must be another sarcoglycanopathy ***(46)***.

3.3.5. Calpain Deficiency in LGMD2A

The gene encoding the 94-kDa, muscle-specific, calcium-activated, neutral proteinase calpain 3 is located on chr 15, and is causally involved in LGMD2A (*47*; *see* Chapter 16). ICC studies of this protein are at an early stage, and diagnosis is currently indicated by means of immunoblotting. Unlike other proteins involved in the MDs, calpain is an enzymatic, rather than a structural, protein. Its location is thought to be cytosolic, but it has been shown to bind to the myofibrillar protein, titin (connectin), by the yeast two-hybrid system ***(48)***.

3.3.6. Dysferlin in LGMD2B and Miyoshi Myopathy

LGMD2B and Miyoshi myopathy (MM) are both associated with dysferlin deficiency; this 237-kDa protein is located at the plasma membrane and shows moderate decrease to total absence in the affected patients ***(49)***. Both LGMD2B, and MM, which is predominantly distal myopathy, can occur in the same kindred and ICC Studies have failed to detect any significant differences in labelling patterns; immunoblotting showed similar decreases in abundance. The currently-used antibodies label only weakly in normal tissue sections so very careful reading of ICC results is necessary. Histological examination may give a preliminary suspicion of LGMD2B since inflammatory infiltrates are more common in this disorder than in other forms of LGMD.

3.3.7. Telethonin in LGMD2G

LGMD2G is a predominantly distal muscular dystrophy and "rimmed vacuoles" have been reported to occur in some cases ***(50)***. The protein encoded by the LGMD2G gene has been named telethonin; it is a 19-kDa sacomeric protein associated with the Z-disc and a substrate of titin, which phosphorylates its C-terminal domain. The protein is expressed in skeletal and cardiac muscle only. The ICC labelling of telethonin in transverse skeletal muscle sections shows the usual "moiré" pattern characteristic of proteins with a sarcomeric distribution.

3.3.8. Lamin A/C in LGMD1B

LGMD1B is associated with chr 1 and affects both skeletal and cardiac muscle; it is thought to be allelic with the autosomal dominant form of Emery-Dreifuss (EDMD2), but though the latter disorder shows skeletal muscle contractures, there is no cardiac involvement ***(51)***.

3.3.9. Caveolin-3 in LGMD1C

Muscle membranes contain specialized indentations called "caveoli," and mutations in the gene for the 18-kDa protein, caveolin-3, have recently been shown in patients with a form of dominant LGMD *(52)*. Caveolin-3 is localized to the sarcolemma, like dystrophin and the Sgs, but it is not thought to be an integral member of that complex. Reduced caveolin-3 labeling has been reported in two LGMD1C families with missense and microdeletion mutations *(52)*. One other missense mutation resulted in near-normal expression of caveolin 3 in a patient who developed muscle weakness in her first decade *(53)*. Clearly, there is not yet sufficient data available to comment on the potential usefulness of caveolin-3 ICC in the diagnosis of this disease entity.

3.3.10. Laminin Abnormalities in LGMD

To date, no form of LGMD has been associated with primary mutations in any of the genes encoding laminin chains (*see* **Note 8** for details of the laminin family). Nevertheless, various secondary abnormalities in chain expression have been reported. For example, a group of sarcoglycanopathy patients showed a severe decrease in laminin β_1-chain, accompanied by an upregulation of β_2-light chain, which is usually expressed rather faintly at the skeletal muscle basal lamina *(54)*. Another subgroup of LGMD patients showing laminin β_1 deficiencies are autosomal dominant myopathies of early onset, with contractures and spinal rigidity *(55)*. Only older family members seemed to demonstrate the labeling deficiency, and not younger individuals, suggesting an acquired, and therefore secondary, process of laminin β_1 decrease. The deficiency was confined to skeletal muscle, with the laminin β_1-light chain in the muscle vasculature unaffected. This secondary reduction in laminin β_1 expression is not uncommon in adult LGMD cases; the authors also have studied a LGMD patient whose initial biopsy showed normal β_1-light chain expression, but whose second biopsy, taken 13 yr later, showed a significant decrease in laminin β_1 labeling. A decrease in laminin β_1 expression has also been reported in LGMD patients with different clinical features *(56)*.

A further group of adult LGMD patients (including two sib pairs) have shown a secondary reduction of laminin α_2-chain expression on blots, but not sections *(57)*. It is possible that these patients share a predisposition to α_2-chain fragility, which is exposed by the tissue-processing required to perform the immunoblot analysis. The α_2 chain is prone to fragmentation, and the 400-kDa polypeptide is normally found as 300-kDa and 80-kDa fragments on blots.

3.4. Congenital Muscular Dystrophies and Merosinopathies

Congenital muscular dystrophies (CMD) are characterized by muscle weakness and wasting, which is present at, or shortly after, birth. They are progres-

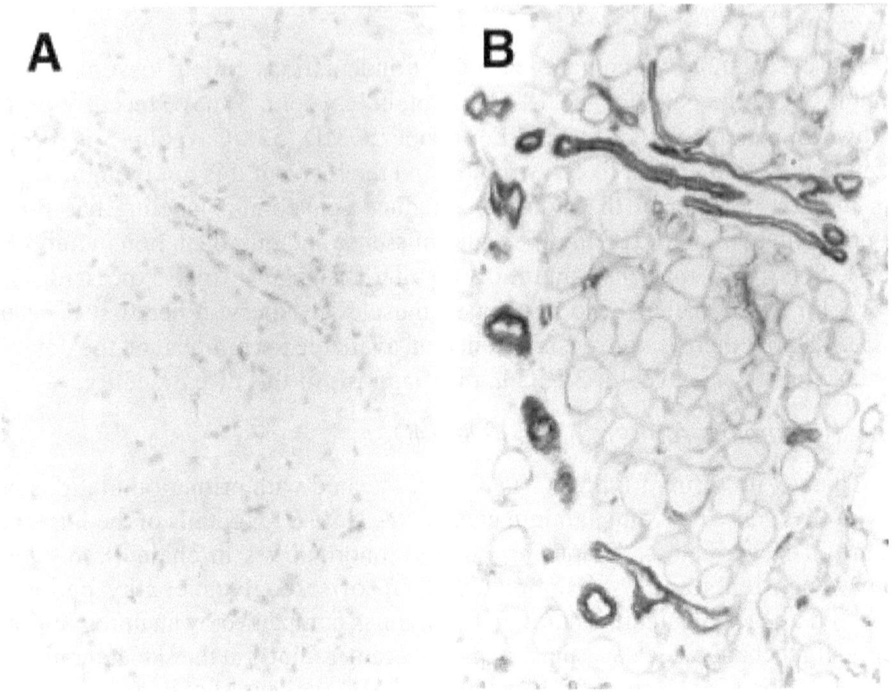

Fig 7. **(A)** CMD: patient aged 3 mo, showing complete absence of laminin-α_2 (merosin) labeling. Laminin-α_2/immunoperoxidase ×200. **(B)** Serial section to 7, showing upregulation of laminin-α_5 at the surface of muscle fibers and the normal labeling of small blood vessels. Laminin-α_5/immunoperoxidase ×200.

sive, and characterized by muscle fiber necrosis and regeneration. In contrast, congenital myopathies may be nonprogressive, and muscles from affected patients show little necrosis and regeneration. A predominant form of CMD in Europe and America is that associated with merosin (laminin-2) deficiency ***(58)***, caused by defects of the *LAMA2* gene on chr 6 (*see* Chapter 12). It has been shown that merosin-deficient CMD patients have significant white matter changes, and also a more severe myopathy, than CMD patients with normal merosin expression ***(59)***, so that immunolabeling studies play an important role in diagnosis and prognosis. In Japan, the Fukuyama type of congenital MD (FCMD) predominates. Although some abnormalities of white matter are seen on CT scans in FCMD, the major central nervous system abnormality is micropolygyria of cerebrum and cerebellum, with severe mental retardation and speech defects as invariable concomitant features ***(60)***.

3.4.1. Merosin-Deficient CMD

The major isoform expressed in the basal lamina of skeletal muscle is laminin-2 (merosin). In total merosin deficiency (**Fig. 7A**) caused by absence of the α_2-heavy chain, considerable upregulation of the α_5-homolog (**Fig. 7B**) is demonstrable by immunolabeling on the muscle fiber population as a whole ***(61)***. If only partial deficiency of the α_2-chain is seen, then the overexpression of the laminin α_5-heavy chain is correspondingly moderate. There is thus a broadly reciprocal relationship between the two molecules. The observation of upregulated laminin α_5-heavy chain can be helpful in instances in which the decrease of α_2 immunolabeling is equivocal, but caution must be exercised when assessing biopsies that contain numerous regenerating fibers in which high α_1 expression is a normal manifestation of myogenesis.

Recently, it has been shown that Abs to different fragments of the laminin α_2-heavy chain may give different results regarding severity of merosin deficiency ***(62)***. Most laboratories have used a commercially available Ab that recognizes a C-terminus 80-kDa fragment; Abs to a 300-kDa fragment have been used only comparatively recently. Some patients' biopsies that showed only minimal laminin α_2 decrease, using the anti-80-kDa fragment Ab, showed a severe decrease when the anti-300-kDa fragment Ab was used (*see* **Note 9**). Confirmation of these patients as being compatible with defects at the *LAMA2* locus was given by haplotype analysis in three informative families. This study also drew attention to the widening range of clinical phenotypes associated with merosin deficiency, and advocated the investigation of laminin α_2 expression with more than one Ab. This approach played a significant part in the identification of a family with a late-onset LGMD caused by partial merosin deficiency ***(63)***, with one member of the family showing white matter changes on MRI scan.

No abnormalities of laminin light chain expression (β_1 and γ_1) are seen in the majority of merosin deficiencies, but a proportion of biopsies, in which the α_2-chain appears totally absent, also show a significant decrease in β_1 labeling ***(61)***. This appeared to be specific to muscle fiber surface labeling, because the labeling intensity of capillaries was unaltered.

Although most immunolabeling studies of CMD have concentrated on the laminin-2 constituents, α_2-heavy chain and β_1- and γ_1-light chains, it has been shown that normal skeletal muscle basal lamina also contains some β_2-light chain. This is present at significantly lower labeling intensity than the β_1-homolog. A marked decrease in β_2 labeling was seen in four cases of total α_2-chain deficiency and a moderate decrease in four cases of partial α_2 deficiency, as well as in two cases of merosin-positive CMD ***(64)***. Because the precise nature of the laminin isoform containing the β_2-light chain, which is subject to these decreases in CMD, is conjectural, the specificity of the association of α_2 and β_2 decrease is not yet proven.

Skin biopsies have been used as an alternative to muscle biopsy for the investigation of laminin-2 deficiency. Biopsy samples are orientated so that transverse sections of the full thickness of the biopsy are obtained. Immunolabeling of normal skin shows laminin α_2-chain localized to the epithelial cells of hair follicles, as well as in a continuous layer at the dermal/epidermal junction, associated with the basement membrane. A similar labeling pattern was seen with both 80-kDa and 300-kDa α_2 Abs. In patients whose muscle biopsies were totally merosin-deficient, no labeling was seen in skin biopsies with either anti-α_2 Ab ***(65)***.

The problem of prenatal detection of CMD has prompted investigation of merosin expression in placenta ***(66)***. Chorionic villous samples (CVS) from placentas of 8–23 wk gestational age were found to react strongly with antilaminin α_2 chain Abs, and with Abs to the other heterotrimer components, β_1 and γ_1. Localization was to basement membranes of trophoblasts: dissection of CVS needs to be done carefully, to eliminate any associated endometrium. This is obviously crucial if the sample is also to be used for DNA analysis ***(67)***. Dissected CVS samples are usually processed by floating them on a drop of cryoembedding medium prior to freezing, which allows the full depth of these small samples to be utilized. When CVS samples are used in prenatal diagnosis, gestational age is 11–13 wk. Total merosin deficiency, in one CVS sample studied, correlated with total absence demonstrated in the fetal muscle after termination. In cases in which the fetus has been shown to be heterozygote, laminin α_2-chain immunolabeling in CVS samples was found to be indistinguishable from normal in a majority of instances, although the carrier state may be associated with some decrease in α_2 labeling of trophoblasts ***(67)***. The difficulties attendant upon the interpretation of ICC results, other than total deficiency, prompt considerable caution and parallel investigation of all CVS samples by haplotype analysis.

3.4.2. Integrin α_7 and Congenital Myopathy

Among the laminin receptors in muscle basal lamina is integrin $\alpha_7\beta_1$D. Integrin β_1 is expressed throughout the body; α_7 is more muscle-specific. Pathogenic mutations in the α_7 gene have recently been identified in three patients with a congenital myopathy and delayed motor milestones ***(68)***. Labeling for integrin α_7 was undetectable in these patients, accompanying a mild reduction in β_1D. A secondary reduction in α_7-protein expression was also found in four more patients with laminin-2 deficiency (in two of these cases, mutations were found in the *LAMA2* gene). An apparent increase in α_7-chain expression has been reported in dystrophin-deficient humans and mice ***(69)***. Targetted disruption of the murine α_7 gene resulted in a condition reported to be a progressive cCMD ***(70)***, but was thought to more resemble a congenital myopathy ***(68)***. There is currently insufficient data to determine how useful the immunoanalysis of integrin α_7 will be in the differential diagnosis of the congenital muscle disorders.

3.4.3. Fukuyama CMD

FCDM is predominant in Japan and is caused by a 3 kb retrotransposal insertion into the 3' noncoding region of the fukutin gene on chr 9q31 *(71)*. Fukutin protein contains an N-terminal signal sequence and is thought to be a secreted extracellular protein. Attempts to localize fukutin in muscle sections by ICC using monoclonal and polyclonal antibodies have been unsuccessful, though the protein has been detected by ICC in tranfected cells. The function of fukutin has vbeen speculated as stabilizing the association of basal lamina (BL) and plasma membrane (PM) in skeletal muscle and other affected tissues. There are also demonstrable decreases in laminin subunits, particularly the α_2-chain *(72)*, but, since FCMD is known to be localized to the chr 9q31 genetic locus, it is clear that these decreases must be of a secondary nature. Excessive variability in dystrophin immunolabeling has also been recorded *(73)*, together with abnormalities of β-spectrin labeling. In at least some patients, there appeared to be a parallel decrease in dystrophin and β-spectrin in fibers that were neither acutely necrotic nor regenerating. Non-FCMD patients' biopsies showed a very low incidence of abnormal immunolabeling for both dystrophin and β-spectrin. Investigations of β-dystroglycan labeling in tissue sections *(74,75)* have given rather conflicting results, but, if present, are certainly secondary in nature.

3.5. Suggested Ab Panels

All of the Abs mentioned in this chapter are commercially available (with the exception, at the time of writing, of the integrin α_7 Abs). Dystrophin Abs are available from Novocastra Laboratories (Newcastle upon Tyne, UK) and Sigma (St. Louis, MO); Abs to all the SGs, laminin α_2-chain, and to emerin are also available from Novocastra. Antibodies to the 80-kDa fragment of laminin α_2-chain are available from Chemicon (El Segundo, AC), and to caveolin-3 from Transduction Laboratories.

3.5.1. First Screening Panel

A preliminary screening panel might be composed of the following Abs: dystrophin: N-terminus, C-terminus, rod domain; Sgs: α-SG, γ-SG; laminins: α_2 80 kDa, 300 kDa; α_5 β-spectrin.

A primary use of this panel will be to identify DMD and BMD biopsies, as effectively as possible; note the use of multiple dystrophin Abs to avoid false-negative results in BMD patients with deletions that remove an Ab-binding site. Immunoblotting will be necessary to distinguish BMD biopsies with near-normal ICC labeling from genuine non-Xp21-linked disorders. The inclusion of Abs to the two SGs most frequently involved in LGMDs initiates investigation of the underlying defects in juvenile and adult LGMD phenotypes. The inclusion of laminin α_2-chain Abs in an initial screening panel should ensure that atypical merosinopathy phenotypes are not missed. Labeling for β-spectrin is included to monitor membrane integrity.

3.5.2. Secondary Ab Panels

1. A secondary LGMD panel might include: SGs: α-SG, β-SG, γ-SG, δ-SG; laminins: β_1, γ_1; emerin, lamin A/C, caveolin-3. dysferlin, and telethonin.

   It is important to re-screen biopsies showing abnormalities of α- and γ-SG labeling, with a full SG panel to clarify their status. As well as Abs to α-, β-, γ-, and δ-Sgs, this panel could usefully include Abs to laminin β_1-light chain, which is decreased in some cases of LGMD (both recessive and dominant), and also to laminin β_2, which may be upregulated when β_1 is decreased. Since patients with the form of LGMD associated with laminin β_1 deficiency often have contractures, labeling for emerin might also be advised. If no defects are identified, biopsies from patients with LGMD phenotypes are screened via calpain 3 immunoblotting.
2. A separate laminins ICC protocol is often used for CMD biopsies, which is an acceptable procedure, as long as provision is made for the atypical phenotypes. A suitable laminins panel might consist of: laminins: α_5 (upregulated in α_2 deficiency), α_2 (both 80-kDa and 300-kDa fragments), β_1 (decreased in a minority of CMD biopsies), β_2, γ_1 (generally unaltered).

The pattern of usage of screening panels will be influenced by the prevalence of phenotypes being investigated; this is particularly true of laboratories working with biopsies from predominantly adult or juvenile patients. The investigation protocols have constantly evolved over the past decade, and will continue to do so, at least until the utopia of 100% detection has been achieved.

4. Notes

1. Immunolabeling patterns are commonly misinterpreted as normal on sections that are too thick. Sections of 10 μm or more lose sensitivity, so that labeling that is variable appears uniform.
2. Selection of the most valid control for variation in labeling intensity, against which BMD biopsies may be compared, is a matter of debate. The uniform dystrophin labeling seen in totally normal muscle offers one standard of comparison, but it may be argued that a more meaningful comparison is that made between a BMD biopsy and a non-Xp21-linked disorder of equivalent histological severity. Labeling intensity, not only of dystrophin, but of a whole range of muscle membrane-associated proteins, is influenced by the presence of histopathological abnormalities. Supranormal intensity of labeling is associated with

hyaline fibers; and regenerating fibers show lower levels of dystrophin expression than fully differentiated fibers.

3. Rupture of muscle plasma membranes may occur in overstressed muscle fibers, and all plasma membrane proteins will be lost from necrotic fibers in the terminal stages of the degradation process. It is important to verify that any dystrophin-negative fibers are not merely necrotic, by using a control Ab, such as anti-β-spectrin, on serial sections, to monitor the integrity of the muscle plasma membrane. This practice is useful and normally valid, since β-spectrin is very rarely involved in the MDs, although there are a few reported exceptions *(76)*.
4. Some sarcoglycanopathy patients show a reduction in dystrophin labeling, particularly of the C-terminus *(37)*. In Newcastle, for example, two patients originally diagnosed as being manifesting carriers of an Xp21-linked condition, on this basis *(22)*, are now known to have mutations in the genes for α- or γ-SG. Similarly, one severe BMD patient *(1)* is now known to have γ-sarcoglycanopathy.
5. Normal-appearing emerin has recently been demonstrated by blot analysis in leucocytes and lymphoblastoid cell lines from a patient with a 22-bp deletion in the promoter region *(77)*. Muscle was not available for analysis from this patient, so that the implications of this finding are not clear-cut.
6. In order to optimize the process of identifying predominantly affected SGs by ICC, it is important that low levels of glycoprotein are detectable, thus distinguishing total absence from severe decrease, and that moderate decreases are not masked by overamplification or other technical factors. As in all applications of ICC in which these are used in a semiquantitative manner, it is recommended that checkerboard titrations are done to define the optimal concentrations of both primary and secondary Abs.
7. Because Abs to α-SG (adhalin) were the first ICC probes to be used in the investigation of sarcoglycanopathies, some patients were tentatively designated as adhalin deficient, only to be reclassified as having a more general sarcoglycanopathy, when probes to the other Sgs became available. Genetic analysis of all four SG genes is required to definitively resolve the diagnostic dilemma.
8. Laminins are cruciform molecules, with a heterotrimeric structure of one heavy chain and two light chains, which span the basal lamina. Laminin nomenclature has changed several times in recent years *(78)*; the new names of relevant laminin chains and their associated genes are listed below.

Gene	Laminin chain	Previous name
LAMA1	α_1	A
LAMA2	α_2	M
LAMB1	β_1	B1
LAMB2	β_2	S
LAMC1	γ_1	B2

Laminin type	Trimer	Previous name
Laminin-1	$\alpha_1\beta_1\gamma_1$	EHS laminin
Laminin-2	$\alpha_2\beta_1\gamma_1$	Merosin
Laminin-3	$\alpha_1\beta_2\gamma_1$	S-laminin
Laminin-4	$\alpha_2\beta_2\gamma_1$	S-merosin

9. The merosin Ab sold by Novocastra Laboratories has the same sensitivity as the 300-kDa one (C. Sewry, personal communication). Note also that the Chemican Ab to laminin in α_5 was originally designated as α_1.

References

1. Nicholson, L. V. B., Johnson, M. A., Bushby, K. M. D., Gardner-Medwin, D., Curtis, A., Ginjaar, H. B., et al. (1993) Trilogy: integrated study of 100 patients with Xp21-linked muscular dystrophy using clinical, genetic, immunochemical, and histopathological data. Part 1: Trends across the clinical groups. Part 2: Correlations within individual patients. Part 3: Differential diagnosis and prognosis. *J. Med. Genet.* **30,** 728–751.
2. Nicholson, L. V. B., Johnson, M. A., Davison, K., O'Donnell, E., Falkous, G., Barron, M., and Harris, J. B. (1992) Dystrophin or a "related protein" in Duchenne muscular dystrophy? *Acta Neurol. Scand.* **86,** 8–14.
3. Klein, C. J., Coovert, D. D., Bulman, D. E., Ray, P. N., Mendell, J. R., and Burghes, A. H. M. (1992) Somatic reversion/supression in Duchenne muscular dystrophy (DMD): evidence supporting a frame-restoring mechanism in rare dystrophin-positive fibers. *Am. J. Hum. Genet.* **50,** 950–959.
4. Nicholson, L. V. B. (1993) The "rescue" of dystrophin synthesis in boys with Duchenne muscular dystrophy. *Neuromusc. Disord.* **3,** 525–532.
5. Wallgren-Pettersson, C., Jasani, B., Rosser, L. G., Lazarou, L. P., Nicholson, L. V. B., and Clarke, A. (1993) Immunohistological evidence for second or somatic mutations as the underlying cause of dystrophin expression by isolated fibers in Xp21 muscular dystrophy of Duchenne-type severity. *J. Neurol. Sci.* **118,** 56–63.
6. Fanin, M., Danieli, G. A., Cadaldini, M., Miorin, M., Vitiello, L., and Angelini, C. (1995) Dystrophin-positive fibers in Duchenne dystrophy: origin and correlation to clinical course. *Muscle Nerve* **18,** 1115–1120.
7. Morandi, L., Mora, M., Gussoni, E., Tedeschi, S., and Cornelio, F. (1990) Dystrophin analysis in Duchenne and Becker muscular dystrophy carriers: correlation with intracellular calcium and albumin. *Ann. Neurol.* **28,** 674–679.
8. Nicholson, L. V. B., Johnson, M. A., Bushby, K. M. D., and Gardner-Medwin, D. (1993) The functional significance of dystrophin-positive fibers in Duchenne muscular dystrophy. *Arch. Dis. Child.* **68,** 632–636.
9. Pons, F., Augier, N., Léger, J. O. C., Robert, A., Tomé, F. M. S., Fardeau, M., et al. (1991) A homologue of dystrophin is expressed at the neuromuscular junctions of normal individuals and DMD patients, and of normal and *mdx* mice: immunological evidence. *FEBS Lett.* **282,** 161–165.

10. Helliwell, T. R., Man, N. T., Morris, G. E., and Davies, K. E. (1992) The dystrophin-related protein, utrophin, is expressed on the sarcolemma of regenerating human skeletal muscle fibers in dystrophies and imflammatory myopathies. *Neuromusc. Disord.* **2,** 177–184.
11. Ervasti, J. M., Ohlendieck, K., Kahl, S. D., Gaver, M. G., and Campbell, K. P. (1990) Deficiency of a glycoprotein component of the dystrophin complex in dystrophic muscle. *Nature* **345,** 315–319.
12. Matsumura, K., Tomé, F. M. S., Collin, H., Azibi, K., Chaouch, M., Kaplan, J.-C., Fardeau, M., and Campbell, K. P. (1992) Deficiency of the 50K dystrophin associated glycoprotein in severe childhood autosomal recessive muscular dystrophy. *Nature* **359,** 320–322.
13. Nicholson, L. V. B., Johnson, M. A., Gardner-Medwin, D., Bhattacharya, S., and Harris, J. B. (1990) Heterogeneity of dystrophin expression in patients with Duchenne and Becker muscular dystrophy. *Acta Neuropathol.* **80,** 239–250.
14. Morandi, L., Mora, M., Confalonieri, V., Barresi, R., Di Blasi, C., Brugnoni, R., et al. (1995) Dystrophin characterization in BMD patients: correlation of abnormal protein with clinical phenotype. *J. Neurol. Sci.* **132,** 146–155.
15. England, S., Nicholson, L. V. B., Johnson, M. A., Forrest, S. M., Love, D. R., Zubrzycka-Gaarn, E. E., Bulman, D. E., Harris, J. B., and Davies, K. E. (1990) Very mild muscular dystrophy associated with the deletion of 46% of dystrophin. *Nature* **343,** 180–182.
16. Angelini, C., Beggs, A. H., Hoffman, E. P., Fanin, M., and Kunkel, L. M. (1990) Enormous dystrophin in a patient with Becker muscular dystrophy. *Neurology* **40,** 808–812.
17. Wada, Y., Itoh, Y., Furukawa, T., Tsukagoshi, H., and Arahata, K. (1990) Quadriceps myopathy: a clinical variant form of Becker muscular dystrophy. *J. Neurol.* **237,** 310–312.
18. Sunohara, N., Arahata, K., Hoffman, E. P., Yamada, H., Nishimiya, J., Arikawa, E., et al. (1990) Quadriceps myopathy: forme fruste of Becker muscular dystrophy. *Ann. Neurol.* **28,** 634–639.
19. Lyon, M. F. (1962) Sex chromatin and gene action in the mammalian X-chromosome. *Am. J. Hum. Genet.* **14,** 135–148.
20. Bonilla, E., Schmidt, B., Samitt, C. E., Miranda, A. F., Hays, A. P., de Oliveira, A. B. S., et al. (1988) Normal and dystrophin-deficient fibers in carriers of the gene for Duchenne muscular dystrophy. *Am. J. Pathol.* **133,** 440–445.
21. Glass, I. A., Nicholson, L. V. B., Watkiss, E., Johnson, M. A., Roberts, R. G., Abbs, S., Brittain-Jones, S., and Boddie, H. G. (1992) Investigation of a female manifesting Becker muscular dystrophy. *J. Med. Genet.* **29,** 578–582.
22. Bushby, K. M. D., Goodship, J. A., Nicholson, L. V. B., Johnson, M. A., Haggerty, I. D., and Gardner-Medwin, D. (1993) Variability in clinical, genetic and protein abnormalities in manifesting carriers of Duchenne and Becker muscular dystrophy. *Neuromusc. Disord.* **3,** 57–64.
23. Hoffman, E. P., Arahata, K., Minetti, C., Bonilla, E., and Rowland, L. P. (1992) Dystrophinopathy in isolated cases of myopathy in females. *Neurology* **42,** 967–975.
24. Bione, S., Maestrini, E., Rivella, S., Mancini, M., Regis, S., Romeo, G., and Toniolo, D. (1994) Identification of a novel X-linked gene responsible for Emery-Dreifuss muscular dystrophy. *Nature* **8,** 323–327.

25. Nagano, A., Koga, R., Ogawa, M., Kurano, Y., Kawada, J., Okada, R., et al. (1996) Emerin deficiency at the nuclear membrane in patients with Emery-Dreiffus muscular dystrophy. *Nature Genet.* **12,** 254–259.
26. Manilal, S., Man, N. t., Sewry, C. A., and Morris, G. E. (1996) The Emery-Dreifuss muscular dystrophy protein, emerin, is a nuclear membrane protein. *Hum. Mol. Genet.* **5,** 801–808.
27. Manilal, S., Sewry, C. A., Man, N. t., Muntoni, F., and Morris, G. E. (1997) Diagnosis of X-linked Emery-Dreifuss muscular dystrophy by protein analysis of leucocytes and skin with monoclonal antibodies. *Neuromusc. Disord.* **7,** 63–66.
28. Ben Hamida, M., Fardeau, M., and Attia, N. (1983) Severe childhood muscular dystrophy affecting both sexes and frequent in Tunisia. *Muscle Nerve* **6,** 469–480.
29. Somer, H., Voutilanen, A., Knutila, S., Kaitila, I., Rapola, J., and Leinonen, H. (1985) Duchenne-like muscular dystrophy in two sisters with normal kayotypes: evidence for autosomal recessive inheritance. *Clin. Genet.* **28,** 151–156.
30. McNally, E. M., Passos-Bueno, M. R., Bönnemann, C. G., Vainzof, M., de Sá Moreira, E., Lidov, H. G. W., et al. (1996) Mild and severe muscular dystrophy caused by a single γ-sarcoglycan mutation. *Am. J. Hum. Genet.* **59,** 1040–1047.
31. Eymard, B., Romero, N. B., Leturcq, F., Piccolo, F., Carrié, A., Jeanpierre, M., et al. (1997) Primary adhalinopathy (α-sarcoglycanopathy): clinical, pathologic, and genetic correlation in 20 patients with autosomal recessive muscular dystrophy. *Neurology* **48,** 1227–1234.
32. Barresi, R., Confalonieri, V., Lanfossi, M., Di Blasi, C., Torchiana, E., Mantegazza, R., et al. (1997) Concomitant deficiency of β- and γ-sarcoglycans in 20 α-sarcoglycan (adhalin)-deficient patients: Immunohistochemical analysis and clinical aspects. *Acta Neuropathol.* **94,** 28–35.
33. McGuire, S. A. and Fischbeck, K. H. (1991) Autosomal recessive Duchenne-like muscular dystrophy: molecular and histochemical results. *Muscle Nerve* **14,** 1209–1212.
34. Anderson, L. V. B. (1996) Optimised protein diagnosis in the autosomal recessive limb-girdle muscular dystrophies. *Neuromusc. Disord.* **6,** 443–446.
35. Ettinger, A. J., Feng, G. P., and Sanes, J. R. (1997) ε-Sarcoglycan, a broadly expressed homologue of the gene mutated in limb-girdle muscular dystrophy 2D. *J. Biol. Chem.* **272,** 32,534–32,538.
36. Bönnemann, C. G., Modi, R., Noguchi, S., Mizuno, Y., Yoshida, M., Gussoni, E., et al. (1995) β-sarcoglycan (A3b) mutations cause autosomal recessive muscular dystrophy with loss of the sarcoglycan complex. *Nature Genet.* **11,** 266–273.
37. Vainzof, M., Passos-Bueno, M. R., Canovas, M., de Sá Moreira, E., Pavanello, R. C. M., Marie, S. K., et al. (1996) The sarcoglycan complex in the six autosomal recessive limb-girdle muscular dystrophies. *Hum. Mol. Genet.* **5,** 1963–1969.
38. Roberds, S. L., Leturcq, F., Allamand, V., Piccolo, F., Jeanpierre, M., Anderson, R. D., et al. (1994) Missense mutations in the adhalin gene linked to autosomal recessive muscular dystrophy. *Cell* **78,** 625–633.
39. Duggan, D. J., Gorospe, J. R., Fanin, M., Hoffman, E. P., and Angelini, C. (1997) Mutations in the sarcoglycan genes in patients with myopathy. *New Engl. J. Med.* **336,** 618–624.

40. Carrié, A., Piccolo, F., Leturcq, F., De Toma, C., Azibi, K., Beldjord, C., et al. (1997) Mutational diversity and hot spots in the α-sarcoglycan gene in autosomal recessive muscular dystrophy (LGMD2D). *J. Med. Genet.* **34,** 470–475.
41. Duggan, D. J., Fanin, M., Pegoraro, E., Angelini, C., and Hoffman, E. P. (1996) α-Sarcoglycan (adhalin) deficiency: complete deficiency patients are 5% of childhood-onset dystrophin-normal muscular dystrophy and most partial deficiency patients do not have gene mutations. *J. Neurol. Sci.* **140,** 30–39.
42. Lim, L. E., Duclos, F., Broux, O., Bourg, N., Sanada, Y., Allamand, V., et al. (1995) β-Sarcoglycan: characterization and role in limb-girdle muscular dystrophy linked to 4q12. *Nature Genet.* **11,** 257–265.
43. Bönnemann, C. G., Passos-Bueno, M. R., McNally, E. M., Vainzof, M., de Sá Moreira, E., Marie, S. K., et al. (1996) Genomic screening for β-sarcoglycan gene mutations: Missense mutations may cause severe limb-girdle muscular dystrophy type 2E (LGMD 2E). *Hum. Mol. Genet.* **5,** 1953–1961.
44. Ben Othmane, K., Ben Hamida, M., Pericak-Vance, M. A., Ben Hamida, C., Blel, S., Carter, S. C., et al. (1992) Linkage of Tunisian autosomal recessive Duchenne-like muscular dystrophy to the pericentromeric region of chromosome 13q. *Nature Genet.* **2,** 315–317.
45. Duggan, D. J., Manchester, D., Stears, K. P., Matthews, D. J., Hart, C., and Hoffman, E. P. (1997) Mutations in the γ-sarcoglycan gene are a rare cause of autosomal recessive limb-girdle muscular dystrophy (LGMD2). *Neurogenetics* **1,** 49–58.
46. Passos-Bueno, M. R., de Sá Moreira, E., Vainzof, M., Marie, S. K., and Zatz, M. (1996) Linkage analysis in autosomal recessive limb-girdle muscular dystrophy (AR LGMD) maps a sixth form to 5q33-34 (*LGMD2F*) and indicates that there is at least one more subtype of AR LGMD. *Hum. Mol. Genet.* **5,** 815–820.
47. Richard, I., Broux, O., Allamand, V., Fougerousse, F., Chiannilkulchai, N., Bourg, N., et al. (1995) Mutations in the proteolytic enzyme calpain 3 cause limb-girdle muscular dystrophy type 2A. *Cell* **81,** 27–40.
48. Sorimachi, H., Kimura, S., Kinbara, K., Kazama, J., Takahashi, M., Yajima, H., et al. (1996) Structure and physiological functions of ubiquitous and tissue-specific calpain species; Muscle-specific calpain, p94, interacts with connectin/titin. *Adv. Biophys.* **33,** 101–122.
49. Anderson, L. V. B., Davison, K., Moss, J. A., Young, C., Cullen, M. J., Walsh, J., et al. (1999) Dysferlin is a plasma membrane protein and is expressed earlyin human development. *Hum. Mol. Genet.* **8,** 855–861.
50. Moreira, E. S., Wiltshire, T. J., Faulkenr, G., Nilforoushan, A., Vainzof, M., Suzuki, O. T., et al. (2000) Limb-girdle muscular dystrophy type 2G is caused by mutation in the gene encoding the sarcomic protein telethonin. *Nat. Genet.* **24,** 163–166.
51. Bonne, G., Di Barletta, M. R., Varnous, S., Becane, H. M., Hammouda, E. H., Merlini, L., et al. (1999) Mutations in the gene encoding lamin A/C cause autosomal dominant Emery-Dreifuss muscular dystrophy. *Nat. Genet.* 21, 285–288.
52. Minetti, C., Sotgia, F., Bruno, P., Scartezzini, P., Broda, P., Bado, M., et al. (1998) Mutations in the caveolin-3 gene cause autosomal dominant limb-girdle muacular dystrophy. *Nature Genet.* **18,** 365–368.

53. McNally, E. M., de Sá Moreira, E., Duggan, D. J., Bönnemann, C. G., Lisanti, M. P., Lidov, H. G. W., et al. (1998) Caveolin-3 in muscular dystrophy. *Hum. Mol. Genet.* **7,** 871–877.
54. Yamada, H., Tomé, F. M. S., Higuchi, I., Kawai, H., Azibi, K., Chaaoch, M., et al. (1995) Laminin abnormality in severe childhood autosomal recessive muscular dystrophy. *Lab. Invest.* **72,** 715–722.
55. Taylor, J., Muntoni, F., Robb, S., Dubowitz, V., and Sewry, C. (1997) Early onset autosomal dominant myopathy with rigidity of the spine: a possible role for laminin β1? *Neuromusc. Disord.* **7,** 211–216.
56. Li, M., Dickson, D. W., and Spiro, A. J. (1997) Abnormal expression of laminin β_1 chain in skeletal muscle of adult-onset limb-girdle muscular dystrophy. *Arch. Neurol.* **54,** 1457–1461.
57. Bushby, K. M. D., Anderson, L. V. B., Pollitt, C., Naom, I., Muntoni, F., and Bindoff, L. (1998) Abnormal merosin in adults: a new form of late onset muscular dystrophy not linked to chromosome 6q2. *Brain* **121,** 581–588.
58. Tomé, F. M. S., Evangelista, T., Leclerc, A., Sunada, Y., Manole, E., Estournet, B., et al. (1994) Congenital muscular dystrophy with merosin deficiency. *C. R. Acad. Sci. Paris* **317,** 351–357.
59. Philpot, J., Sewry, C., Pennock, J., and Dubowitz, V. (1995) Clinical phenotype in congenital muscular dystrophy: correlation with expression of merosin in skeletal muscle. *Neuromusc. Disord.* **5,** 301–305.
60. Kamoshita, S., Konishi, Y., Segawa, M., and Fukuyama, Y. (1976) Congenital muscular dystrophy as a disease of the central nervous system. *Arch. Neurol.* **33,** 513–516.
61. Sewry, C. A., Philpot, J., Mahony, D., Wilson, L. A., Muntoni, F., and Dubowitz, V. (1995) Expression of laminin subunits in congenital muscular dystrophy. *Neuromusc. Disord.* **5,** 307–316.
62. Sewry, C. A., Naom, I., D'Alessandro, M., Sorokin, L., Bruno, S., Wilson, L. A., Dubowitz, V., and Muntoni, F. (1997) Variable clinical phenotype in merosin-deficient congenital muscular dystrophy associated with differential immunolabeling of two fragments of the laminin α2 chain. *Neuromusc. Disord.* **7,** 169–175.
63. Tan, E., Topaloglu, H., Sewry, C., Zorlu, Y., Naom, I., Erdem, S., et al. (1997) Late onset muscular dystrophy with cerebral white matter changes due to partial merosin deficiency. *Neuromusc. Disord.* **7,** 85–89.
64. Cohn, R. D., Herrmann, R., Wewer, U. M., and Voit, T. (1997) Changes of laminin β2 chain expression in congenital muscular dystrophy. *Neuromusc. Disord.* **7,** 373–378.
65. Sewry, C. A., Philpot, J., Sorokin, L. M., Wilson, L. A., Naom, I., Goodwin, F., et al. (1996) Diagnosis of merosin (laminin-2) deficient congenital muscular dystrophy by skin biopsy. *Lancet* **347,** 582–584.
66. Voit, T., Fardeau, M., and Tomé, F. M. S. (1994) Prenatal detection of merosin expression in human placenta. *Neuropediatrics* **25,** 332–333.
67. Naom, I., Sewry, C., D'Alessandro, M., Topaloglu, H., Ferlini, A., Wilson, L., Dubowitz, V., and Muntoni, F. (1997) Prenatal diagnosis in merosin-deficient congenital muscular dystrophy. *Neuromusc. Disord.* **7,** 176–179.

68. Hayashi, Y. K., Chou, F. L., Enguall, E., et al. (1998) Mutations in the Integrin α7 gene cause congenital myopathy. *Nature Genet.* **19,** 94–97.
69. Hodges, B. L., Hayashi, Y. K., Nonaka, I., Wang, W., Arahata, K., and Kaufman, S. J. (1997) Altered expression of the α7β1 integrin in human and murine muscular dystrophies. *J. Cell Sci.* **110,** 2873–2881.
70. Mayer, U., Saher, G., Fässler, R., Bornemann, A., Echtermeyer, F., Von der Mark, H., et al. (1997) Absence of integrin α7 causes a novel form of muscular dystrophy. *Nature Genet.* **17,** 318–323.
71. Kobayahi, K., Nakahori, Y., Miyake, M., Matsumura, K., Kondo-Iida, E., Nomura, Y., et al. (1998) An acient retrotransposal insertion causes Fukuyama-type congenital muscular dystrophy. *Nature* **394,** 388–392.
72. Hayashi, Y. K., Engvall, E., Arikawa-Hirasawa, E., Goto, K., Koga, R., Nonaka, I., Sugita, H., and Arahata, K. (1993) Abnormal localization of laminin subunits in muscular dystrophies. *J. Neurol. Sci.* **119,** 53–64.
73. Arikawa, E., Ishihara, T., Nonaka, I., Sugita, H., and Arahata, K. (1991) Immunocytochemical analysis of dystrophin in congenital muscular dystrophy. *J. Neurol. Sci.* **105,** 79–87.
74. Matsumura, K., Nonaka, I., and Campbell, K. P. (1993) Abnormal expression of dystrophin-associated proteins in Fukuyama-type congenital muscular dystrophy. *Lancet* **341,** 521–522.
75. Arahata, K., Hayashi, K., Mizuno, Y., Yoshida, M., and Ozawa, E. (1993) Dystrophin-associated glycoprotein and dystrophin co-localisation at sarcolemma in Fukuyama congenital muscular dystrophy. *Lancet* **342,** 623–624.
76. Minetti, C., Tanji, K., Rippa, P. G., Morreale, G., Cordone, G., and Bonilla, E. (1994) Abnormalities in the expression of β-spectrin in Duchenne muscular dystrophy. *Neurology* **44,** 1149–1153.
77. Manilal, S., Recan, D., Sewry, C. A., Hoeltzenbein, M., Llense, S., Leturcq, F., et al. (1998) Mutations in Emery-Dreifuss muscular dystrophy and their effects on emerin protein expression. *Hum. Mol. Genet.* **7,** 855–864.
78. Burgeson, R. E., Chiquet, M., Deutzmann, R., Ekblom, P., Engel, J., Kleinman, H., et al. (1994) A new nomenclature for the laminins. *Matrix Biol.* **14,** 209–211.

22

Multiplex Western Blot Analysis of Muscular Dystrophy Proteins

Louise V. B. Anderson

1. Introduction

Protein analysis usually requires the application of immunological techniques, and, in the preceding chapter, the use of antibodies (Abs) to label proteins in tissue sections has been described. Proteins in unfixed frozen sections are in near native form, and analysis of proteins in these circumstances represents a close approximation to the situation in vivo. In contrast, analysis of tissue proteins by denaturing polyacrylamide gel electrophoresis (PAGE) and Western blot analysis represents a very artificial situation, in which the nature of the technique requires each protein to be completely denatured: subunits dissociated, and each polypeptide chain unfolded. Basically, the polypeptides in a complex mixture are solubilized and sieved through a PAG matrix (under the influence of an electric current), in which they separate according to size. Large polypeptides remain near the top of the gel; smaller species pass further down the matrix. If the gel is stained with a nonspecific protein stain, such as Coomassie blue, it can be seen that each polypeptide chain is represented by a band at a different position down the gel; a sample of skeletal muscle could be separated into several hundred different bands, many overlapping. Such a large number of overlapping bands is very difficult to analyze, so that the separated polypeptides are often electrophoresed out of the gel and blotted onto charged paper (usually nitrocellulose). Unlike the fragile gel, this paper (or Western blot) is easily handled, and can be labeled with specific Abs, so that single bands or groups of bands can be visualized in each sample lane. Furthermore, the size and intensity of band label (i.e., how broad and dark it is) is related to the abundance of the protein labeled by the Ab. Thus, Western blot analysis can provide three types of information about the proteins present in a tissue

From: *Methods in Molecular Medicine, vol. 43: Muscular Dystrophy: Methods and Protocols*
Edited by: K. M. D. Bushby and L. V. B. Anderson © Humana Press Inc., Totowa, NJ

sample mixture: Is a particular protein present (band visible or not)? What size is it (migration distance down gel)? Approximately how much of it is present (density of labeled band)? Usually, the answers to these questions are not provided in absolute units, but in comparative terms, i.e., in relation to normal control samples run on the same gel/blot.

There are many excellent reviews and textbooks that describe methods for PAGE and Western blotting ***(1–4)***. The methods described in this chapter are by no means the only way that such analysis may be performed, but they do represent the current system that the author uses ***(5)***, and they are methods that have evolved over many years of experience with the specific problems presented by diagnostic blotting for the muscular dystrophy (MD) proteins.

2. Materials

2.1. Apparatus

The basic system used is the Bio-Rad (Hercules, CA) Protean II 16-cm system with 1.5-mm spacers (= thickness of gel), and PowerPac 1000 power supply; plus their Transblot Western blotting system with plate electrodes, supercooling coil, and PowerPac 200 power supply. All the components, spare parts, and power packs can be purchased separately. Other equipment, such as the peristaltic pump, gradient mixer, and gel drier, can be purchased from Bio-Rad, or any other supplier. The thermocirculator the author uses is no longer supplied by Bio-Rad, but is similar to the Grant RC400G chilling circulator supplied by many companies. The microcentrifuge, rocking table, magnetic stirrers, and Ika Ultra Turrax homogenizer T25 with 8-mm tool can also be purchased from general laboratory suppliers. Gilson Pipetmen (Gilson, Middletown, WI) are used for volume accuracy throughout. The densitometric software used by the author is not available commercially, but Bio-Rad does supply a Model GS-700 Imaging Densitometer with software and SCSI card for use with a PC computer.

2.2. Chemicals

Generally, it is a case of the purer the better for electrophoresis purposes. This means Analar-grade whenever possible, or good quality non-Analar chemicals supplied for electrophoresis (e.g., sodium dodecyl sulphate (SDS) and acrylamide from Bio-Rad, Electran-grade chemicals from Merck, Trizma base from Sigma) (*see* **Note 1**). Diaminobenzidine (DAB) is also of variable quality: That supplied by Merck dissolves well. Most of the Abs to the current MD proteins (dystrophin, α-, β-, γ-, δ-sarcoglycan (SG), calpain 3, and emerin, plus β-dystroglycan as a control) are available from Novocastra Laboratories (note that the Novocastra Ab to the laminin α_2-chain of merosin only works on sections); Abs to laminin α_2-chain are also available from Chemicon, and Abs to caveolin 3 are available from Transduction Laboratories.

2.3. Solutions and Buffers

The method presented is for a denaturing SDS-discontinuous system of electrophoresis. The method is based on the system of Laemmli *(6)*, with the author's modifications (*see* **Note 2**).

1. Acrylamide: 30.0% acrylamide, 0.8% *bis*-acrylamide (**Caution:** *see* **Note 3**). This should be stored in the dark, where it will be stable for up to 2 mo at 4°C.
2. Stacking gel buffer: 1.25 *M* Tris-HCl, pH 6.8, at 20°C.
3. Resolving gel buffer: 1.875 *M* Tris-HCl, pH 8.8, at 20°C.
4. 10X Concentrated electrophoresis tank buffer: 3.0% Tris, 14.4% glycine, 2% SDS (pH will be ~8.3 when diluted).
5. Stock solutions: 25% SDS (stable for several weeks at room temperature (RT) but precipitates in the cold), 8 *M* urea (stable for several weeks), 0.2% bromophenol blue, 15 mg/mL ammonium persulphate (APS) (must be made fresh daily). Commercial solutions of *N,N,N',N'*-tetramethylethylenediamine (TEMED) and mercaptoethanol (both used undiluted) should be stored in the dark at 4°C.
6. Treatment buffer: 125 m*M* Tris-HCl (0.5 mL stock 1.25 *M*), 4% SDS (0.8 mL stock 25% SDS), 4 *M* urea (2.5 mL stock 8 *M* urea), 5% mercaptoethanol (0.25 mL), 10% glycerol (0.5 mL), 0.001% bromophenol blue (0.025 mL stock 0.2% bromophenol blue), pH to 6.8 with HCl, final volume 5 mL. Prepared as required (*see* **Note 4**).
7. Resolving gel overlay: 5.0 mL resolving gel buffer, 0.2 mL stock 25% SDS, 19.8 mL H_2O. Interface rinsing buffer: 2.5 mL stacking gel buffer, 0.2 mL stock 25% SDS, 0.75 mL glycerol, 21.55 mL H_2O.
8. Gel fixation solution: 20% trichloracetic acid in H_2O. Coomassie blue protein stain: 1.15 g R-250 salt, dissolved in 1 L of 25% industrial methylated spirit/10% acetic acid in H_2O (filter before using each new batch of stain), destain with 10% industrial methylated spirit/10% acetic acid in H_2O.
9. 5X Concentrated Western blot transfer buffer: 3.% Tris, 14.40% glycine, 0.05% SDS (add 20% Analar methanol when diluting, i.e., 400 mL conc. transfer buffer + 400 mL methanol + 1200 mL H_2O).
10. Ponceau S reversible protein stain (if required): 0.2% Ponceau S stain in 1% acetic acid, destain - water. Amido black permanent protein stain (if required): 5 g amido black stain in 1 L of 50% methanol/10% acetic acid in H_2O, destain - 45% methanol/10% acetic acid in H_2O.
11. Blot washing buffer (TBST): 10 m*M* Tris-HCl, 150 m*M* NaCl, 0.05% Tween-20 detergent (~pH 8.0). Blocking buffer: 5% nonfat dried milk powder (from supermarket) in TBST buffer.
12. DAB visualization solution: When required, dissolve 50 mg DAB in 4 mL H_2O and add to 96 mL phosphate-buffered saline (*see* **Note 5**). Just before use, add 87.5 µL commercial 30% hydrogen peroxide solution (*see* **Note 6**). Many other

visualization methods are available *(4)*, but the author has found the DAB–H_2O_2 system to be very robust.

3. Methods

3.1. Gel Electrophoresis

The following recipe is for one biphasic gel, 16 cm × 14 cm × 1.5 mm, with a 4–5.5% gradient above a plain 7% gel. This biphasic system is optimized to resolve all the currently known MD proteins on a pair of gels/blots. Thus, the lower half of the gel contains 7% acrylamide (for resolving calpain 3, merosin, the SGs, emerin, and caveolin-3, in the molecular mass range of 17–100 kDa); the upper half contains a gradient of 5.5–4% (for resolving myosin heavy chain and dystrophin in the range 200–400 kDa). A 3% stacking gel is used above the resolving gel.

1. Clean inner surfaces of glass plates with alcohol. Put a mark 4.5 cm from top on the outside surface with a felt pen (= 2 cm deep stacking gel). Assemble cassettes, and place in casting stand.
2. Prepare gel mixtures as follows (*see* **Note 7**):

	7%	5.5%	"4"% (*see* **Note 8**)
Resolving gel buffer	5.00 mL	3.00 mL	3.00 mL
Acrylamide	5.83 mL	2.75 mL	1.67 mL
Glycerol	2.50 mL	1.125 mL	0.45 mL
H_2O (distilled or deionized)	10.96 mL	7.62 mL	9.375 mL

   Degas the solutions (*see* **Note 9**).
3. Complete 7% step mixture as follows: 0.20 mL stock 25% SDS, 0.50 mL APS, and 10 µL TEMED. Mix well, and pipet 18 mL into the gel cassette. The gradient must be poured immediately.
4. Complete gradient mixtures as follows:

	5.5%	"4"%
Stock 25% SDS	0.12 mL	0.12 mL
APS	0.375 mL	0.375 mL
TEMED	10 µL	10 µL

   Mix well.
5. Take the gradient mixer, put 10 mL 5.5% gel mixture into the chamber nearest the outlet and 10 mL 4% gel mixture in the other chamber. Start the stirrer under the gradient mixer. Start the peristaltic pump on maximum speed, until the mixture runs to waste. Alter the pump speed so that it runs at about 4 mL/min, open the valve between the chambers, and pump the gel gradient into the cassette, observing the interface between the 7% and gradient layers, to avoid turbulence

at the boundary. Switch off the pump when the liquid reaches the felt pen mark. Clean pump tubing by pumping water through to waste, on maximum speed.

6. Gently layer 2–3 mL resolving gel overlay across the top of the gel mixture with a plastic pipet. Allow to set for at least 3 h at RT.
7. Repeat the preceding steps for other gel.
8. Prepare samples. Weigh muscle (**keep frozen**; *see* **Note 10**), add 19 vol (e.g., 20 mg + 380 µL) of treatment buffer, and immediately homogenize (Ultra-turrax 2 × 15 s). For normal control muscle, this 1:20 dilution will give a protein loading of approx 200 µg in 30 µL *(7)*.
9. Place samples in boiling water for 5 min, then spin in a microcentrifuge (1300 rpm, 9500*g*) for 5 min.
10. When ready, pour off the overlay from the gels, rinse the top of the gels 3× with interface rinsing buffer, and drain with folded filter paper. Stand the cassettes upright, and insert combs to form 10 × 1-cm wells.
11. Prepare the 3% stacking gel mixture for both gels as follows: 2.5 mL stacking gel buffer, 2.5 mL acrylamide, 0.75 mL glycerol, and 17.78 mL H_2O. Degas under vacuum, and add: 0.20 mL stock 25% SDS, 1.25 mL APS, and 20 µL TEMED. Mix well.
12. Fill the cassettes, jiggling the comb to disturb any air bubbles. Allow to set for about 45 min (no longer than 2 h, or the buffer systems between the stacking and resolving gels will start to diffuse into each other).
13. Dilute the tank buffer 1:10 with deionized H_2O. Put 4 L into the Protean II tank, and measure a further 2 L into a cylinder for the upper chamber.
14. Remove the comb from the stacking gel, and rinse out the wells 3× with tank buffer. Fit the cassettes to the central core of the electrophoresis tank, and fill the upper chamber with tank buffer.
15. Carefully apply the samples, 30 µL per lane, to the bottom of the wells. Remember to put treatment buffer in any blank lanes.
16. Place the cassettes/upper tank unit in the main tank, top up with buffer, and put on the lid. Attach the leads to power unit. Run at 21 mA (2 gels) overnight (*see* **Note 11**), with the thermocirculator set at 10°C. In the morning, turn off the power supply, remove, and open the gel cassettes, then proceed to staining or blotting steps.
17. Gel staining: Fix in TCA for 30 min, stain overnight, destain with several changes (*see* **Subheading 2.3.8.**). Gel drying: Soak gel in H_2O for 30 min before drying on a vacuum gel dryer.

3.2. Western Blotting

The blotting buffer is based on the Otter system *(8)*, and includes both methanol and SDS (*see* **Note 12**).

1. On the day before, put 2 L diluted transfer buffer into the blotting tank, and leave it at +4°C overnight, together with a further 2 L transfer buffer in a measuring cylinder.
2. As soon as the gels are removed from the electrophoresis tank, equilibrate them in a dish of transfer buffer for 15 min, with gentle agitation.

3. Meanwhile, set up the blotting tank with the supercooling coil, and the thermo-circulator set at –20°C (maximum). Immerse the nitrocellulose sheets in the tank for at least 15 min to get the air out of the paper (*see* **Note 13**).
4. Assemble each blotting sandwich as follows, on the black (negative) side of a cassette: soaked fiber pad, soaked three sheets of Whatman no. 3 filter paper, soaked one sheet of Whatman no. 50 filter paper, equilibrated gel, soaked nitro-cellulose paper, soaked three sheets of Whatman no. 3 filter paper, and soaked fiber pad. Ensure close contact, and the absence of air bubbles between the gel and the nitrocellulose, by gently rolling a glass rod over the top of the last filter paper layer.
5. Insert the cassettes into the blotting tank, with the black side of the cassette to the black (negative) terminal marker. Top to the marker with cooled transfer buffer, and close the lid. Reduce the themocirculator setting to –13.5°C. Connect to the power supply: 200 V, 1 A current (limiting) for 6–7 h.
6. Switch off the power supply. Open each cassette, and remove the nitrocellulose blots. Immerse the blots briefly in water, and dry between paper towels (*see* **Note 14**).
7. Fix and stain the postblotted gels with Coomassie blue (*see* **Subheading 3.1., step 17**). If required, compare with an unblotted gel, to estimate the efficiency of transfer.
8. The blots can be stained with total protein stains like Ponceau S (reversible) or amido black (permanent) (*see* **Subheading 2.3., step 10**) but the MD proteins cannot be visualized without immunolabeling.

Figure 1 shows lanes of normal human skeletal muscle from a Coomassie-blue-stained gel before (panel A) and after (panel B) blotting. Panel C shows lanes from a blot that has been stained with amido black.

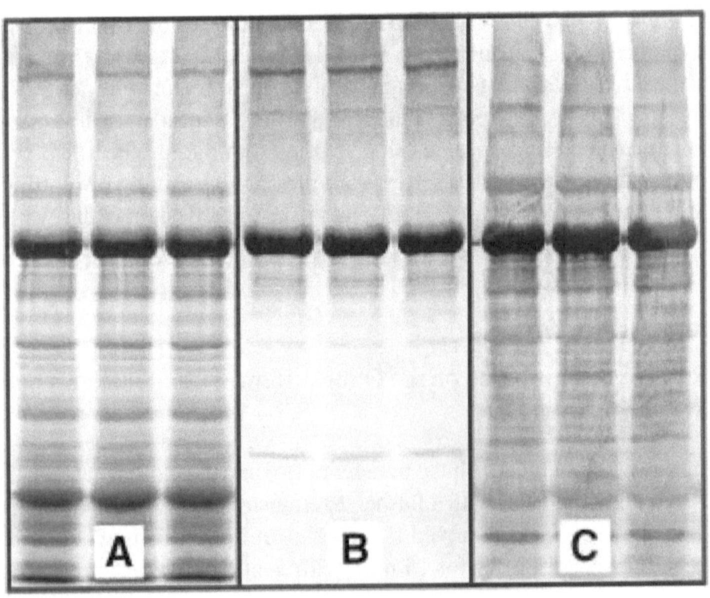

3.3. Immunolabeling

1. Block unreacted binding sites on the nitrocellulose blots by incubation in blocking buffer (*see* **Note 15**). This and all subsequent incubation steps are performed for 1 h at RT, with gentle agitation. Pour off the blocking buffer, and retain.
2. Incubate the blots for 1 h with a cocktail of primary monoclonal Abs (dystrophin, merosin, SGs, and so on, appropriately diluted with each other, and with TBST). The Abs may be used in any combination, so long as the size of all the immunoreactive bands is taken in to consideration (*see* **Notes 16** and **17**), and attempts are not made to analyze proteins of the same size on the same blot (*see* **Table 1**).
3. Suitable multiplex Ab combinations are as shown in **Table 2** andin **Fig. 2**. The dilutions suggested are for guidance: Higher dilutions may well give good results, depending on the visualization method used. β-Dystroglycan is repeated on both blots as an internal control.
4. Pour off the primary Abs, rinse blot with TBST, and wash in TBST for 15 min, with gentle agitation. The second wash step is for 15 min with milk blocking buffer, as used in **Subheading 3.3., step 1**. The third wash step is in TBST for a further 15 min.
5. Incubate blot for 1 h with horseradish peroxidase-conjugated secondary Ab (e.g., Dako P260 diluted 1:300 in TBST.
6. Pour off the second Ab, rinse blot with TBST, and wash in TBST for 3 × 15 min.
7. During the last wash cycle, prepare the DAB visualization solution (*see* **Subheading 2.3., step 12**). When ready, drain the blot, add the DAB solution, and gently agitate for 2–5 min, until bands are fully visualized.
8. Rinse the blot well with cold tap water, dry between paper towels, and store in the dark. Blots can be stuck onto Whatman no. 3 filter paper with glue sticks.

3.4. Analysis of Results

3.4.1. Presence of Proteins

For diagnostic purposes, when protein expression is being used to guide mutation analysis, it is sufficient to put the blot result in one of three categories: whether a protein band appears normal, appears abnormal (of unusual size or reduced labeling intensity for the amount of muscle protein loaded), or is absent. If other bands are indistinguishable from normal, the absence of one particular protein band usually indicates a primary problem in the gene for that protein. If labeling for a protein appears to be reduced, this may still usefully indicate where to start the search for gene mutations, provided that protein

---

Fig. 1. *(opposite page)* **(A)** Lanes of human skeletal muscle on a biphasic PAG stained with the protein stain Coomassie blue. **(B)** Similar lanes after blotting. Note the preferential transfer of the lower-molecular-mass bands. **(C)** Lanes from the blot stained with the protein stain amido black. Gel and blot lanes provided by courtesy of Elizabeth E. Bull.

Table 1
Muscular Dystrophy Proteins and Their Sizes

Protein	Approx size (kDa)	
Dystrophin	400	(300–400, if using rod Ab NCL-DYS1)
Dysferlin	230	
Myosin heavy chain	200	(stained on gel, not immunolabeled)
?	120	(additional band with NCL-g-SG)
Calpain 3	94	
Merosin	80	(Chemicon/Gibco Ab)
Calpain 3	60–45	(breakdown products with exon 8 Ab)
α-SG	50	
β-Dystroglycan	43	
β-SG	43	
γ-SG	35	
δ-SG	35	(doublet)
Emerin	34	
Calpain 3	30	(N-terminal fragment)
Caveolin-3	18	

Table 2
Possible Multiplex Anibody Combinations for a Pair of Blots

Combination A	Combination B
1/50 NCL-DYS2 (dystrophin C-term)	1/50 NCL-DYS1 (dystrophin rod)
1/300 NCL-hamlet (dysferlin)	1/10 NCL-CALP-12A2 (calpain 3 exon 8)
1/10 NCL-CALP-2C4 (calpain 3 exon 1)	1/1000 Chemicon 1922 anti-merosin
1/10 NCL-a-SG (α-sarcoglycan)	1/200 NCL-b-DG (β-dystroglycan)
1/200 NCL-b-DG (β-dystroglycan)	1/2 NCL-g-SG (γ-sarcoglycan)

breakdown is not an issue ***(9)***. The situation is more complicated in the sarcoglycanopathies, in which the reduction in one member of the SG complex of proteins usually affects them all ***(10,11)***. However, in some cases, particularly γ-sarcoglycanopathy (LGMD2C), one protein may be missing, and the others reduced in labeling intensity. In these cases, the most severely affected protein is the one most likely to harbor the underlying gene mutation ***(12–14)***. Similarly, in Duchenne dystrophy, dystrophin may be absent and labeling for the associated proteins is reduced.

3.4.2. Size

The SDS–protein complexes have identical charge densities, and migrate during electrophoresis, according to their size. The relative mobility (R_f) of a protein is determined by measuring the distance from the top of the resolving gel to the protein band, and dividing by the total distance from the top to the bottom of the gel run (as indicated by the electrophoresis dye front). Formal estimates of molecular mass normally require bands to be visualized in nongradient gels, alongside a standard series of proteins or polypeptides of known sizes. Under these conditions, a plot of $\log_{10}$ polypeptide molecular mass vs R_f is a straight line, and the molecular masses of unknown proteins can be read from the linear standard curve *(2,3)*. Unfortunately, this cannot be undertaken for proteins that are undetectable with ordinary protein stains. The MD proteins are only detectable on immunolabeled blots, and, although prestained molecular mass standards are available for transfer onto blots (Sigma, Bio-Rad), the sizes are not accurate, and are really only suitable as a guide. Nevertheless, the size of a protein on a blot (for example, of dystrophin in a Becker muscular dystrophy (BMD) patient with a gene deletion that removes several exons) could be estimated using the multiplex protein bands as the molecular mass standards (*see* **Fig. 3**), although the accuracy of this approach is limited by the biphasic construction of the resolving gel. For diagnostic purposes, however, the abnormal-sized protein expressed in most BMD patients is diagnostic in itself, making further analysis unnecessary (*see* **Fig. 4**). Bands of normal size, but reduced abundance, may be observed in some cases with presumed point mutations (e.g., lanes 1 and 9 in **Fig. 4**).

3.4.3. Abundance

3.4.3.1. Image Acquisition

Dried gels and blots are scanned at 400 dpi, using an Epson GT8000 flatbed scanner: White light is used for gels, and blue for blots. Each image is stored as a bit-map, in which 8 bits = 1 byte = 1 pixel. Each pixel is graded from 0 (pure black) to 255 (pure white) on a 256 greyscale. Greyscale is not proportional to concentration, but optical density (OD) is according to Beer's law, and therefore OD is the proper measure for use in quantitation. It is possible to modify Optimas v5.2 image analysis software (Cybernetics) for use with a flatbed scanner (*see* **Note 18**). For this, greyscale values are converted to OD units by scanning a specially constructed strip with known OD values (e.g., the Kodak SR-37 step-wedge has 37 steps, with OD values from 0.05 to 1.85). The greyscale values measured for each step are then plotted against the true OD values, so that the scanner is calibrated as a true densitometer. Subsequently, the greyscale value for each pixel is automatically converted to an OD value.

3.4.3.2. Densitometry

Ideally, one would want to sum the OD values for each pixel within the band, but this number would be too unwieldy. Mean pixel density is a function

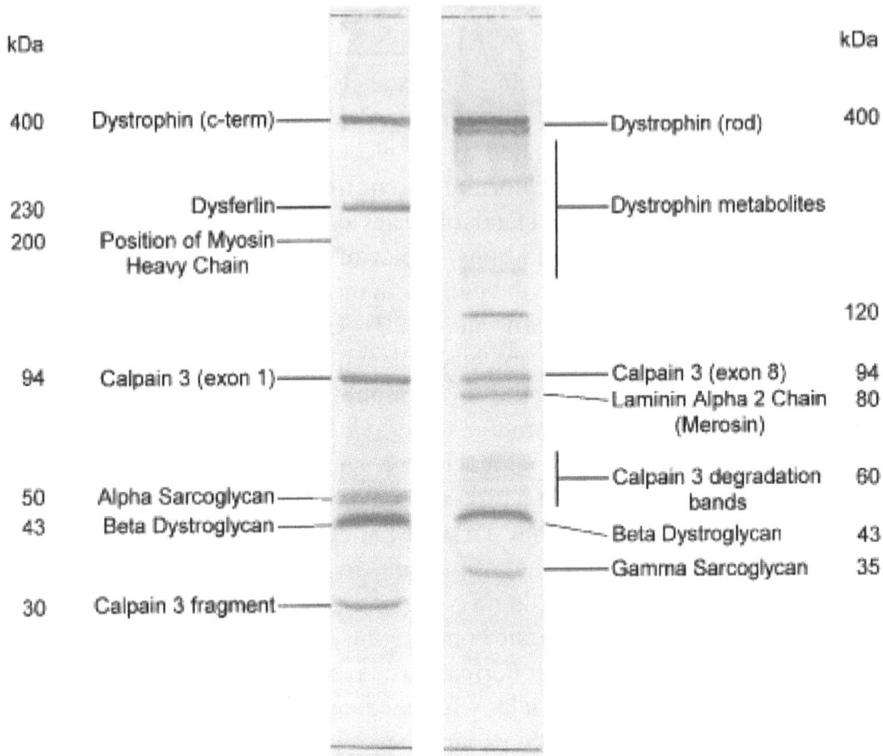
kDa
400
230
200
94
50
43
30
Dystrophin (c-term)
Dysferlin
Position of Myosin Heavy Chain
Calpain 3 (exon 1)
Alpha Sarcoglycan
Beta Dystroglycan
Calpain 3 fragment
Dystrophin (rod)
Dystrophin metabolites
Calpain 3 (exon 8)
Laminin Alpha 2 Chain (Merosin)
Calpain 3 degradation bands
Beta Dystroglycan
Gamma Sarcoglycan
kDa
400
120
94
80
60
43
35

Fig. 2

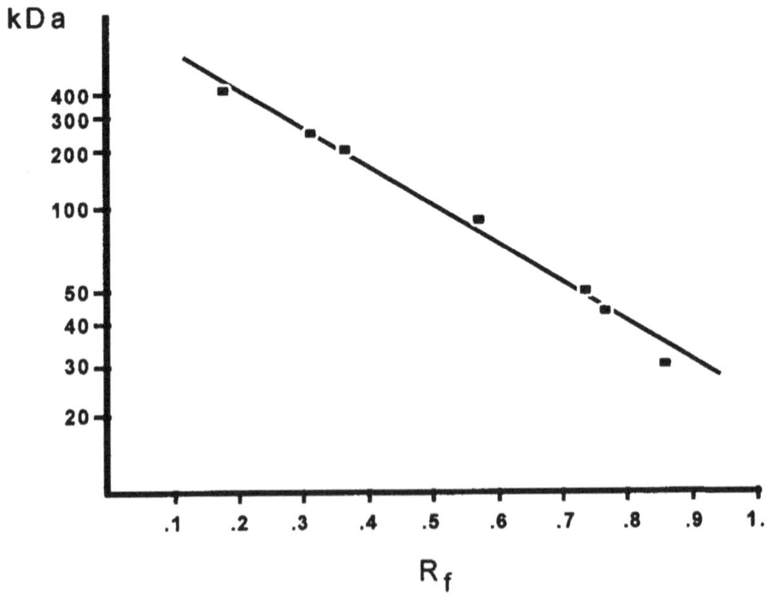
kDa
400
300
200
100
50
40
30
20
.1
.2
.3
.4
.5
.6
.7
.8
.9
1.0
Rf

Fig. 3

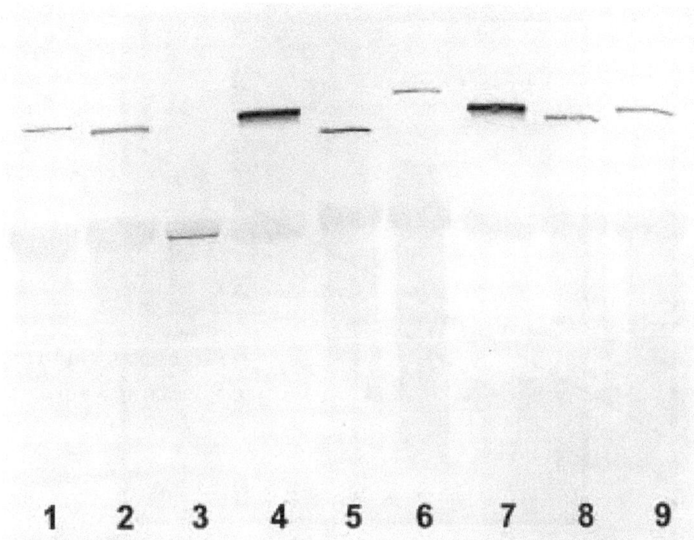

Fig. 4. Western blot of muscle from some BMD patients labeled with an Ab to the C-terminus of dystrophin. Lane: 1 = BMD no deletion detected, 2 = BMD exons 45–47 deleted, 3 = BMD exons 13–47 deleted, 4 = control muscle, 5 = BMD exons 45–53 deleted, 6 = BMD exons 14–26 duplicated, 7 = control muscle, 8 = BMD exons 45–47 deleted, 9 = BMD no deletion detected.

obtainable from the Optimas software, however. The outline of each band is defined by a programmed software algorithm involving background measurements, to obtain a value for volume OD in which:

Volume OD = (sum of the OD for every pixel/number of pixels) × band area in cm^2

Most commercial densitometry packages (e.g., Bio-Rad) produce a density profile obtained by averaging pixel density across a path of adjustable width down the gel lane. In the system described above, however, each band is outlined and surveyed individually, so that even the most distorted band can be analyzed, regardless of its shape (*see* **Note 19**).

Fig. 2. *(opposite page)* Two lanes from a multiplex Western blot labeled with a variety of monoclonal Abs to MD proteins (*see* **Table 2**).

Fig. 3. *(opposite page)* Example of a standard curve for estimating molecular masses, using the immunolabeled protein bands in the left hand lane of Fig. 2. The ghost of the myosin heavy-chain band at 200 kDa is also used as a standard: Although not labeled by Abs, it is usually discernible on blots as an outline of a band where the nitocellulose is a different color.

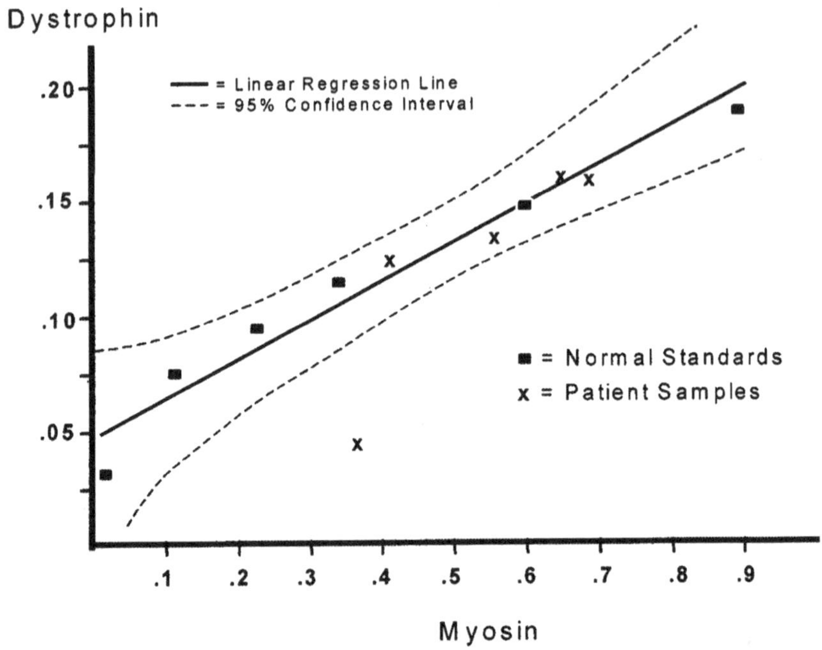

Fig. 5. Estimation of dystrophin abundance: linear regression line of the volume OD values for myosin heavy chain and the corresponding values for dystrophin (labeled with the C-terminal Ab Dy8/6C5 or NCL-DYS2), using dilutions of normal muscle. Four of the five patients fall within the 95% confidence interval for the line, but the fifth is clearly an outlier. This patient had a myosin value of 0.38, and this would normally correspond to a dystrophin value of 0.106 (read from the standard curve). However, the actual value measured was 0.04, indicating that the dystrophin levels are reduced to approx 38% of normal. Analysis performed with GraphPad InStat version 3.00 for Windows 95.

3.4.3.3. Analysis

Pathological muscle samples can contain a variable amount of fat and fibrous connective tissue. Therefore, myosin heavy-chain staining on the postblotted gel is used as an indication of how much true muscle protein is loaded in each sample. Thus, for a single sample, the volume OD for the particular protein band is divided by the corresponding value for myosin heavy chain in that sample, to produce a density value that is adjusted for the amount of muscle protein present. For comparative measurements (to determine whether the abundance of a particular protein is abnormally reduced), 5–6 dilutions of normal muscle homogenate should be run on the same blot as a group of unknown clinical samples. After densitometric analysis of the postblotted gel and the

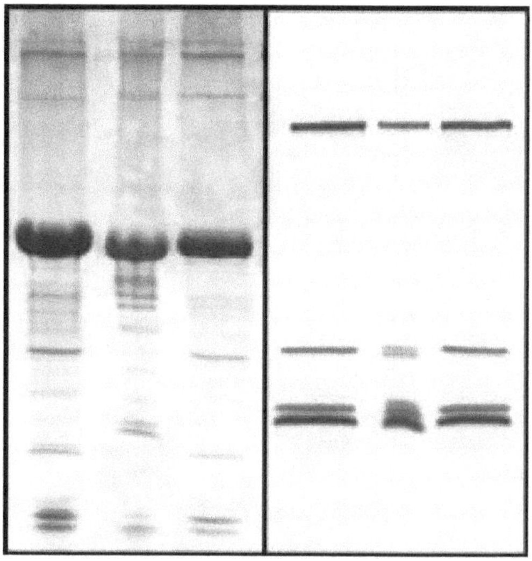

Fig. 6. Distortion in the middle lane of a gel (on left) and corresponding blot (on right) caused by a different concentration of SDS in the middle sample.

immunolabeled blot, a standard curve (regression line) can be calculated, where x = volume OD values for myosin heavy chain, and y = volume OD values for the protein of interest. For the clinical samples, the measured values of x (myosin) are used to read calculated values of y (MD protein of interest) from the standard curve. The calculated value is then compared with the actual measured value, to determine whether the protein abundance is reduced, compared to normal. Many software packages will also calculate the 95% confidence interval for the regression line (*see* **Fig. 5**). Since Western blot analysis is not really meant to be a quantitative technique, the breadth of the regression line's 95% confidence interval is a useful indication of the inaccuracy in any particular blot. Visual inspection of the graph will also indicate whether the xy values for an unknown clinical sample fall inside or outside the 95% confidence interval for the normal muscle samples run on the same blot (*see* **Note 20**).

3.5. Troubleshooting

A common source of disappointing results is a change in buffer composition between adjacent lanes. If a sample has a low myosin content, so that all the protein bands are faint, it is not feasible to simply double the volume of sample applied. This results in an imbalance in the SDS and urea content between adjacent lanes, so that the lanes become skinny and distorted (**Fig. 6**). If a sample has a low myosin content, a further sample may be homogenized with a 1:10, rather than 1:20, vol of treatment buffer. Alternatively, the sample volume may be

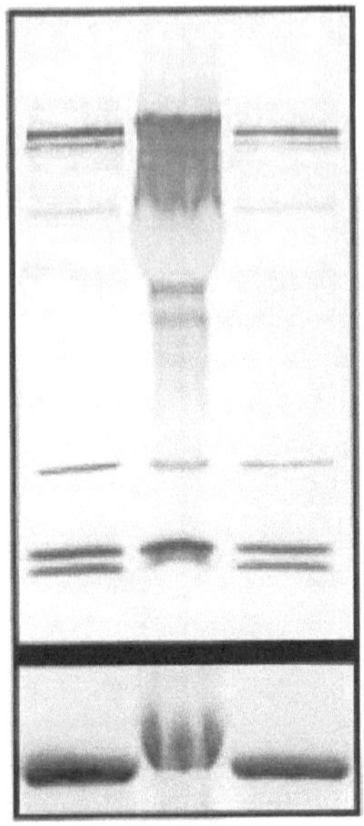

Fig. 7. Distortion in the middle lane of a blot (upper panel) and corresponding gel (lower panel showing myosin band only), caused by contamination of the muscle sample with mountant. The tissue block had previously been oriented for sectioning and the mountant was not removed before the sample was homogenized.

doubled, so long as an extra volume of treatment buffer is added in all the other sample wells. Too large a volume will result in poor band resolution, however.

The other common problem arises from using muscle samples that have been set in mountant for sectioning. Contamination with mountant results in band smearing (**Fig. 7**), and this should be avoided by slicing off as much mountant as possible, while the tissue is frozen. As a last resort, the muscle sample may need to be thawed and the mountant quickly wiped off on a tissue before homogenization, but this situation should be avoided, if at all possible.

4. Notes

1. The quality of SDS, acrylamide, *bis*-acrylamide (*N,N'*-methylene *bis*-acrylamide), APS and TEMED may vary from company to company, and may be a source of unsatisfactory results.
2. PAG results from the polymerization of acrylamide monomer into long chains and the crosslinking of these by bifunctional compounds, such as *bis*-acrylamide, reacting with free functional groups at chain termini. The author has tried piperazine diacrylamide as an alternative crosslinking agent, but found it was much less stable than *bis*-acrylamide on storage. Polymerization is initiated by the addition of APS, and accelerated by adding TEMED. The gel pore size is influenced by

the total acrylamide concentration in the polymerization mixture: the higher the percentage of acrylamide, the smaller the pore size *(2,3)*. In a discontinuous system, a stacking gel is used above the resolving gel, to effectively concentrate relatively large volumes of dilute samples and sharpen the resulting bands. The stacking gel has a lower pH than the resolving gel, and a very low percentage of acrylamide, so that it does not exert a sieving effect. In addition, the sample treatment buffer, stacking buffer, and resolving gel buffers need to contain chloride (leading) ions; the electrode reservoir buffer contains glycinate (trailing) ions. The stacking phenomenon is described in detail in ref. ***3***. In a denaturing system, heat is used in the presence of excess SDS and a thiol reducing agent, such as 2-mercaptoethanol or dithiothreitol (to break the crosslinking disulphide bonds among or between polypeptide chains). Under these conditions, most polypeptides bind SDS in a constant weight ratio (1.4 g SDS: 1 g protein), so that they have essentially identical charge densities, and migrate in the gels according to size alone *(2,3)*. The author uses more SDS in the gel and in the electrophoresis treatment buffer than is usual, because this has been found to improve extraction and solubility of very high molecular mass proteins. A gradient of glycerol is used throughout the resolving and stacking gel, which stabilizes the acrylamide gradient and the two phases of the resolving gel. The addition of glycerol to the stacking gel seems to improve the appearance of the (essentially overloaded) myosin heavy-chain band.

3. **Caution:** Unpolymerized acrylamide is a neurotoxin, and may be absorbed through the skin, or inhaled. For this reason, it is best if acrylamide and *bis*-acrylamide powders are weighed in a fume hood. At the very least, the operator should always wear a face mask that incorporates a filter, and safety goggles and protective gloves. Gloves must also be worn when handling unpolymerized acrylamide solutions. Once polymerization has occurred, the resulting gel is relatively nontoxic. However, a small proportion of monomer may remain unpolymerized, and it is wise to wear gloves at all times when handling gels.
4. Urea is added to the treatment buffer to aid the dissociation and solubility of large protein complexes in skeletal muscle, particularly those of myosin and laminin. However, cyanate ions can accumulate in stock solutions of urea as a result of chemical isomerization. These ions can react with amino groups to form carbamylated derivatives, which could lead to proteins with anomalous electrophoretic properties. Heating protein samples in urea solutions is also not normally recommended, because this increases the potential problem of carbamylation. Nevertheless, these problems are reduced by not keeping the urea stock solution for more than a month, and by using the urea in Tris buffers, which have free amido groups to neutralize the cyanate ions.
5. **Caution:** DAB is a potential carcinogen, and gloves should be worn when handling it. DAB dissolves better in water than in PBS. It is easiest to weigh out 50 mg samples of DAB in 5-mL plastic bijou bottles, and store them dry at –20°C.
6. H_2O_2 is the substrate for the peroxidase enzyme attached to the secondary Ab; DAB is the chromogen that allows the enzymatic reaction to be followed.

7. Gilson P20, P200, P1000, and P5000 pipets are used to measure the volumes.
8. This is actually 3.34%, but some gel is left in the chambers and tubing; hence, the gradient actually poured is 4–5.5%.
9. Oxygen inhibits polymerization, so the gel mixtures are usually degassed prior to use.
10. One of the best ways to keep samples frozen before homogenization is to place the tubes in a square metal rack (Denley) wedged in a polystyrene Igloo ice bucket (Jencons), with some liquid nitrogen underneath.
11. The gel is run slowly overnight (for about 16 h), to improve the resolution of the high molecular mass bands.
12. Methanol is added to a transfer buffer to counteract the swelling of the gel ***(15)***, and to increase the capacity and affinity of nitrocellulose for proteins. It also has the effect of removing the detergent from SDS–protein complexes. The addition of SDS counteracts this, and improves the elution from the gel of high molecular mass proteins, such as dystrophin.
13. We have found that Protran nitrocellulose from Schleicher and Schuell gives excellent results. Always handle nitrocellulose with gloves, to avoid binding finger proteins.
14. Always store nitrocellulose in the dark (e.g., in brown envelopes in a drawer): This applies before and after labeling with Abs.
15. Nitrocellulose has a high binding capacity for proteins (approx 80–100 μg/cm^2). Any binding sites not occupied by transferred proteins need to be blocked prior to incubation with Ab. This blocking step is also repeated briefly after incubation with the primary Abs, during the second washing step.
16. Ab NCL-DYS1 detects a number of dystrophin metabolites ***(7)***; different Abs to merosin detect protein fragments of different sizes, the two commonest being 80 kDa and 300 kDa; NCL-g-SG labels an additional unidentified band ***(13)***; NCL-d-SG labels a doublet that makes it difficult to use in combination with NCL-emerin, and the calpain 3 Abs NCL-CALP-2C4 and NCL-CALP-12A2, also react with a number of gene products of different sizes ***(16)***.
17. Daltons or kDa are the units of molecular mass. Molecular weight and M_r (relative molecular mass) describe a ratio, and, as such, have no units. It is a common error to describe a protein as having a molecular weight of kDa.
18. Optimas software can be modified by programming in ALI (analytical language for images), but this is not a novice undertaking.
19. Among the commercial analysis packages available, the "1D Advanced" gel analysis software of Phoretix International (Newcastle, UK) is suitable for use with data generated from a multipurpose desktop scanner, while Bio-Rad sells a complete hardware and software system. Both products produce good results, so long as the grayscale values are converted to OD units using a gray-scale step-wedge.
20. Western blot analysis is not a reliable quantitative technique, and many of the statistical assumptions normally required for regression analysis cannot be met. The analysis described is therefore more of a guide than a gospel.

Acknowledgment

All the work described in this chapter has been performed by Keith Davison, without whose legendary attention to detail the multiplex blotting system would not have been possible.

References

1. Bjerrum, O. J. and Hegarty, B. T. (1988) *CRC Handbook of Immunoblotting of Proteins*, vol 1: *Technical Descriptions*, CRC, Boco Raton, FL.
2. Hames, B. D. and Rickwood, D. (1998) *Gel Electrophoresis of Proteins: A Practical Approach*, 2 IRL/Oxford University Press, Oxford.
3. Dunn, M. J. (1993) *Gel Electrophoresis of Proteins*, Bios, Oxford.
4. Dunbar, B. S. (1994) *Protein Blotting: A Practical Approach*, IRL/Oxford University Press, Oxford.
5. Anderson, L. V. B. and Davison, K. (1999) A multiplex western blotting system for the analysis of muscular dystrophy proteins. *Am. J. Pathol.* **154,** 1017–1022.
6. Laemmli, U. K. (1970) Cleavage of structural proteins during the assembly of the head of bacteriophage T4. *Nature* **227,** 680–685.
7. Nicholson, L. V. B., Davison, K., Falkous, G., Harwood, C., O'Donnell, E., Slater, C. R., and Harris, J. B. (1989) Dystrophin in skeletal muscle: I. Western blot analysis using a monoclonal antibody. *J. Neurol. Sci.* **94,** 125–136.
8. Otter, T., King, S. M., and Witman, G. B. (1987) A two-step procedure for efficient electrotransfer of both high-molecular-weight (>400,000) and low-molecular-weight (<20,000) proteins. *Anal. Biochem.* **162,** 370–377.
9. Anderson, L. V. B. (1996) Optimised protein diagnosis in the autosomal recessive limb-girdle muscular dystrophies. *Neuromusc. Disord.* **6,** 443–446.
10. Nigro, V., de Sá Moreira, E., Piluso, G., Vainzof, M., Belsito, A., Politano, L., et al. (1996) Autosomal recessive limb-girdle muscular dystrophy, LGMD2F, is caused by a mutation in the δ-sarcoglycan gene. *Nature Genet.* **14,** 195–198.
11. Bönnemann, C. G., Passos-Bueno, M. R., McNally, E. M., Vainzof, M., de Sá Moreira, E., Marie, S. K., et al. (1996) Genomic screening for β-sarcoglycan gene mutations: Missense mutations may cause severe limb-girdle muscular dystrophy type 2E (LGMD 2E). *Hum. Mol. Genet.* **5,** 1953–1961.
12. Vainzof, M., Passos-Bueno, M. R., Canovas, M., de Sá Moreira, E., Pavanello, R. C. M., Marie, S. K., et al. (1996) The sarcoglycan complex in the six autosomal recessive limb-girdle muscular dystrophies. *Hum. Mol. Genet.* **5,** 1963–1969.
13. Sewry, C., Taylor, J., Anderson, L. V. B., Ozawa, E., Pogue, R., Piccolo, F., et al. (1996) Abnormalities in α-, β- and γ-sarcoglycan in patients with limb-girdle muscular dystrophy. *Neuromusc. Disord.* **6,** 467–474.
14. Eymard, B., Romero, N. B., Leturcq, F., Piccolo, F., Carrié, A., Jeanpierre, M., et al. (1997) Primary adhalinopathy (α-sarcoglycanopathy): Clinical, pathologic, and genetic correlation in 20 patients with autosomal recessive muscular dystrophy. *Neurology*, **48,** 1227–1234.

15. Towbin, H., Staehelin, T., and Gordon, J. (1979) Electrophoretic transfer of proteins from polyacrylamide gels to nitrocellulose sheets: procedure and some applications. *Proc. Natl. Acad. Sci. USA* **76,** 4350–4354.
16. Anderson, L. V. B., Davison, K., Moss, J. A., Richard, I., Fardeau, M., Tomé, F. M. S., et al. (1998) Characterization of monoclonal antibodies to calpain 3 and protein expression in muscle from patients with limb-girdle muscular dystrophy type 2A. *Am. J. Pathol.* **153,** 1169–1179.

23

Fetal Muscle Biopsy

Eric P. Hoffman and Mark Evans

1. Introduction

The large majority of situations in which prenatal diagnosis is applied in the muscular dystrophies (MDs) is for Duchenne muscular dystrophies (DMD). Hence, discussion of fetal muscle biopsy in this chapter is limited to DMD, although, in principle, it should be applicable to any other primary protein deficiency that is expressed in fetal life (e.g., sarcoglycanopathies).

Prenatal diagnosis in DMD, as in most inherited disorders, is typically done through DNA analysis of amniocytes or chorionic villus sampling. As described in detail in this volume, direct mutation detection, or genetic linkage analysis, or both, generally provides an accurate diagnosis to the fetus at risk for DMD *(1)*. However, in certain situations, a clear cut affected or unaffected diagnosis cannot be assigned to the fetus (so-called "ambiguous risk"). This typically occurs when the family does not have a deletion mutation, and linkage analysis must be used for carrier detection and prenatal diagnosis. Linkage analysis is often capable of providing a definitive diagnosis for a fetus, but two things complicate the interpretation of linkage analysis in some families. First, recombination between intragenic polymorphic markers in the dystrophin gene occurs in about 10% of meioses, in which only a part of the at-risk dystrophin gene is inherited by a family member. Because the causative mutation typically cannot be visualized in nondeletion families, it may be impossible to determine whether the mutation was inherited or not, when recombination occurs. For example, linkage analysis can show that the mother of a fetus shares half the at-risk dystrophin gene with her affected brothers, and that her male fetus inherits this recombinant at-risk dystrophin gene. This scenario would lead to a 50% risk carrier risk assigned to the mother, and similarly a 50% assigned to the fetus (an ambiguous risk). Second, the high mutation rate of the dystrophin

From: *Methods in Molecular Medicine, vol. 43: Muscular Dystrophy: Methods and Protocols*
Edited by: K. M. D. Bushby and L. V. B. Anderson © Humana Press Inc., Totowa, NJ

gene dictates that a relatively large proportion of DMD patients represents new mutations. For example, the mother of an isolated case of DMD may or may not be a carrier. If the patient does not have a deletion, and his mother becomes pregnant with another male, this male fetus has only a 33% risk of being affected, but 66% if the fetus receives the same dystrophin gene as his affected brother. In this manner, the high mutation rate of the dystrophin gene, and the resulting preponderance of isolated cases, results in a proportion of prenatal diagnostic situations in which the risk to the fetus is ambiguous.

Here, it is important to discuss what is meant by significant risk. In the scenarios above, the fetus can have a 33, 50, or 66% risk of having DMD. Most would agree that such a high risk is significant. However, in the authors' experience, pregnant women who have had a brother succumb to DMD, can find even a 1% risk to be significant (i.e., unacceptable). Thus, the authors have done fetal muscle biopsies on fetuses with only a 1% risk, despite the fact that the morbidity risk of the procedure may be as high as 10%. This is because the mother considers 1% risk too high, and is willing to accept the morbidity risk of the procedure, in order to bring the risk to the fetus to population risk (1/10,000). Risk to a fetus can never be brought to 0%, because the 1/10,000 new mutation rate could still be considered, by some, as significant.

In cases in which the risk to the fetus is unacceptable to the parents (anywhere from 1% upwards, depending on the parents), dystrophin testing of fetal muscle biopsy should be considered for a more definitive diagnosis ***(2–10)***. The accuracy and sensitivity of fetal muscle biopsy relies on the presumption that all individuals with DMD have little or no dystrophin in their muscle, and that this biochemical phenotype is present from fetal life onwards ***(11,12)***. Thus, in nondeletion cases, dystrophin testing of fetal muscle can provide a definitive diagnosis, despite ambiguities of DNA testing.

Dystrophin testing of fetuses can be done on abortuses (fetopsies), or on viable fetuses through fetal muscle biopsy. In the former, dystrophin testing of the abortus can often dramatically alter the risk to future pregnancies. For example, the mother of a son with DMD is pregnant with a male fetus. Her affected son has no detectable deletion mutation, and there is no previous family history (isolated case). By linkage analysis, the male fetus inherits the at-risk dystrophin gene; the risk to the fetus is approx 66% in the absence of serum creatine kinase (SCK) data. In this scenario, the mother decides to terminate the pregnancy. It is critical in such scenarios that the abortus be tested for dystrophin content in the muscle, because the findings will substantially alter the mother's carrier risk, and will dramatically lower the ambiguity in future pregnancies. If the fetus tests negative for dystrophin, then it can be assumed that the mother is in fact a carrier, and the risk to future male pregnancies with the at-risk dystrophin gene increases from 66 to 100%. On the other hand, if the abortus tests positive for dystrophin, then a future male pregnancy with the at-risk dystrophin gene drops from 66 to 20% (gonadal mosaicism risk for the at-risk X). The authors find that women are more likely to opt for prenatal muscle biopsy, if available, than fetopsy testing of the abortus.

An important issue to discuss with the consultant, when offering fetal muscle biopsy, is the morbidity risk of the procedure. Fetal muscle biopsy, as practiced in the majority of cases to date, involves ultrasound-guided fetoscopy, in which the gluteus or quadriceps of the fetus is visualized, then a subcutaneous biopsy is taken using a kidney biopsy gun (or some other tool able to sample under the skin of the fetus) ***(10,13)***. Sample sizes are typically on the order of milligrams, and, despite the use of kidney biopsy guns, the majority of the sample may still be cutaneous tissue. The authors have received samples that show thousands of muscle fibers, and samples in which only a few fetal muscle fibers were detectable in multiple biopsies from a single case. Of the 20 cases that the authors have tested to date, two were unsuccessful in obtaining testable muscle fibers. However, other cases required multiple attempts to obtain muscle, rarely on multiple-procedure days. No fetus has been spontaneously aborted during or after the procedure, when testing for DMD, but one fetus was aborted after a procedure, to obtain a biopsy for mitochondrial muscle disorders. Thus, the 10% morbidity risk that the authors quote is a conservative estimate, based on muscle biopsy in general. The procedure requires experience and skill, and the morbidity risk may vary considerably from physician to physician.

The authors have processed fetal muscle biopsies from four different referring services, most of which have been from Mark Evans, MD (Hutzel Hospital Detroit), and Mitchell Golbus, MD (University of California, San Francisco) ***(13)***. Of these 20 muscle biopsies done, 13 tested normal for dystrophin, and were born with normal SCK levels (unaffected), five tested dystrophin-negative, and two were inadequate samples. One of these biopsies was from a female with a *de novo* translocation at Xp21, which was diagnosed as dystrophin-positive, and born with no abnormalities and normal SCK ***(5)***.

2. Materials

1. Phosphate buffered saline (PBS).
2. Horse serum (Sigma).
3. Superfrost + microscope slides (Fisher, Pittsburgh, PA).
4. Tissue Tek embedding media (VWR Scientific).
5. Antidystrophin antibodies (ABs) (60 kd, d10).
6. Antimyosin heavy-chain (F59, provided by Frank Stockdale), or other control Ab.
7. Cy3-conjugated second Abs (antimouse or antisheep immunoglobulin G).
8. Gel/Mount (Biomeda, Foster City, CA).
9. Fluorescent microscope.

3. Method

3.1. Fetal Muscle Biopsy

This is done by ultrasound-guided fetoscopy, as previously described *(10,13)*. Tissue is placed on the side of a glass vial, sealed, and frozen in liquid nitrogen. The biopsy can be stored in an airtight container at –80°C until analyzed. If the biopsy is to be stored long-term, then it is best to place some ice in the storage tube to keep the sample hydrated.

3.2. Immunofluorescence

1. Cryosections are cut at 4–5 μ, and thawed onto room temperature Superfrost+ slides. Sections are air-dried for approximately 15 s, then covered in blocking solution (350 μL PBS containing 10% horse serum). Slides are placed in a hydrated chamber until all slides are cut.
2. Primary Abs are diluted in PBS with 10% horse serum, spun in a microcentrifuge at 3,000 RPM, and the pellet avoided.
3. The blocking solution is shaken off the tissue sections, then the sections incubated with 100 μL diluted primary Ab in PBS with 10% horse serum. Slides are incubated in a hydrated chamber at room temperature.
4. Sections are incubated with the primary Ab for 2–3 h, then the primary Ab solution shaken off.
5. Slides are washed 3×, for 5 min each, with 350 μL of PBS with 10% horse serum.
6. Slides are then incubated with 100 μL of Cy3-conjugated second Ab (1:1000 dilution in PBS with 10% horse serum, centrifuged for 5 min at 3,000 RPM in a microcentrifuge to eliminate aggregates), for 15 min.
7. Slides are washed 3× with PBS with 10% horse serum.
8. Tissue sections are cover-slipped with Gel/Mount, and visualized with a fluorescent microscope.

4. Notes

1. The authors use fetal muscle controls, both normal fetal muscle and DMD fetal muscle.
2. Occasionally, the authors have encountered uterine tissue that was biopsied along with the fetal tissue. This can complicate the analysis, because uterine smooth muscle will stain positive for dystrophin, and the small smooth muscle cells may appear similar to fetal myofibers to the untrained eye. Depending on the control Abs used, smooth muscle can be distinguished from fetal skeletal muscle (F59 myosin heavy-chain Ab does not stain smooth muscle cells).
3. The fetal muscle biopsies can be extremely small and difficult to handle. It may take considerable skill to mount and section the small fetal biopsies.
4. It is not uncommon for the biopsied fetal tissue to consist primarily of skin or other nonmuscle tissue. Often, a number of biopsies are taken, to provide some assurance that one or more contains fetal muscle.

5. Some dystrophin Abs crossreact with a protein expressed in hair follicles. Because fetal skin is frequently included in the fetal biopsy, one must be able to distinguish between fetal muscle fibers and dystrophin-positive hair follicles. This is best done with a control Ab (like myosin heavy chain).

References

1. Miller, R. G. and Hoffman, E. P. (1994) Molecular diagnosis and modern management of Duchenne muscular dystrophy. *Neurolog. Clin.* **12,** 699–725.
2. Gustavii, B., Lofberg, L., and Henriksson, K. G. (1983) Fetal muscle biopsy. *Acta Obstet. Gynecol. Scand.* **62,** 369–371.
3. Guo, Y. (1990) [Prenatal diagnosis of Duchenne muscular dystrophy by fetoscopic muscle biopsy. Report of a case]. *Chung Hua Shen Ching Ching Shen Ko Tsa Chih.* **23,** 35–37, 63.
4. Evans, M. I., Greb, A., Kunkel, L. M., Sacks, A. J., Johnson, M. P., Boehm, C., Kazazian, H. H., Jr., and Hoffman, E. P. (1991) In utero fetal muscle biopsy for the diagnosis of Duchenne muscular dystrophy. *Am. J. Obstet. Gynecol.* **165,** 728–732.
5. Evans, M. I., Farrell, S. A., Greb, A., Ray, P., Johnson, M. P., and Hoffman, E. P. (1993) In utero fetal muscle biopsy for the diagnosis of Duchenne muscular dystrophy in a female fetus "suddenly at risk". *Am. J. Med. Genet.* **46,** 309–312.
6. Evans, M. I., Krivchenia, E. L., Johnson, M. P., Quintero, R. A., King, M., Pegoraro, E., and Hoffman, E. P. (1995) In utero fetal muscle biopsy alters diagnosis and carrier risks in Duchenne and Becker muscular dystrophy. *Fetal Diagn. Ther.* **10,** 71–75.
7. Evans, M. I., Quintero, R. A., King, M., Qureshi, F., Hoffman, E. P., and Johnson, M. P. (1995) Endoscopically assisted, ultrasound-guided fetal muscle biopsy. *Fetal Diagn. Ther.* **10,** 167–172.
8. Kuller, J. A., Hoffman, E. P., Fries, M. H., and Golbus, M. S. (1992) Prenatal diagnosis of Duchenne muscular dystrophy by fetal muscle biopsy. *Hum. Genet.* **90,** 34–40.
9. Benzie, R. J., Ray, P., Thompson, D., Hunter, A. G., Ivey, B., and Salvador, L. (1994) Prenatal exclusion of Duchenne muscular dystrophy by fetal muscle biopsy. *Prenat. Diagn.* **14,** 235–238.
10. Heckel, S., Favre, R., Flori, J., Koenig, M., Mandel, J., Gasser, B., and Chaigne, D. (1999) In utero fetal muscle biopsy: a precious aid for the prenatal diagnosis of duchenne muscular dystrophy. *Fetal Diagn. Ther.* **14,** 127–132.
11. Bieber, F. R., Hoffman, E. P., and Amos, J. (1989) Dystrophin analysis in duchenne muscular dystrophy: use in diagnosis and in genetic counseling. *Am. J. Hum. Genet.* **45,** 362–367.
12. Clerk, A., Strong, P. N., and Sewry, C. A. (1992) Characterisation of dystrophin during development of human skeletal muscle. *Development* **114,** 395–402.
13. Evans, M. I., Hoffman, E. P., Cadrin, C., Johnson, M. P., Quintero, R. A., and Golbus, M. S. (1994) Fetal muscle biopsy: collaborative experience with varied indications. *Obstet. Gynecol.* **84,** 913–917.

IV

Future Perspectives

24

Use of Animal Models to Understand Human Muscular Dystrophy

Mark M. Rich, Rita J. Balice-Gordon, and Sita Reddy

1. Introduction

In the decade following the identification of mutations in the dystrophin genein Duchenne *(1)* and Becker *(2)* muscular dystrophies (DMD/BMD), defects in components of the dystrophin–glycoprotein complex (DGC), which links F-actin in the cytoskeleton with laminin in the extra cellular matrix, have been shown to result in several human MD syndromes *(3)*. Defects in α-, β-, γ-, and δ-sarcoglycans, which are components of the DGC, are associated with limb-girdle MDs (LGMD) 2D, E, C, and F, respectively; laminin α_2-chain mutations have been shown to result in congenital MD *(4)*. Defects in non-DGC components that cause include the calpain 3 in LGMD2A *(4)*, expansion of a CTG repeat in the 3' untranslated region of a serine threonine kinase (myotonic dystrophy protein kinase [DMPK]) in myotonic dystrophy (DM) *(5)*, and mutations in a novel nuclear protein in Emery-Dreifuss MD *(6)*.

One or more muscle functions are altered as a consequence of such defects, some or all of which may be critical to the development of dystrophic changes. Alterations in DGC and laminin α2 has been shown to alter the mechanical properties of muscle cell surfaces *(7)*, modify ion channel function *(8)*, and perturb the transduction of growth signals *(9,10)*. Loss of calpain 3 may have a widespread effect on several signal transduction pathways mediated by intracellular calcium levels *(11)*. CTG repeat expansion in DM results in the nuclear accumulation of the mutant *DMPK* mRNA encoding the expanded CUG repeat track *(12)*. Accumulation of CUG repeats within the nucleus causes Myotonia and several histological features of DM skeletal *(13)*. Additionally nuclear accumulation of the mutant allele results in decreased DMPK protein levels,

From: *Methods in Molecular Medicine, vol. 43: Muscular Dystrophy: Methods and Protocols*
Edited by: K. M. D. Bushby and L. V. B. Anderson © Humana Press Inc., Totowa, NJ

which contributes to decreased skeletal muscle force production *(14)*. Insight into key steps contributing to the dystrophic process in skeletal muscle can be obtained by the sequential evaluation of the integrity of the signaling process from the nerve to the muscle in animal model systems. Although dystrophic dogs, cats, and hamsters have provided useful insights into the disease process *(15)*, the mouse has become the animal model of choice for the evaluation of the etiology of human muscular dystrophies, both for the ease of manipulation of their genomes and for the relatively low cost of maintenance. Strains of mice in common use include the naturally occurring mdx strain in which a nonsense mutation abolishes dystrophin expression *(16)*. Novel strains of mice carrying mutations in Utrophin *(17,18)*, laminin α2 *(19)*, and DMPK *(14,18)* have been generated via homologous recombination in embryonic stem cells. Other strains of mice expressing transgenes using muscle-specific promoters include those expressing (TG repeats *[13]*)dystrophin *(21,22)*, and utrophin *(23)*, which have been useful both in evaluating the function of such transgenes in vivo, and, for their ability to rescue the dystrophic phenotype in the mdx mouse model. Construction of such strains of mice is not part of this review, and the reader is referred to several excellent sources *(24,25)* for details of such procedures.

Despite the significant advantages afforded by the ability to make specific targeted mutations in mice, evaluation of causal relationships between the mutations and the pathology may be complicated by differences between mouse and human physiology. Such differences are perhaps most clearly illustrated using the mdx mouse model of DMD. Loss of dystrophin in DMD patients causes progressive dystrophic changes in muscle, leading to death, usually by the second decade in life. In contrast, the mdx mouse, although showing severe necrotic changes and weakness beginning at approx 3 wk of age, is able to regenerate muscle more efficiently, thus resulting in normal life spans of approx 2 yr *(26,27)*.

These differences may be attributable to the reduced life-span of mice, compared to humans, combined with a similar rate of progression and/or to differences in structure, composition, or compensatory mechanisms, such as regenerative capacity. For example, because the surface-to-volume ratio is inversely proportional to fiber diameter, human muscle fibers could be subject to greater stress per unit area when compared to mouse fibers, which may result in a more severe phenotype in humans, compared to mice, even when all other parameters are equal. Thus, such differences should be kept in mind when causal relationships are being established between genotype and the observed phenotype.

However, although all phenotypic changes may not manifest as a consequence of identical mutations in humans and mice, individual aspects of signal transduction can be assessed using the scheme described in this chapter. Such schemes have been useful in evaluating the integrity of several independent features of nerve and muscle function *(14)*, and evaluation of differences between mouse and human muscles can lead to important insights that could have significant therapeutic value. One example of such differences is the possible use of utrophin to rescue dystrophic changes in DMD *(23)*.

2. Materials: Choice of Mice

1. The choice of mice to be sampled should include considerations of the strain, sex, and age of the control and test animals. The use of inbred mice, age- and sex-matched between control and test animals, decreases variability and increases the sensitivity of the assays described. In the authors' experience, 129sv was found to be a more sensitive background to assay for DMPK loss, compared to C57Bl/6J (unpublished observations).
2. A second example of such strain-specific differences, which could alter the progression of necrotic skeletal muscle disease, is the variability in skeletal muscle regenerative potential. Such differences include the increased regenerative potential of skeletal muscle in Swiss SJL/J mice, compared to BALBc, AKR, C3H, and C57B mice *(28,29)*.
3. The authors have noticed significant differences in the phenotype associated with DMPK loss, when the mutation is studied in male, compared to female, mice *(14)*. Similar differences have also been noted by Grounds and McGeachie *(29)*, who found muscle regeneration to be much more vigorous in male mice, compared to female mice.
4. Last, when studying progressive late-onset disorders, the age at which detailed analyses are performed can be critical, and are therefore best chosen in conjunction with simple noninvasive testing of muscle function to determine a time-frame when dystrophic changes become significant. One such test evaluating proximal muscle weakness is the coat hanger test described by Lalonde et al. (***30***; *see* **Note 1**). The use of this and similar tests can help define a window of time when the pathological phenotype is best studied.

3. Methods: Evaluation of Nerve and Muscle Function

Progressive muscle weakness is a hallmark of myopathies, and can be the result of functional defects in one or several steps in the process of force generation. Described below is a relatively straightforward paradigm for evaluating the integrity of consecutive physiological events, including nerve conduction analysis, electromyography, parameters of force development, and histological evaluation of neuromuscular junctions and muscle fibers. These studies can be used to determine whether there is a primary neuropathic defect, myopathic defect, or both *(31)*. Such studies help define the rate-limiting steps in the development of a muscle disease, and allow mechanistic models to be built and facilitate the design of rational therapy (*see* **Note 2**). The authors indicate a possible progression in the analysis scheme that allows the test animal to be utilized in a fashion that allows maximum information to be obtained.

3.1. Nerve Conduction Studies

Nerve conduction studies (*see* **Note 3**) allow for a rapid screening of defects in nerve conduction velocity, axon loss, and defects in neuromuscular transmission. All of these defects can cause weakness in mice that appears similar to that seen in myopathy. It is important to rule out defects in nerve and neuromuscular junction transmission prior to analysis of myopathy, via measurement of muscle force generation and contractile properties.

3.1.1. Performing Nerve Conduction Studies

1. Adult mice are anesthetized with a ketamine–xylazine mixture injected intraperitoneally (*see* **Note 4**). Nerve conduction studies are performed by stimulating either the brachial plexus, located in the armpit of the mouse, or the sciatic nerve at the sciatic notch. Two subdermal electrodes are used to stimulate the nerve. For stimulating the brachial plexus, the cathode electrode is placed near the plexus, and the anode electrode is placed over the sternum. A ground electrode is placed at the extensor surface of the elbow, where little muscle is present. Two recording electrodes are used. The active electrode is placed in the flexor surface of the forepaw, where flexor muscles are located, and the reference electrode is placed over the extensor surface of the forepaw, where no muscle is present.
2. For stimulating the sciatic nerve in the leg, the cathode is placed over the sciatic notch, and the anode is placed in the midline over the spine. The ground electrode is placed at the ankle, where little muscle is present. The active recording electrode is placed in the flexor surface of the hindpaw, where flexor muscle of the foot are located, and the reference electrode is placed over the extensor surface of the hindpaw, where no muscle is present.
3. The stimulus strength is increased gradually, until a compound muscle action potential (CMAP) is recorded, which represents the sum of the action potentials of all the muscle fibers in a muscle(s). A response can usually be first detected with several milliamperes of current. As the current is increased further, the amplitude of the CMAP response gradually increases. Finally, at a current strength of 10–30 mA, the CMAP amplitude no longer increases. This is the supramaximal response, and represents the sum of all the action potentials from all the muscle fibers firing when all axons innervating the muscle are stimulated.
4. Nerve conduction velocity can be measured in the sciatic nerve by varying placement of the stimulus along the length of the nerve. To do this, the first stimulation is performed with both the cathode and anode placed across the ankle. A response is obtained at the ankle, then a second response is obtained by stimulating at the sciatic notch. The difference in time between the onset of the two responses is measured, which is the time it takes the impulse to travel along the nerve from the sciatic notch to the ankle. The distance along the course of the sciatic nerve is

then measured with the leg extended, and a velocity can be obtained by dividing distance by time: In control mice, this should be between 30 and 45 m/s. If values other than this are obtained, either the method of stimulation or recording of the response are incorrect. In the forelimb, it is more difficult to accurately measure nerve conduction velocity, because the distance is less than in the hindlimb.

5. Another measure that can be performed is the distal latency, which is done by simply measuring the time to the onset of the CMAP from stimulation performed at a distal site in the nerve. In the sciatic nerve, the distal latency is measured on stimulations performed at the ankle. The distal latency is a combination of the time it takes for the impulse to conduct along the distal nerve trunk, the time of neuromuscular transmission, and the time of the muscle fiber action potentials to sweep past the recording electrode.

3.1.2. Interpreting Nerve Conduction Studies

Interpretation of the results of nerve conduction studies can shed light on the underlying processes, and can be used to rule in or rule out alternative mechanisms (**Fig. 1**).

3.1.2.1. Demyelinating Neuropathy

When myelination is disrupted, there is a slowing of conduction along the nerve. This manifests as slowing of nerve conduction in two ways: first is a prolongation of distal latency, which occurs secondary to slowed conduction along the distal nerve branches; the second finding is a slowing of conduction velocity in the proximal nerve, which can be measured directly.

3.1.2.2. Axonal Neuropathy

When axons die, the primary finding is a reduction in the CMAP amplitude, which occurs without a significant increase in the distal latency, and without much slowing of nerve conduction velocity. Before concluding that a reduced CMAP amplitude is secondary to axonal neuropathy, however, it is important to rule out defects of neuromuscular transmission or severe myopathy (*see* **Subheading 3.1.2.3.**).

3.1.2.3. Defects of Neuromuscular Transmission

With defects in neuromuscular transmission, nerve conduction velocity is normal. CMAP amplitudes can be either normal or reduced. The primary way to identify defects of neuromuscular transmission is to perform repetitive nerve stimulation while recording the CMAP. At slow rates of stimulation (2–3 Hz), all causes of defects in neuromuscular transmission lead to a decrement in the CMAP amplitude of greater than 10%, by the third stimulus. To determine whether the defect in neuromuscular transmission is pre- or postsynaptic, high rates (30–50 Hz) of repetitive stimulation can be performed. If the defect is

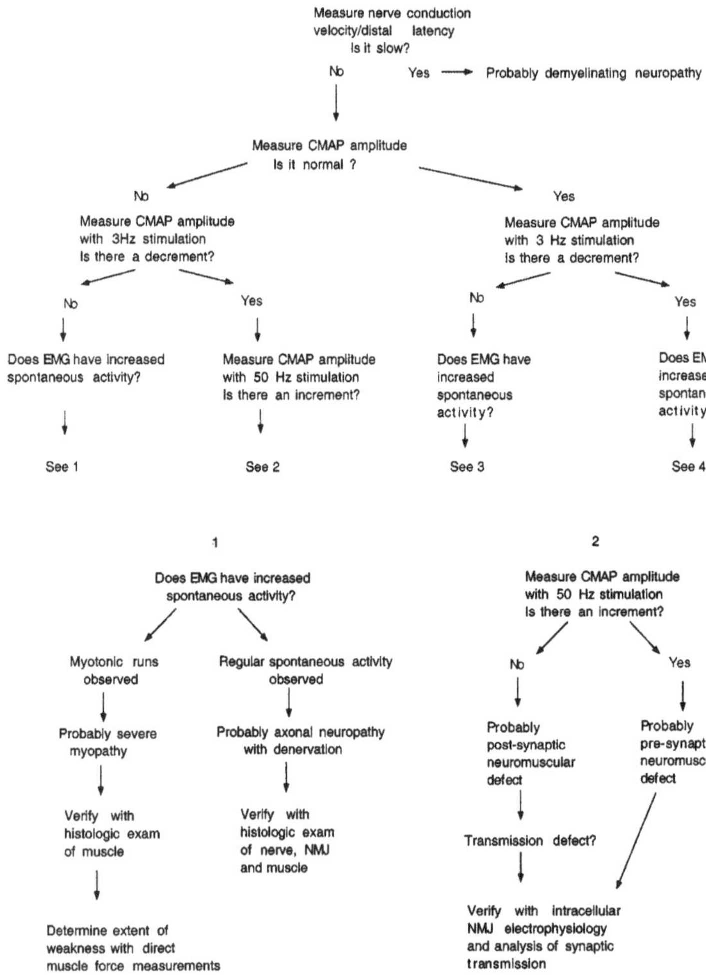

Fig. 1. *(This and opposite page)* Flow chart for the analysis of nerve, neuromuscular junction, and muscle function.

presynaptic, the initial CMAP is less than normal, and a large increase in the CMAP amplitude (greater than 100%) is seen with fast repetitive stimulation. If the defect is postsynaptic, the CMAP is usually normal or minimally reduced in amplitude and little increase in amplitude is seen (<100%) with fast repetitive stimulation.

3.1.2.4. Myopathy

In myopathy, the nerve conduction velocity and distal latency are normal. CMAP amplitude is normal, except in severe myopathy, and repetitive stimu-

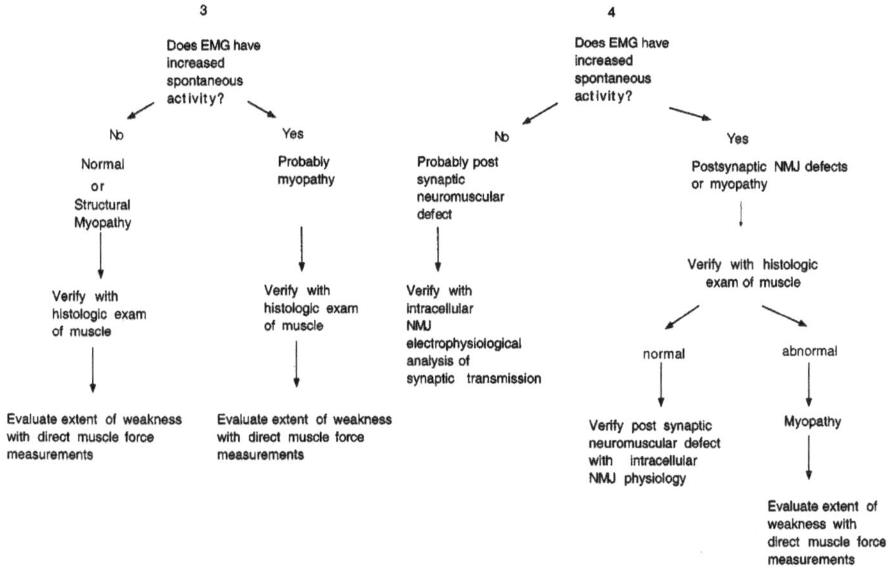

Fig. 1. *(continued)*

lation is usually unremarkable, although mild decrements can occur with slow rates of stimulation.

3.2. Electromyography

An important adjunct to the nerve conduction studies is electromyography (EMG), in which small regions of muscle are sampled to look at abnormal spontaneous activity of muscle fibers.

3.2.1. Performing EMG Studies

To perform EMG, a ground electrode is placed near the midline of the back (placement is not crucial). An EMG needle is then inserted into muscles one at a time: Typical muscles to study include the gastrocnemius, tibialis anterior, quadriceps, biceps, intrinsic paw muscles, and paraspinal muscles. The electrode is moved throughout different regions of each muscle studied. In normal muscle, with each movement of the electrode, there is a brief burst of muscle fiber action potentials, known as insertional activity. Otherwise, no electrical activity is present in muscle of anesthetized mice. In denervated muscle, in addition to insertional activity, there is spontaneous activity, which is regular in rhythm, and sounds like a ticking or the beating of a heart. This represents the spontaneous activity of denervated muscle fibers. Similar spontaneous activity can occur in myopathy. In addition, in some myopathies, muscle can be hyperexcitable and have rapid runs of action potentials, known as myotonia (*see* **Note 5**). When visualized, rapid runs of action potentials, which vary in rate and amplitude, are seen.

3.2.2. Interpreting EMG Studies

1. When comparing nerve conduction responses from affected and control animals, reproducible placement of electrodes for both stimulating and recording nerves is very important in both groups. Make sure reproducible values are obtained in control mice before moving to study experimental mice.
2. The amplitude of the CMAP is affected by placement of electrodes. Both sides of an animal should be studied. If one side gives a much smaller CMAP response than the other side, misplacement of electrodes should be considered, and the side with the small response should be restudied.
3. Stimulus artifacts can obscure CMAP responses, when stimulation is performed at the ankle. In this situation, it may not be possible to obtain a supramaximal response without obscuring the CMAP. Use as large a stimulus strength as possible, and record distal latency using that stimulus strength.
4. With repetitive stimulation, it is important to make sure that changes in CMAP amplitude are not caused by movement occurring during the stimulation. Movement shows up as a change in the baseline. When the baseline is not stable, it is very difficult to conclude whether a real change in CMAP amplitude is occurring.
5. Finally, nerve conduction and EMG tests are meant to guide in diagnosis. Although **Fig. 1** lays out the most likely diagnosis for each set of electrophysiologic findings, there are exceptions, and caution must be exercised when interpreting results.

3.3. Measuring Muscle Force Generation

Should the in vivo analysis of the etiology of muscle weakness described above suggest a primary myopathy, it is useful to further evaluate the extent and progression of muscle weakness. For this purpose, in vitro analyses of muscle twitch and tetanic force generation are performed. In addition, muscle force generated by nerve stimulation can be compared to that elicited by direct muscle stimulation, to further characterize defects in muscle fiber activation.

3.3.1. Analysis of Muscle Contractile Properties

2. To characterize muscle contractile properties, animals are deeply anesthetized and individual muscles are dissected. Muscles are placed in a tissue chamber filled with oxygenated Ringer's solution (typically 119 m*M* NaCl, 4.7 m*M* KCl, 2.5 m*M* $CaCl_2$, 1.2 m*M* KH_2PO_4, 1.2 m*M* $MgSO_4$, 25 m*M* HEPES, pH 7.4).
2. Both ends of the muscle are tied with silk thread (size 6–0). The rostral end of the muscle is fixed with silk thread to a fixed-point platform, and can be oriented vertically in a jacketed heart chamber (Kontes), or horizontally in a perfusion

chamber containing continuously oxygenated Ringer's solution maintained at 25°C. The caudal end is attached to the lever arm of a dual mode servomotor system (such as Cambridge Tech., model 300B).

3. Direct stimulation of the muscle is provided via a pair of platinum wire electrodes running the length of the muscle, to allow the measurement of muscle force produced during directly evoked isometric contractions. Using pulses of 0.2 ms duration, delivered at 1 Hz, muscle length is adjusted to obtain the length at which maximal twitch force is elicited (Lo). Voltage is adjusted between 8 and 12 V, to give supramaximal stimulation with 1.2–1.5× the current required to elicit maximal twitch force. These parameters are verified and adjusted, if necessary, several times during the experiment, so that maximal twitch force is maintained.
4. The mean value of five twitches is used to determine twitch contraction time (time to peak force) and half relaxation time (time for force to decrease to one-half its peak value). These values can be indicative of a relative slowing of muscle fiber contraction.
5. The force–frequency relationship and maximal isometric tetanic force are established by stimulating the muscle at frequencies of 10, 20, 40, 60, 80, and 100 Hz for 1 s, with approx 5 min between contractions.
6. Fatiguability is assessed from the decline of peak isometric force following repetitive stimulation over a period of 3 min (30–40 Hz, 0.33 duty cycle, 90 trains/min). Muscle force can be displayed on a storage oscilloscope (Hewlett Packard 54600), and recorded with software using an A-D converter.
7. Following these measurements, muscle can then be removed from the tissue chamber, blotted dry, weighed, frozen, and processed for morphometry and fiber-type immunohistochemistry. Total muscle cross-sectional area was calculated as wet muscle mass divided by muscle length times density (1.06 g/cm^{-3}) ***(32)***. In this way, force is calculated and expressed as gm/cm^{-2}.

3.3.2. Analysis of Muscle Fatiguability and Force–Frequency Relationships

Muscle fatigue properties are assessed as an indicator of the relative integrity of oxidative and glycolytic pathways for energy production. Muscles composed primarily of fast-twitch, glycolytic fibers (IIa and IIb) typically show a greater decline in force generation over time, compared to muscles composed primarily of type I, oxidative fibers ***(33)***. In addition, muscles compromised in disease states, such as mitochondrial myopathies, often have markedly altered fatigue properties ***(34)***

1. Muscle fatiguability is evaluated by measuring the peak tetanic force following repetitive stimulation at 30 Hz for 3 min. If no differences in the percent decline in tetanic tension are observed among groups, this would suggest that the relative integrity of glycolytic pathways is in the normal range.
2. Analysis of the relationship between direct muscle stimulation frequency and force generation can show whether muscles from different animals develop maxi-

mum tetanic forces at the same rate and in the same range of stimulation (80–100 Hz) as age-matched control mice. If, at stimulation rates that result in maximal force production, tetani are completely fused, this would suggest that the contractile apparatus is likely to be functioning at saturating levels of Ca^{2+}. Changes in the relationship between frequency of stimulation and amount of force generated (force–frequency relationships) are often indicative of alterations in the amount of Ca^{2+} release, and thus the amount of activation of the contractile apparatus at a given stimulus frequency.

3.3.3. Relationship Between Functional Studies and Histological Studies

This functional analysis of skeletal muscle contractile properties can be combined with a histological analysis of the same muscles, to determine whether there is altered fiber degeneration, regeneration, atrophy, or fiber composition.

3.4. Example: Evaluating the Role of DMPK in Skeletal Muscle Function

The authors have used a similar paradigm (**Fig. 2**) to analyze age-matched, wild-type, *Dmpk+/–*, and *Dmpk–/–* mice ***(14)***. These analyses have shown that, in these mutant mice, the 30–50% deficit in force generation in skeletal muscles is the result of impaired excitation/contraction coupling (**Fig. 2**). Histological analysis of *Dmpk–/–* skeletal muscle structure showed increased fiber degeneration and regeneration, fiber-size variation, and loss of sarcomeric organization, compared to age-matched, wild-type controls. On ultrastructural evaluation, abnormal mitochondria, dilation of the sarcoplasmic reticulum, and Z line loss were observed. Thus, although the precise mechanism underlying the decreased force production remains to be determined, the authors' data shows that impaired excitation/contraction, and/or abnormalities of the contractile apparatus *per se,* are likely to underlie the progressive muscle weakness observed in DMPK–/– mice. Thus this series of experiments performed on *Dmpk–/–* mice serve to illustrate the utility of the described approach in the functional analysis of nerve, neuromuscular junction, and the muscle in mice.

4. Notes

1. In this test, the mouse is placed in the middle of a thin (2-cm diameter) horizontal bar (40-cm length) of a triangular coat hanger. The coat hanger is suspended (so that it cannot sway) 80 cm above a padded desk. This distance normally provides mice with a strong incentive not to fall. Muscle function can be studied by measuring the following latencies: time until two paws touch a side bar, time until three paws touch the side bar, time until four paws touch the side bar, and time to fall. Because this test is simple to perform, and should not take more than 5 min/animal, it can be performed on control and test animals at set time intervals in the study, to evaluate progressive muscle weakness.

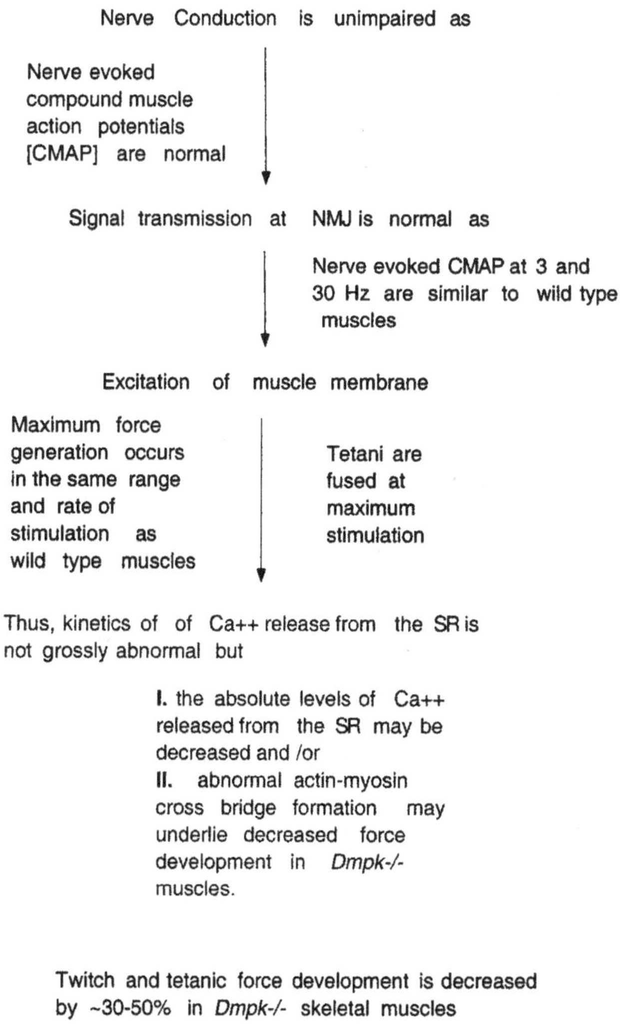

Fig. 2. Physiological analyses of Dmpk–/– skeletal muscle.

2. Insight into the rate limiting steps is facilitated by evaluating the integrity of several physiological steps on a single animal, rather than when such analyses are scattered over several test animals.
3. Nerve conduction tests and EMG can be easily performed using an EMG machine from either Dantec or Nicolet.
4. For mice that are sick or weak, a lower dose should be used, to prevent overdose.
5. The sound created by myotonia has been described as similar to the sound of a dive bomber or a revving motorcycle.

References

1. Koenig M., Hoffman E. P., Bertelson C. J., Monaco A. P., Feener C., and Kunkel L. M. (1987) Complete cloning of the Duchenne muscular dystrophy (DMD) cDNA and preliminary genomic organization of the DMD gene in normal and affected individuals. *Cell* **50,** 509–517.
2. Monaco A. P., Bertelson C. J., Liechti-Gallati S., Moser, H., and Kunkel L. M. (1988) An explanation for the phenotypic differences between patients bearing partial deletions of the DMD locus. *Genomics* **2,** 90–95.
3. Michalak, M. and Opas, M. (1997) Functions of dystrophin and dystrophin associated proteins. *Curr. Opin. Neurol.* **10,** 436–442.
4. Bonnemann C. G., McNally E. M., and Kunkel L. M. (1996) Beyond dystrophin: current progress in the muscular dystrophies. *Curr. Opin. Pediatr.* **8,** 569–582.
5. Brook, J. D., McCurrach, M. E., Harley, H. G., Buckler, A. J., Church, D., Aburtani, H., et al. (1992) Molecular basis of myotonic dystrophy: Expansion of a trinucleotide (CTG) repeat at the 3' end of a transcript encoding a protein kinase family member. *Cell* **68,** 799–808.
6. Bione S., Maestrini E., Rivella S., Mancini M., Regis S., Romeo G., and Toniolo, D. (1994) Identification of a novel X-linked gene responsible for Emery-Dreifuss muscular dystrophy. *Nature Genet.* **8,** 323–327.
7. Petrof, B. J., Shrager, J. B., Stedman, H. H., Kelly, A. M., and Sweeney, H. L. (1993) Dystrophin protects the sarcolemma from stresses developed during muscle contraction. *Proc. Natl. Acad. Sci. USA* **90,** 3710–3714.
8. Franco-Obregon, A. Jr. and Lansman, J. B. (1994) Mechanosensitive ion channels in skeletal muscle from normal and dystrophic mice. *J. Physiol.* **481,** 299–309.
9. Brown, S. C. and Lucy, J. A. (1993) Dystrophin as a mechanochemical transducer in skeletal muscle. *Bioessays* **15,** 413–419.
10. Aumailley, M. and Krieg, T. (1996) Laminins: a family of diverse multifunctional molecules of basement membranes. *Invest. Dermatol.* **106,** 209–214.
11. Melloni, E., Salamino, F., and Sparatore, B. (1992) Calpain-calpastatin system in mammalian cells: properties and possible functions. *Biochimie* **74,** 217–223.
12. Taneja, K. L., McCurrach, M., Schalling, M., Housman, D., and Singer, R. H. (1995) Foci of trinucleotide repeat transcripts in nuclei of myotonic cells and tissues. *J. Cell Biol.* **128,** 995–1002.
13. Mankodi, A., Logigian, E., Callahan, L., McClain, C., White, R., Henderson, D., Krym, M., and Thornton, C. A. (2000) Myotonic dystrophy in transgenic mice expressing an expanded CUG repeat. *Science* **289,** 1769–1773.
14. Reddy, S., Smith, D. B. J., Rich, M. M., Leferovich, J. M., Reilly, P., Davis, B. D., et al. (1996) Mice lacking the myotonic dystrophy kinase develop a late onset myopathy. *Nature Genet.* **13,** 423–442.
15. Nonaka I. (1998) Animal models of muscular dystrophies. Lab. Anim. Sci. **48,** 8–17.
16. Bulfield, G., Siller, W. G., Wight, P. A. L., and Moore, K. J. (1984) X chromosome-linked muscular dystrophy (mdx) in the mouse. *Proc. Natl. Acad. Sci. USA* **81,** 1189–1192.

17. Grady, R. M., Merlie, J. P., and Sanes, J. R. (1997) Subtle neuromuscular defects in utrophin deficient mice. *J. Cell. Biol.* **136,** 871–882.
18. Deconnick, A. E., Potter, A. C., Tinsley, J. M., Wood, S. J., Vater, R., Young, C., Metzinger, L., Vincent, A., Slater, C. R., and Davies, K. E. (1997) Post synaptic abnormalities at the neuromuscular junctions of utrophin deficient mice. *J. Cell. Biol.* **136,** 883–894.
19. Miyagoe, Y., Hanaoka, K., Nonaka, I., Hayasaka, M., Nabeshima, Y., Arahata, K., Nabeshima, Y., and Takeda, S. (1997) Laminin alpha$_2$ chain-null mutant mice by targeted disruption of Lama$_2$ gene: a new model of merosin (laminin 2)-deficient congenital muscular dystrophy. *FEBS Lett.* **415,** 33–39.
20. Jansen, G., Groenen, P. J. T. A., Bachner, D., Jap, P. H. K., Coerwinkel, M., Oerlemans, F., Broek, W., Gohlsch, B., Pette, D., Plomp, J. J., Molenaar, P. C., Nederhoff, M. G. J., Echteld, C., Dekker, M., Berns, A. Hameister, H. and Weiriringa, B. (1996) Abnormal myotonic dystrophy protein kinase levels produce only mild myopathy in mice. *Nature Genet.* **13,** 423–442.
21. Wells, D. J., Wells, K. E., Asante, E. A., Turner, G., Sunada, Y, Campbell, K. P., Walsh, F. S., and Dickson, G. (1995) Expression of human full-length and minidystrophin in transgenic mdx mice: implications for gene therapy of Duchenne muscular dystrophy. *Hum. Mol. Genet.* **4,** 1245–1250.
22. Cox, G. A., Cole, N. M., Matsumura, K, Phelps, S. F., Hauschka, S. D., Campbell, K. P., Faulkner, J. A., and Chamberlin, J. S. (1993) Overexpression of dystrophin in transgenic mdx mice eliminates dystrophic symptoms without toxicity. *Nature* **364,** 725–729.
23. Tinsley, J. M., Potter, A. C., Phelps, S. R., Fisher, R., Trickett, J. I., and Davies, K. E. (1996) Amelioration of the dystrophic phenotype of mdx mice using the truncated utrophin transgene. *Nature* **384,** 349–353.
24. Hogan, B., Bedington, R., Constantini, F., and Lacy, E. (1994) *Manipulating the Mouse Rmbryo: A Laboratory Manual.* Cold Spring Harbor Laboratory, Cold Spring Harbor, NY.
25. Joyner, A. L., ed. (1993) Gene Targeting: A Practical Approach, IRL.
26. Carnwath, J. W. and Shotten, D. M. (1987) Muscular dystrophy in the mdx mouse: histopathology of the soleus and extensor digitorum longus muscles. *J. Neurol. Sci.* **80,** 39–54.
27. Dimario, J. X., Uzman, A., and Strohman, R. C. (1991) Fiber regeneration is not perisitent in dystrophic (MDX) mouse skeletal muscle. *Dev. Biol.* **148,** 314–321.
28. Grounds, M. D. (1987) Phagocytosis of necrotic muscle in muscle isografts is influenced by the strain, age and sex of host mice. *J. Pathol.* **153,** 71–82.
29. Grounds, M. D. and McGeachie, J. K. (1989) Comparison of muscle precursor replication in crush injured skeletal muscle of Swiss and Balbc mice. *Cell Tissue Res.* **255,** 385–391.
30. Lalonde, R., Botez, M. I., Joyal, C. C. and Caumartin, M. (1992) Motor abnormalities in lurcher mutant mice. *Physiol. Behavior* **51,** 523–525.
31. Kimura, J. (1989) *Electrodiagnosis in Diseases of Nerve and Muscle: Principles and Practice,* 2nd ed., F. A. Davis.

32. Close, K. (1972) Dynamic properties of mammalian skeletal muscle. *Phys. Rev.* **52,** 129–197.
33. Burke, R. E. (1994) Physiology of motor units, in *Myology,* 2nd ed. (Engel, A. G. and Franzini-Armstrong, C., eds.), McGraw-Hill, New York, pp. 464–483.
34. Morgan-Huges, J. A. (1994) Mitochondrial diseases, in *Myology,* 2nd ed. (Engel, A. G. and Franzini-Armstrong, C., eds.), McGraw-Hill, New York, pp. 1610–1660.

25

Options for Development of Gene-Based Therapy for Muscular Dystrophy

Matthew G. Dunckley and George Dickson

1. General Introduction

1.1. History

The gene involved in Duchenne and Becker muscular dystrophies (DMD/BMD) was the first human gene to be successfully identified by the approach of reverse genetics, or positional cloning *(1)*, leading to the recognition of this approach as a valid and useful way of identifying genes for which the biochemical product is unknown. Since then, the genes causing the majority of other MDs have also been mapped, sequenced, and their protein products identified *(2)*. Meanwhile, the development of the necessary tools for incorporating genetic material into living cells (gene transfer) has moved from the first attempts to express synthetic reporter genes in cultured cells, through in vivo studies in animal models, to the onset of clinical trials. Indeed, DMD was one of the first inherited diseases thought likely to benefit from gene therapy (GT) *(3)*. Although it is now accepted that DMD may be more difficult to treat in this way than some other single-gene disorders, this and other MDs remain suitable candidates for GT for a number of reasons.

1.1.1. Genetic Basis Known and Genes Cloned

Most MDs have now been mapped to at least a chromosomal locus *(4)*, and many have been extensively characterized by methods described elsewhere in this volume *(2)*. Moreover, the cloning of full-length recombinant (cDNA) versions of these genes into expression vectors is enhancing the understanding of the pathogenesis of these MDs *per se,* as well as providing the starting material for potential genetic therapies.

From: *Methods in Molecular Medicine, vol. 43: Muscular Dystrophy: Methods and Protocols*
Edited by: K. M. D. Bushby and L. V. B. Anderson © Humana Press Inc., Totowa, NJ

1.1.2. Recessive, Loss-of-Function Disorders

Most MDs are associated with an absence or reduction of the normal gene product in skeletal muscle. Hence, it is likely that the addition of synthetic functional copies of the appropriate gene will restrict progression of these disorders, provided such genes are expressed at sufficient levels, at the right subcellular location, and for enough time.

1.1.3. No Alternative Therapeutic Options

Muscular dystrophies are generally severe, progressive disorders, and none are effectively treatable with existing drugs. The introduction of specific functional genes into dystrophic muscle can potentially correct the cause of disease at the most fundamental level possible, and may thus offer treatments that are both effective and permanent.

1.1.4. Animal Models Available.

The benefits of animal models for MDs are covered in Chapter 24. In terms of gene transfer, these animals allow the effectiveness of recombinant gene constructs to be assessed in vivo by both germline (transgenic animals) and somatic gene transfer ***(5,6)***. Currently, gene transfer research for DMD is largely restricted to somatic gene transfer in mdx mice, the mouse model for the disease ***(7)***, although dystrophic dog models may become increasingly valuable for preclinical trials ***(8–10)***. In addition, transgenic animals may in turn be crossed with other animal models to assess compensatory mechanisms. For instance, double-knockout mice, lacking dystrophin and utrophin expression, have a severe MD relative to their mdx parentage, confirming the importance of utrophin in the development of DMD pathology ***(11,12)***.

1.1.5. Muscle is a Stable System.

Healthy mature muscle is in the form of postmitotic, multinucleated myofibers, lined with dormant satellite myoblast precursor cells, which can replicate and repair muscle upon injury ***(13)***. In MD, muscle regeneration cannot apparently keep pace with the extent of chronic injury, is inhibited by the deposition of nonmuscle tissue, and leads to progressive muscular wasting. Nevertheless, regeneration may improve the uptake of genetic material into muscle cell nuclei during cell division, partly because the breakdown of muscle structure may allow free dissemination of gene transfer reagents through the endomysial space, to target maximal numbers of myoblasts and myofibers ***(14,15)***. Furthermore, because no further mitosis occurs following fusion of myoblasts into new myotubes, recombinant genes introduced during regeneration are unlikely to be lost, even if unintegrated in the host genome. Finally, skeletal muscle is also very well vascularized, so that it may in the future be amenable to gene transfer by injection into the systemic circulation.

As advances in understanding MDs and gene transfer have progressed in parallel, it is not surprising that the delivery of recombinant genes to skeletal muscle has received substantial attention. This chapter endeavors to provide a brief overview of the history of gene transfer studies for MD, outline some priorities for developing effective GTs as the authors see them, and consider whether these are likely to be realistic therapeutic options for MD in the future. Because the vast majority of gene transfer studies for MD have involved the *DMD* gene, these form the basis for most of this chapter, but it is likely that many of these strategies will also be applicable to other MDs.

1.2. Requirements for GT of Dystrophic Muscle

Clearly, the primary aim of gene transfer is to deliver a functional synthetic gene construct into the target cell, using some kind of delivery system, or vector. In order for this approach to achieve therapeutic benefit, the following aspects of the process are essential, or at least desirable.

1.2.1. Recombinant Gene Constructs for Expression in Muscle Cells

In the case of DMD, the native dystrophin gene is over 3 million bp in size ***(1)***, precluding the cloning of the whole gene into conventional expression systems. Although yeast artificial chromosomes (YACs) have been constructed that contain the entire gene ***(16)***, and smaller YAC contigs have even been introduced into eukaryotic cells by liposome- or protoplast-mediated gene transfer ***(17,18)***, dystrophin replacement has so far focused on delivering recombinant cDNA-based genes to skeletal muscle cells in vitro and in vivo, either to myoblasts or directly into differentiated muscle cells. Full-length mouse ***(19)*** and human ***(20)*** dystrophin cDNAs derived from the 14-kb major skeletal muscle transcript, have been cloned and expressed in mammalian cells, generating recombinant proteins of the appropriate size (427 kDa). In addition, a severely truncated 6.3-kb mini-dystrophin gene, derived from a mildly affected BMD patient, has been exceptionally valuable in evaluating the effects of recombinant dystrophin expression in dystrophic muscle cells ***(21)***. This gene is deleted for exons 17–48 and expresses a 229-kDa dystrophin protein lacking 46% of the central rod domain. Both the full-length and the smaller mini-dystrophin constructs have been tested for their ability to restore normal muscle phenotype in dystrophic mdx mice, by the production of transgenic mice ***(5,22,23)***.

1.2.2. Sufficient Gene Expression

Whereas germline gene transfer results in transgene expression from every nucleus, it is unlikely that somatic gene transfer will achieve normal expression levels of the appropriate protein in 100% of cells in vivo, especially in multinucleated muscle. Therefore, it is important to ascertain a minimum level beyond which therapeutic benefit is likely to be achieved. Transgenic mdx mice, expressing truncated or full-length human dystrophin, indicate that as low as 30% normal expression levels of even the Becker-type minidystrophin may be sufficient to substantially reduce muscle degeneration *(5)*. This is encouraging, and represents a more realistic goal, but it must be remembered that some dystrophin was expressed by every nucleus in these animals. Of greater relevance to a gene transfer scenario may be the observation that overall dystrophin expression of over 30% endogenous levels in female DMD carriers may still result in a myopathy *(24,25)*. Because these carriers have a mosaic pattern of dystrophin expression, distribution of the protein is also clearly important *(26)*.

1.2.3. Correct Localization and Function of Recombinant Protein

The protein product of recombinant genes must be localized appropriately within the target tissue in order to restore function. The ability of endogenous dystrophin to diffuse along the myofiber from a dystrophin-expressing nucleus is certainly limited, as structural proteins tend to localize in restricted nuclear domains *(27,28)*. Nevertheless, overexpression of dystrophin from a relatively small number of myonuclei may cause dystrophin to diffuse over a wider area of the myofiber than normal, and to compensate for a lack of expression in adjacent nuclei.

1.2.4. Regulation of Gene Expression

The correction of some MDs by gene transfer may be further complicated by the complexity of endogenous gene expression. For instance, transcription of the *DMD* gene occurs from at least seven promoters, and undergoes extensive alternative splicing, to generate a range of tissue- and developmentally regulated isoforms *(29)*. Fortunately, on the basis of animal studies, it seems that dystrophin does not require highly regulated expression in order to correct the muscle features of the disease: Overexpression of recombinant dystrophin corrects the myopathy in mdx mice, with no deleterious effects *(22)*. As a greater basic understanding of gene regulation is achieved, recombinant gene constructs, incorporating tissue-specific promoters, introns, and other untranslated sequences, should be developed, in order to correct all aspects of the MD phenotype.

1.2.5. Long-Term Gene Expression

Persistent gene expression is desirable, in order to avoid additional discomfort, expense, and immune reactions (to transgenes or vectors) likely to result from repeated administration. Immunosuppressive co-treatments may be acceptable, in order to maximize the effectiveness of gene transfer, as in the case of organ transplantation, but the susceptibility of MD patients to immunosuppressive complications, such as respiratory infections, will be a major consideration.

1.2.6. Efficient Vector Systems

Ideally, vectors are required that can accommodate full-length recombinant genes, enter a large proportion of muscle nuclei, give rise to stable gene transfer, and elicit little or no immune response. A wide range of vectors have been used to carry genes into skeletal muscle, and will now be considered under viral and nonviral categories.

2. Gene Transfer

2.1. Gene Transfer to Skeletal Muscle, Using Viral Vectors

The life cycle of viruses depends on entry and expression of their own genetic material within living host cells, so they are already, by definition, gene transfer vectors. In order to create recombinant viral vectors, sequences crucial for viral replication are removed from the wild-type viral genome and replaced by foreign recombinant gene sequences. A number of viruses have now been modified as gene transfer vectors ***(30–33)***, but retroviral and adenoviral (ADV) vectors represent the vast majority used in skeletal muscle (**Table 1**).

2.1.1. Retroviral Gene Transfer to Skeletal Muscle

Retroviral vectors are particularly attractive for gene transfer, because the biology of retroviruses is well understood, the retroviral genome comprises just three open reading frames in a single transcriptional unit, and the majority of viral proteins can be provided *in trans,* allowing the generation of infectious, but replication-defective retroviruses (for review, *see* ref. ***34***). The ability to separate *cis*-acting regulatory domains from viral protein-coding domains of the retroviral genome means that any gene of interest can be placed between the retroviral long terminal repeat, and packaged into infectious retrovirus particles, as long as the excised functions are supplied *in trans* by a packaging cell line ***(35)***. In addition, retroviruses stably integrate their genome into host-cell DNA, utilizing the process of normal cell replication to pass on to all subsequent daughter cells.

At first, retroviral vectors may seem inappropriate for dystrophin gene transfer, because they have a capacity for no more than about 8 kb foreign genetic material, and cannot infect nondividing cells (with the exception of lentiviruses) ***(36)***. However, the authors previously cloned the minidystrophin cDNA described

Table 1
Desirable Features of Viral Vectors and Their Target Tissues for Efficient, Long-Lasting Gene Transfer

Viral vector	Target tissue
Nonpathogenic	High receptor expression
Replication-deficient	Accessible
Large insert capacity	Well vascularized
Nondeleterious integration	Stable
Nonimmunogenic	
High titers	
Stable	

above into a retroviral vector and generated titers up to 10^5 CFU/mL *(37)*. Mdx muscle cells in culture were exposed to vector preparations, and allowed to fuse into myotubes. The Becker-type dystrophin molecule was expressed at the sarcolemma in a pattern identical to normal dystrophin. Having shown that satellite myoblasts can be transduced in culture, the authors then aimed to transduce proliferating satellite cells in regenerating muscle in vivo *(38)*. Because retroviral vectors only infect dividing cells, it was assumed that the best uptake of recombinant virus in vivo would occur at the peak of the regenerative phase of the mdx mouse, at about 2–6 wk of age. Initially, only about 3% of myofibers expressed minidystrophin after a single intramuscular (im) injection of vector. In order to improve the transduction efficiencies, the mdx myofibers were challenged with bupivacaine 48–72 h prior to retroviral injection, inducing a more acute phase of degeneration/regeneration over a larger area of the muscle. This led to expression of recombinant dystrophin in up to 10% of the muscle fibers *(39)*. Subsequently, in order to increase the length of exposure to the vector, retroviral producer cells were themselves implanted into mdx muscle fibers during the regenerative phase, leading to more consistent transduction efficiencies of up to 25% *(40)*. In order to reduce the effects of immunological rejection of the packaging cells, these studies were also carried out in nude mice lacking cell-mediated immunity, resulting in still further increases of dystrophin expression, showing that immunological factors were significant.

A refinement of producer cell implantation has recently been suggested, in order to target widespread sites of muscle regeneration in MD. This involves converting host macrophages into retroviral producer cells generating transgene-carrying retroviral vectors *(41)*. Injection of these cells into the systemic circulation should target areas of inflammation, such as damaged regenerating muscle, and infect satellite cells at the site of greatest activity. This technique thus combines the efficiency of packaging cell implantation for retroviral gene transfer and a natural targeting behavior. Moreover, because macrophages from the recipient would be used as vectors, it is likely that immune responses will be avoided.

Retroviruses infect target cells by an interaction of the surface glycoproteins with receptor molecules on the cell surface *(42)*. These glycoproteins determine the tropism of retroviral infection (restricting or expanding host range), and thus may be modified to bind specific cell- and tissue-specific markers *(43)*. At present, however, although binding to the cell surface has been achieved with comparable efficiency to wild-type virus, subsequent infection has not yet been observed with any significant efficiency *(44)*. Although greatest efficiencies of vector uptake may be achieved by tissue-targeting of vectors, tissue-specific expression of recombinant retroviruses is also possible by replacing the viral promoter and/or enhancer with a tissue-specific eukaryotic element. In this way, nonmuscle cells transduced by the vector would not express the transgene, enhancing vector safety. Studies on the dystrophin promoter, by the authors and other groups, indicate that it is fairly weak at driving gene expression, relative to others *(40,45)*. Instead, muscle-specific retroviral vectors may be created by inserting a muscle creatine kinase (MCK) enhancer element into the U3 region of the 3' viral long terminal repeat, leading to high levels of gene expression only in differentiated muscle cells (myotubes or myofibers) *(45,46)*.

One of the continuing obstacles for direct in vivo gene transfer, especially by retroviral vectors, has been the problem of generating titers high enough for large tissues or systemic injection. However, high-efficiency gene transfer of retroviral vector constructs (e.g., by lipofection), to packaging cell lines expressing high levels of retroviral structural proteins, results in the transient production of high-titer, helper-free retrovirus *(47)*. Another approach to circumvent this problem has been to package the Moloney murine leukemia virus retroviral contents within the more stable envelope from the vesicular stomatitis virus incorporating the G glycoprotein *(48)*. This not only provides a more stable particle and the possibility of titers in excess of 10^9 cfu/mL, compared to normal titers of 10^5–10^6 cfu/mL, but also enables retroviral vectors to infect a wider host range *(49)*. It has been found that murine retroviruses are rapidly inactivated by human complement, if in contact with human serum, because of host cell variations in the glycosylation of retroviral envelope proteins *(50)*. Therefore, in order to improve retroviral gene transfer in human subjects, anticomplement antibodies could be injected prior to injection of the retrovirus preparation, resulting in a window of opportunity for successful infection *(51)*, or retroviral vectors could be produced in species-specific cells *(50)*. Alternatively, conventional immunosuppressive drugs, such as FK506, may be required *(52)*.

Recently, the lentiviral family of vectors, including human (HIV), felive (FIV), and simian immunodeficiency virus, have been explored as vectors suitable for gene transfer to nondividing cells, such as neurons and muscle cells *(53)*. There are obvious concerns about using HIV-based systems, but FIV vectors have already been shown to be safe for gene transfer to nondividing cells *(54)*, including macrophages and neurons, and may offer a promising alternative to murine retroviral vectors. To date, however, lentiviral vectors have not been shown to efficiently transduce skeletal muscle.

2.1.2. ADV Gene Transfer to Skeletal Muscle

The most obvious viral vectors for gene transfer to skeletal muscle are those that are naturally capable of infecting nondividing cells. ADV genetics has been studied for many years, so these were soon adapted as vectors for gene transfer *(55)*. Recombinant ADVs are constructed from plasmid-based shuttle vectors containing at least the 5'- inverse terminal report (ITR), packaging signal, and E1a enhancer, allowing viral replication to be restricted to cells that constitutively express the E1 gene products, activated by nonviral transcription factors *(56)*. The transgene cassette, including a promoter, the gene of interest, and a polyadenylation signal, is cloned into the site of the E1 deletion, and the construct is transfected into an E1-expressing packaging cell line. Here, homologous recombination occurs, to generate replication-defective ADV particles containing the transgene, which are then plaque-purified to produce a high-titer viral preparation *(57)*. Most strains of ADV are: nonpathogenic, especially the recombinant ADVs derived from serotypes 2 and 5 *(58)*; stable, enabling storage for several months at –80°C without significant loss of infectivity *(59)*; nonintegrating, avoiding insertional mutagenesis and transmission in germline cells; capable of production at high titers (>1 10^{12} × PFU/mL); capable of infecting nondividing cells, including skeletal muscle and cardiomyocytes *(60)*. Although the disadvantage of nonintegrating DNA is that extra-chromosomal ADV DNA is lost during cell division, differentiated skeletal and cardiac muscles should retain episomal DNA within the nucleus for the lifetime of the cell. Tissue-specific targeting of ADV gene transfer may be engineered by modifying the properties of the viral envelope *(43,61)*, and incorporating tissue-restricted promoter/enhancer elements in the expression cassette. For instance, a large 1.35-kb MCK promoter/enhancer segment has been used in an ADV vector to generate muscle-specific expression *(62)*. ADV vectors have also been used in an ex vivo approach to gene transfer to dystrophic muscle, which is claimed to create a reservoir of dystrophin-expressing myoblasts, as well as increasing the efficiency of gene transfer *(63)*.

The chief disadvantage of ADV vectors is that most individuals (~80%) are already seropositive for the common strains. It is therefore likely that ADV infections will elicit immune responses, and that these will become increasingly severe, should repeated administration of the vector be required. The efficiency of infection probably varies, depending on the age and immune status of the animal, because ADV gene transfer has been shown to be significantly more efficient in neonates and athymic nude mice than in juvenile and adult muscle (***64–67***; G. Dickson and T. A. Piper, unpublished data). This is probably the result of transactivation of ADV late genes by cellular E1-like factors ***(68)***; also, the strain of mouse and the transgene itself both influence the type of immune response to a particular ADV vector, and thus affect the persistence of gene expression ***(69)***.

Cell-mediated immune responses have been reported in animal experiments and in human clinical subjects ***(69,70)***. These may sometimes be a result of the removal of E3 from first-generation vectors, because proteins expressed by this region appear to be involved in suppressing T-cell-mediated immunosurveillance ***(71)***. In later ADV vectors, only part of the E3 gene is removed. Recently, it has also been shown that repeated ADV-mediated gene transfer can be effectively achieved if recombinant interleukin-12 is administered at the same time as the virus ***(72)***, or by incorporating interleukin-12 into the viral vectors ***(59)***, and that this results from this cytokine diminishing the activation of type 2 helper T-cells. Immunosuppression using agents such as FK506 may also reduce some of these effects ***(52)***. As well as immune responses, ADV gene transfer can be toxic at high dosages, and may later cause cell death, because of host-encoded E1a-like activators, or expression of an E2a-encoded DNA-binding protein. Indeed, vectors bearing a temperature-sensitive mutation in E2a produce a substantially increased longevity of transgene expression in vivo ***(73)***.

ADVs can stably package up to 106% of the normal viral genome (an extra 2 kb), allowing 7–9 kb exogenous DNA to be incorporated in to these vectors ***(74)***. This is still less than the 14-kb full-length dystrophin cDNA, but can accommodate the 6.3-kb Becker-type minidystrophin cDNA previously described. In one of the earliest reports, single im injections of a high titer ADV vector, incorporating a Rous Sarcoma Virus (RSV)-driven minidystrophin gene, were administered to the biceps femoris muscle of neonatal mdx mice, resulting in dystrophin expression in 5–50% of fibers, which persisted for at least 3 mo ***(75)***. An extension of this study by Vincent et al., ***(76)*** illustrated that myofibers expressing recombinant minidystrophin were also protected from the degeneration usually associated with dystrophin deficiency in mdx muscle. A functional correction of MD in mdx mouse muscles has been demonstrated using the minidystrophin gene cloned into a second-generation E1/E3-deleted ADV vector ***(77)***. Isolated muscles were mechanically stressed, and those in regions negative for dystrophin were more damaged than those expressing the minidystrophin from the ADV vector ***(78)***.

Up to 4 kb of extra space can be created in the recombinant ADV genome by variously deleting E1, E3, and E4 ***(77,79)***. In order to compare the effects of genome size on gene transfer, a series of dystrophin minigenes with in-frame deletions of 3.0, 4.4, and 5.7 kb were transferred to dystrophic mdx muscle in vivo by ADV vectors ***(80)***. However, because the only sequences absolutely required for viral replication are the ITRs, it is theoretically possible to remove all but approx 500 bp of the viral genome, allowing insertion of up to 36 kb exogenous DNA. Viral replication and assembly would then only be possible in the presence of a helper virus or complementary helper cell, which provided all proteins *in trans*. Such helper-dependent pseudo-ADV systems have now been developed ***(66,81)***. A major limitation to this approach is the separation of the recombinant virus from the helper, but it may be possible to construct a helper virus that is unable to, or is inefficient at, packaging its own genome (perhaps through size constraints), rather like the helper systems developed for phagemid rescue.

Alternatively, helper viruses may be prevented from contaminating vector preparations by means of a fatal *Cre*-excision system ***(82)***. Initial results suggest that it may also be possible to separate recombinant ADV from the helper on cesium chloride gradients ***(81)***. First, this would mean that inserts of up to ~35 kb would be possible, allowing the inclusion of the full-length cDNA under the control of a muscle-specific promoter, with space to spare. Indeed, pseudo-ADV vectors have allowed delivery and expression of the entire 14-kb dystrophin cDNA to mdx muscle cells in culture ***(83)*** and in vivo ***(84)***, under the control of a muscle-specific promoter. Second, removal of the majority of the viral genome reduces the possibility of replication-competent ADV rescue by recombination with wild-type ADV, thus generating a safer therapeutic reagent. Finally, the problems associated with immunity, e.g., Cytotoxic T-Lymphocytes (CTL) responses to viral proteins produced in vivo, will be greatly diminished. As a result of these developments, ADV gene transfer of dystrophin genes has most recently progressed into preclinical studies in dystrophic dogs ***(10)***, and may even enter early clinical trials in the near future (*see* the MDA web page, http://www.mdausa.org/research/index.html).

2.1.3. Other Viral Vectors for Gene Transfer to Skeletal Muscle

Adenoassociated virus (AAV) vectors have also been reported to give very high efficiency gene transfer to skeletal muscle, over a long period of time ***(85)***, but have a small capacity for foreign DNA, and are difficult to generate in high purity and at high titers. Nevertheless, muscle is particularly susceptible to AAV infection ***(86)***, and, for reasons unknown, no humoral or cellular immune responses are generated ***(32)***. Some genes involved in the limb girdle MDs may be small enough for gene transfer by AAV. As yet, however, it is unclear how much of the dystrophin cDNA can be removed and still generate a functional protein. If such functional microdystrophin cDNAs can be created, AAV vectors may be valuable even for DMD GT. The only other viral vectors with potential for gene transfer to skeletal muscle are based on herpes simplex virus (HSV), because they will infect nondividing cells, and have a large capacity for foreign DNA. Although the full-length human dystrophin cDNA has recently been incorporated in an HSV vector, the control of lysis and latency is still not sufficiently understood to produce stable, safe vectors for GT ***(31,63)***.

2.2. Nonviral Gene Transfer to Skeletal Muscle

In comparison to viral vectors, nonviral, physical/chemical gene transfer methods are much more easily modified, easier to quality control, and generally simpler to prepare in purified formulations. Moreover, the size of DNA construct is virtually unrestricted, and the risk of immune responses is greatly reduced. Because these reagents are entirely synthetic, an almost infinite variety of chemical formulations is possible, and may be designed to have specific characteristics. Obviously, the most important requirements are the ability to form a complex with DNA, and to be able to carry DNA across cell membranes. This is normally satisfied by molecules with a cationic (positive) charge, and a vast array of formulations have now been used. All nonviral transfection methods, however, seem to be considerably more effective in cell culture than in vivo, which currently limits their prospects in clinical therapy.

2.2.1. Direct Injection of Naked DNA into Skeletal Muscle

The simplest nonviral gene transfer approach in skeletal muscle involves directly injecting gene expression constructs as purified plasmid DNA into muscle in vivo. The full-length human dystrophin cDNA was one of the first genes to be expressed in mouse muscle by this technique ***(87)***, but it could be expressed in less than 2% of myofibers. Since then, various improvements to efficiency have been reported, including endotoxin removal, to prevent dose-related toxicity ***(88)***, and the use of strong muscle-specific regulatory elements in the construct ***(89)***. Recently, the application of electric pulses across muscles has also been shown to improve uptake of DNA, presumably via an electroporation-type effect on the cell membranes and T-tubules ***(90)***. Although this approach is still likely to be more relevant to DNA-mediated vaccination and production of secretory proteins than to MDs, it may be highly effective in certain muscle groups, such as the diaphragm ***(91,92)***. It is also very useful experimentally to check the efficacy of a construct in vivo, without requiring the lengthy and laborious process of creating transgenic mice. For instance, direct injection of minidystrophin genes into the diaphragm of mdx4^{cv} (low revertant) mice showed increased sarcolemmal stability *(91)*, as assessed by procion orange staining of muscle preparations after experimental lengthening contractions. Those authors have also demonstrated that both minidystrophin and full-length recombinant dystrophin induces the recovery of neuronal nitric oxide synthase at the sarcolemma of mdx4^{cv} limb muscles injected with plasmid DNA *(92)*. This molecule interacts with a component of the dystrophin–glycoprotein complex, α_1-syntrophin, and this probably indicates recovery of biological function.

2.2.2. Lipid-Mediated Gene Transfer to Skeletal Muscle

The uptake and expression of naked plasmid DNA was discovered serendipitously as part of a control for lipid-mediated gene transfer to skeletal muscle *(93)*. Anionic lipids have been studied for many years as means of delivering drugs by encapsulation in lipid membranes. However, it has been found that cationic lipids, which form a complex with nucleic acids by electrostatic binding at the liposome surface (lipoplex), are more effective at gene transfer. Once recombinant DNA has been carried inside the cell by endocytosis, it must escape from the endosome and pass across the nuclear envelope, in order to be expressed within the nucleus.

Different liposome formulations vary in their transfection efficiency, generally because of differences in their behavior during this process. Schwartz et al. *(94)* have shown that an overall charge close to neutrality was most efficient in vivo; a more positively charged complex gives highest gene transfer efficiency in vitro. This probably results from a reduced interference with anionic serum proteins or components of the extracellular matrix, such as heparan sulphates. In many liposome formulations, the neutral lipid, DOPE, is used to achieve this lower charge differential. Increased DNA concentrations above 1 μg/mL tend to lead to coagulation of complexes, probably decreasing their probability of being taken up by the cell, as well as also potentially contributing to toxicity and tissue damage *(95)*. Polylysine condensation of plasmid DNA enhances liposome-mediated gene transfer efficiency to myoblasts up to 25-fold, even in the presence of serum, probably by protecting against nucleases and improving nuclear localization *(95)*. The authors' studies also suggest that smaller lipoplexes, such as those formed by DOSPER, improve transfection efficiency to skeletal muscle *(96)*. Liposome-mediated transfection of the large (14-kb) full-length dystrophin cDNA has been achieved in cultured muscle cells, and led to widespread gene expression *(97)*. Recently, it has also been reported that lipofection of a dystrophin cDNA lowered intracellular free calcium and calcium leak channel activity in mdx myotubes *(98)*, which also suggests that cDNAs do not need to be integrated into host chromosomes to show a significant physiological effect.

2.2.3. Modified Liposome Methods

Most nonviral gene transfer methods, such as cationic liposome–DNA complexes, have so far been restricted to gene transfer to skeletal muscle cells in vitro, but they may be improved by chemical modification for suitability in vivo. Liposomes incorporating fusogenic peptides of the hemagglutinating virus of Japan (HVJ, or Sendai virus) have been used to improve liposome-mediated gene transfer in vivo and showed uptake and expression of a full-length dystrophin cDNA, after direct injection into mdx quadriceps, in up to 26% of myofibers at the injection site ***(99)***, although only transient gene expression was reported.

Because integrins are frequent targets of entry by viruses, integrin-binding peptides have been developed containing a cyclic RGD sequence bound to 16 lysines. These molecules bind DNA and integrins with high affinity and with an overall neutral charge, and have been shown to improve transfection efficiency, especially in cells that are normally difficult to transfect, such as neurons and cardiomyocytes ***(100)***. These are small ligands, antigenically similar to their naturally occurring counterparts, so that they are also unlikely to induce immune responses in vivo. However, endosomal degradation occurs, unless lipofectin is incorporated in the complex ***(101)***. Relative to viral vectors, liposomes offer the advantage of being poor antigens, so they may be delivered repeatedly via the systemic circulation. Therefore, when liposomal reagents have been developed with improved in vivo gene transfer profiles, a large number of muscle groups could potentially be transfected. The transportation of charged macromolecules, such as DNA, into muscle is probably severely restricted by the basal lamina, and is further restricted in DMD patients by fibrosis, especially in later stages of the disease, indicating that the youngest patients may be the most suitable therapeutic candidates.

2.3. Alternative Gene Correction Strategies for MDs

2.3.1. Overexpression of Utrophin

Dystrophin-related protein, or utrophin, displays extensive homology to dystrophin, especially at the N- and C-termini ***(102)***. However, it is developmentally regulated, with maximal expression occurring at 17–18 wk gestation in humans, which then decreases as dystrophin expression increases ***(103)***. Although utrophin is expressed in adult tissue, in muscle it is concentrated at neuromuscular and myotendinous junctions, where it is associated with the dystrophin–glycoprotein complex, then with agrin at the extracellular surface ***(104,105)***. In regenerating muscle, as in the mdx mouse and DMD patients, utrophin is upregulated at the sarcolemma, and produces a peripheral staining pattern similar to that of dystrophin in normal muscle ***(106)***.

Hence, it may be possible to overexpress utrophin in the muscles of DMD patients, using pharmacological agents as activators of the utrophin promoter ***(107)***. However, no correlation has yet been found between the level of utrophin expressed and the severity of muscle pathology in mdx mice ***(108)***. Indeed, some dystrophin-deficient patients, expressing over 17× normal levels of utrophin, still have a severe Duchenne-type MD, although this could indicate that the timing of utrophin expression may be critical ***(102)***. Double-knockout (DKO) dystrophin/utrophin mice are severely affected by a progressive MD and cardiomyopathy ***(11,12)***. However, skeletal-muscle-specific expression of a utrophin cDNA rescues the pathology ***(109)***, lending support to the hypothesis that overexpression of endogenous utrophin in the skeletal muscle of DMD patients may reduce or prevent the development of MD. Because the discrepancy in the effects of utrophin expression between animals and humans has yet to be resolved, it still remains to be seen whether or not utrophin can functionally substitute for dystrophin in adult human muscle.

2.3.2. Oligonucleotide-Based Correction Strategies.

These encompass several novel alternatives to cDNA gene transfer for MDs, and are still at a relatively early stage of development. The first approach arose directly from the observation that spontaneous dystrophin-positive (revertant) muscle fibers in dystrophic muscle are at least partly the result of exon-skipping during the processing of dystrophin mRNA ***(110)***. It has been shown that addition of synthetic antisense oligoribonucleotides (short, modified RNA oligonucleotides) to mutant β-globin transcripts can correct aberrant splicing ***(111)***, so that a similar method may be used to increase the amount of dystrophin by exon-skipping in DMD. By blocking the binding of splicing factors to specific splice sites around the mdx dystrophin mutation, using antisense oligoribonucleotides, the authors were able to induce exon skipping and generate in-frame dystrophin, expressed at the sarcolemma of cultured mdx muscle cells ***(112)***. The efficiency of this process is currently very low, but may potentially be greatly improved by conjugation with "Trojan" peptides ***(113)***, tissue-targeting peptides, such as antibodies, and better oligonucleotide chemistries. A related strategy involves the use of double-stranded DNA/RNA hybrid oligonucleotides designed to target a specific point mutation in genomic DNA. These are then believed to then correct point mutations via a homologous recombination-type mechanism ***(114)***. Most dystrophin mutations are deletions, but up to one-third may be point mutations affecting splicing, amino acid, or reading frame, and may potentially be corrected in this way.

3. Future Prospects

3.1. What Are the Priorities for Gene Transfer to Dystrophic Skeletal Muscle?

The authors have attempted to show that experimental studies on gene transfer to skeletal muscle have progressed enormously over the past decade. Nevertheless, the efficiency of gene transfer remains considerably below levels likely to achieve therapeutic benefit. How can a greater number of muscle fibers be encouraged to take up and express recombinant DNA? And which muscle groups should be the first to receive GT? The authors believe that the answers to both of these questions lie in improving the tissue-specificity of recombinant gene expression and in the development of vectors capable of homing-in on skeletal muscle cells.

3.1.1. Tissue-Specific Gene Expression in Skeletal Muscle

As discussed in **Subheading 1.2.**, when developing vectors for GT, it is necessary to ensure that the gene under study is expressed at levels high enough, and for long enough, to have a favorable therapeutic effect. It is likely that tissue-specific transcription will ensure that fewer undesirable hazards will be encountered, such as unintentional germline gene transfer or activation of oncogenes, and express the gene of interest at sufficient levels, because of the abundance of endogenous muscle-specific transcription factors. The transgenic mice described above expressed recombinant dystrophin molecules from cDNAs driven by the human α-skeletal actin ***(115)*** and the mouse MCK promoters ***(5,23)***. Expression of the transgenes was limited to skeletal muscle, although some low-level expression was detected in cardiac tissue.

The use of tissue-specific promoters is preferable from the point of view of safety, but these regulatory elements can be relatively large (2–6 kb), and therefore difficult to incorporate in virus-based transfer vectors. Nevertheless, the larger-capacity ADV vectors have ample space in their genome, and combinations of smaller enhancer elements may also lead to substantial tissue-specificity ***(45)***.

Transcriptional control systems are also in development, whereby inducible elements can allow genes to be switched on and off by means of a drug (e.g., *see* ref. ***116***). It may be expected that correct regulation of dystrophin expression would be obtained if the natural muscle-specific promoter region of the gene was used to drive recombinant cDNAs. However, there are several dystrophin promoters, as well as intronic transcriptional regulators, and data obtained to date suggests that small recombinant versions of the native promoter are poor at driving recombinant gene expression in cultured muscle, and in vivo *(117,45)*. Correction of the muscle pathology in DMD may not require precise regulation of dystrophin gene, since both overexpression of the recombinant protein in transgenic mdx muscle and relatively low levels of dystrophin expression (20–30% of endogenous protein at the muscle membrane) can afford substantial protection against muscle fiber necrosis, even when utilizing BMD-based cDNAs *(22,5)*.

3.1.2. Vectors for Targeting Specific Skeletal Muscle In Vivo

One major problem presented, in the case of DMD, is how to target a number of different muscle groups (and possibly the central nervous system) without resorting to local administration of the transgene, requiring multiple im injections in potentially inaccessible sites, e.g., the diaphragm *(118)*. Muscle is highly vascularized and stable, so it is not unreasonable to expect that a systemic delivery system could be utilized for convenient transfer of therapeutic reagents.

Animal experiments have shown that recombinant ADVs introduced intraperitoneally or intravenously are usually deposited in the liver *(119)*. However, Stratford-Perricaudet et al. *(77)* demonstrated reporter gene transfer to skeletal and cardiac muscle by a recombinant ADV delivered through the vascular system in newborn mice, although the efficiency of gene transfer was relatively low. The most comprehensive work, to date, demonstrating that the route of administration is a major determinant of the transduction efficiency of various tissues by recombinant ADVs, was a study in young rats published by Huard et al. *(120)*. Although they showed efficient gene transfer to the heart, diaphragm, and intercostal muscles after intra-arterial administration of the virus, the only delivery technique that resulted in significant transduction of skeletal muscle fibers was im injection. Thus, it seems that more elaborate systems will be needed to deliver recombinant dystrophin genes to muscle, especially the muscles involved in maintaining respiratory and cardiac function. The ability to modify viral tropism, by incorporating ligand-binding moieties on viral envelopes, will undoubtedly prove highly important in gene transfer to skeletal muscle. Moreover, the incorporation of tissue-targeting peptides in nonviral gene transfer formulations and oligonucleotide conjugates could substantially improve the validity of these techniques in a clinical setting, and should be actively pursued *(43)*.

3.1.3. Safety Issues

A requirement of the regulatory agencies is that any reagent, viral or otherwise, destined for use in a clinical environment, must be manufactured to high safety standards *(121)*. In the case of recombinant viruses, it is essential to demonstrate that the viral stock is not contaminated by replication competent

Table 2
DMD as a Target Disorder for Genetic Transfer

Potentials	Problems
Recessive lethal	Muscle is big target
High spontaneous mutation rate	Very large complex gene
Skeletal muscle is stable	Fibrosis may limit gene delivery
Muscle is highly regenerative	Hard to target cardiac muscle
Muscle is highly vascularized	Immune evasion necessary
Cloned genes available	Very efficient delivery required
Good animal models exist	Nervous system involvement

virus. Sensitive detection methods and improved vector designs have combined to minimize this risk, but quality control of such reagents, as with vaccines, must be meticulous. At present, and before GT for DMD or other MDs can fully progress to human clinical trials, it will be necessary to test present procedures in animal models larger than the mdx mouse, such as the xmd dog ***(10)***. Dosage (and related toxicity effects), route of administration, persistence of transgene expression, and efficacy of treatment, are all matters that must be addressed in these animals, to maximize the benefit of phase 1 trials, and in order to avoid jeopardizing clinical trials in the future.

3.2. Will GT ever Work for MDs?

Although considerable progress has been made in addressing requirements for GT in skeletal muscle, a clinically useful genetic medicine is still some distance away (**Table 2**). Nevertheless, as soon as increases in gene transfer efficiency are achieved, limited-priority muscle groups, such as respiratory and postural muscles, could lead to improvements to quality of life in early clinical trials. However, because cardiomyopathies and cognitive defects affect many patients, gene transfer to cardiac myocytes and neural tissue remain significant challenges for GT of DMD. Meanwhile, the gene transfer methods developed for DMD will continue to provide extensive data into the mechanisms of gene expression and pathology in muscle tissues. Neurological features of DMD and some other MDs may require earlier intervention, such as *in utero* gene transfer. Clearly, a greater understanding of basic biological processes will improve the prospects for an effective GT. Steroid treatments are still used in limited circumstances and for restricted periods in the MDs, and a number of these are currently being evaluated in a carefully performed clinical trial. Cardiac features are also amenable to treatment by ACE inhibitors, and surgery, with subsequent mechanical support, are still vital options in the maintenance of ambulation and quality of patients' lives. These more conventional supports, combined with GT, may gradually develop an effective paradigm for therapeutics of the MDs.

References

1. Koenig, M., Hoffman, E. P., Bertelson, C. J., Monaco, A. P., Feener, C., and Kunkel, L. M. (1987) Complete cloning of the Duchenne muscular dystrophy (DMD) cDNA and preliminary genomic organisation of the DMD gene in normal and affected individuals. *Cell* **50,** 509–517.
2. Ozawa, E., Noguchi, S., Mizuno, Y., Hagiwara, Y., and Yoshida, M. (1998) From dystrophinopathy to sarcoglycanopathy: evolution of a concept of muscular dystrophy. *Muscle Nerve* **21,** 421–438.
3. Verma, I. M. and Naviaux, R. K. (1991) Human gene therapy. *Curr. Opin. Genet. Dev.* **1,** 54–59.
4. Kaplan, J.-C. and Fontaine, B. (1999) Neuromuscular disorders: gene location. *Neuromusc. Disord.* **9,** I-XIV.
5. Wells, D. J., Wells, K. E., Asante, E. A., Turner, G., Sunada, Y., Campbell, K. P., Walsh, F. S., and Dickson, G. (1995) Expression of human full-length and minidystrophin in transgenic mdx mice: implications for gene therapy of Duchenne Muscular Dystrophy. *Hum. Mol. Genet.* **4,** 1245–1250.
6. Fassati, A., Wells, D. J., Sgro-Serpente, P. A., Walsh, F. S., Brown, S. C., Strong, P. N., and Dickson, G. (1997) Genetic correction of dystrophin deficiency and skeletal muscle remodelling in adult mdx mouse via transplantation of retroviral producer cells. *J. Clin. Invest.* **100,** 620–628.
7. Bulfield, G., Siller, W. G., Wight, P. A. L., and Moore, K. J. (1984) X chromosome-linked muscular dystrophy (mdx) in the mouse. *Proc. Natl. Acad. Sci. USA* **81,** 1189–1192.
8. Kornegay, J. N., Tuler, S., Miller, D. M., and Levesque, D. C. (1988) Muscular dystrophy in a litter of golden retriever dogs. *Muscle Nerve* **11,** 1056–1064.
9. Cooper, B. J., Winand, N. J., Stedman, H., et al. (1988) The homologue of the Duchenne locus is defective in X-linked muscular dystrophy of dogs. *Nature* **334,** 154–156.
10. Howell, J. M., Lochmuller, H., O'Hara, A., Fletcher, S., Kakulas, B. A., Massie, B., Nalbatoglu, J., and Karpati, G. (1998) High level dystrophin expression after adenoviral-mediated dystrophin minigene transfer to skeletal muscle of dystrophic dogs: prolongation of expression with immunosuppression. *Hum.Gene Ther.* **9,** 629–634.
11. Deconinck, A. E., Rafael, J. A., Skinner, J. A., Brown, S. C., Potter, A. C., Metzinger, L., et al. (1997) Utrophin-dystrophin-deficient mice as a model for Duchenne muscular dystrophy. *Cell* **90,** 717–727.
12. Grady, R. M., Teng, H., Nichol, M. C., Cunningham, J. C., Wilkinson, R. S., and Sanes, J. R. (1997) Skeletal and cardiac myopathies in mice lacking utrophin and dystrophin: a model for Duchenne muscular dystrophy. *Cell* **90,** 729–738.
13. Grounds, M. D. and Yablonka-Reuveni, Z. (1994) Molecular and cell biology of skeletal muscle regeneration, in *Molecular and Cell Biology of Muscular Dystrophy* (Partridge, T., ed.), Chapman and Hall, London, pp. 210–238.

14. Wolff, J. A., Dowty, M. E., Jiao, S., Repetto, G., Berg, R. K., Ludtke, J. J., and Williams, P. (1992) Expression of naked plasmids by cultured myotubes and entry of plasmids into T tubules and caveolae of mammalian skeletal muscle. *J. Cell Sci.* **103,** 1249–1259.
15. Morgan, J. E. (1994) Cell and gene therapy in Duchenne muscular dystrophy. *Hum. Gene Ther.* **5,** 165–173.
16. DenDunnen, J. T., Grootscholten, P. M., Dauwerse, J. G., Walker, A. P., Monaco, A. P., Butler, R., et al. (1992) Reconstruction of the 2.4 Mb human DMD-gene by homologous YAC recombination. *Hum. Mol. Genet.* **1,** 19–28.
17. Gnirke, A. and Huxley, C. (1991) Transfer of the human HPRT and GART genes from yeast to mammalian cells by microinjection of YAC DNA. *Somat. Cell Mol. Genet.* **17,** 573–580.
18. Strauss, W. M. and Jaenisch, R. (1992) Molecular complementation of a collagen mutation in mammalian cells using yeast artificial chromosomes. *EMBO J.* **11,** 417–421.
19. Lee, C., Pearlman, J., Chamberlain, J., and Caskey, C. (1991) Expression of recombinant dystrophin and its localization to the cell membrane. *Nature* **349,** 334–336.
20. Dickson, G., Love, D. R., Davies, K. E., Wells, K. E., Piper, T. A., and Walsh, F. S. (1991) Human dystrophin gene transfer: production and expression of a functional recombinant DNA-based gene. *Hum. Genet.* 88, 53–58.
21. England, S. B., Nicholson, L. V. B., Johnson, M. A., Forrest, S. M., Love, D. R., Zubrzycka-Gaarn, E. E., et al. (1990) Very mild muscular dystrophy associated with deletion of 46% of dystrophin. *Nature* **343,** 180–182.
22. Cox, G. A., Cole, N. M., Matsumura, K., Phelps, S. F., Hauschka, S. D., Campbell, K. P., Faulkner, J. A., and Chamberlain, J. S. (1993) Overexpression of dystrophin in transgenic mdx mice eliminates dystrophic symptoms without toxicity. *Nature* **364,** 725–729.
23. Phelps, S. E., Hauser, M. A., Cole, N. M., Rafael, J. A., Hinkle, R. T., Faulkner, J. A., and Chamberlain, J. S. (1995) Expression of full-length and truncated dystrophin mini-genes in transgenic mdx mice. *Hum. Mol. Genet.* **4,** 1251–1258.
24. Sewry, C. A., Sansome, A., Clerk, A., Sherratt, T. G., Hasson, N., Rodillo, E., et al. (1993) Manifesting carriers of Xp21 muscular dystrophy; lack of correlation between dystrophin expression and clinical weakness. *Neuromusc. Disord.* **3,** 141–148.
25. Bushby, K. M. D., Goodship, J. A., Nicholson, L. V. B., Johnson, M. A., Haggerty, I. D., and Gardner-Medwin, D. (1993) Variability in clinical, genetic and protein abnormalities in manifesting carriers of Duchenne and Becker muscular dystrophy. *Neuromusc. Disord.* **3,** 57–64.
26. Bonilla, E., Schmidt, B., Samitt, C. E., Miranda, A. F., Hays, A. P., DeOliveira, A. B. S., et al. (1988) Normal and dystrophin-deficient muscle fibers in carriers of the gene for Duchenne muscular dystrophy. *Am. J. Pathol.* **133,** 440–445.
27. Pavlath, G. K., Rich, K., Webster, S. G., and Blau, H. M. (1989) Localisation of muscle gene products in nuclear domains. *Nature* **337,** 570–573.
28. Noursadeghi, M., Walsh, F. S., Heiman-Patterson, T., and Dickson, G. (1993) Trans-activation of the murine dystrophin gene in human-mouse hybrid myotubes. *FEBS Lett.* **320,** 155–159.

29. Ahn, A. H. and Kunkel, L. M. (1993) The structural and functional diversity of dystrophin. *Nature Genet.* **3,** 283–291.
30. Kaufman, H., Schlom, J., and Kantor, J. (1991) A recombinant vaccinia virus expressing human carcinoembryonic antigen (CEA). *Int. J. Cancer* **48,** 900–907.
31. Huard, J., Goins, W. F., and Glorioso, J. C. (1995) Herpes simplex virus type 1 vector mediated gene transfer to muscle. *Gene Ther.* **2,** 385–392.
32. Xiao, X., Li, J., and Samulski, R. J. (1996) Efficient long-term gene transfer into muscle of immunocompetent mice by adeno-associated virus vector. *J. Virol.* **70,** 8098–8108.
33. Feero, W. G., Rosenblatt, J. D., Huard, J., Watkins, S. C., Epperly, M., Clemens, P. R., et al. (1997) Viral gene delivery to skeletal muscle: insights on maturation-dependent loss of fiber infectivity for adenovirus and herpes simplex type 1 viral vectors. *Hum. Gene Ther.* **8,** 371–380.
34. Fassati, A., Dunckley, M. G., and Dickson, G. (1995) Retroviral vectors, in *Molecular and Cell Biology of Human Gene Therapeutics* (Dickson, G., ed.), Chapman and Hall, London, pp. 1–19.
35. Miller, A. D. and Buttimore, C. (1986) Redesign of retrovirus packaging cell lines to avoid recombination leading to helper virus production. *Mol. Cell. Biol.* **6,** 2895–2902.
36. Hajihosseini, M., Iavechev, L., and Price, J. (1993) Evidence that retroviruses integrate into post-replication host DNA. *EMBO J.* **13,** 4969–4974.
37. Dunckley, M. G., Love, D. R., Davies, K. E., Walsh, F. S., Morris, G. E., and Dickson, G. (1992) Retroviral-mediated transfer of a dystrophin minigene into mdx mouse myoblasts *in vitro. FEBS Lett.* **296,** 128–134.
38. Salminen, A., Elson, H. F., Mickley, L. A., Fojo, A. T., and Gottesman, M. M. (1991) Implantation of recombinant rat myocytes into adult skeletal muscle: a potential gene therapy. *Hum. Gene Ther.* **2,** 15–26.
39. Dunckley, M. G., Wells, D. J., Walsh, F. S., and Dickson, G. (1993) Direct retroviral-mediated transfeur of a dystrophin minigene into mdx mouse muscle *in vivo. Hum. Mol. Genet.* **2,** 717–723.
40. Fassati, A., Wells, D. J., Walsh, F. S., and Dickson, G. (1996) Transplantation of retroviral producer cells for *in vivo* gene transfer into mouse skeletal muscle. *Hum. Gene Ther.* **7,** 595–602.
41. Parrish E. P., Cifuentes-Diaz C., Li Z. L., Vicart P., Paulin D., Dreyfus P. A., et al. (1996) Targeting widespread sites of damage in dystrophic muscle: engrafted macrophages as potential shuttles. *Gene Ther.* **3,** 13–20.
42. Kavanaugh, M. P., Miller, D. G., Zhang, W., Law, W., Kozak, S. L., Kabat, D., and Miller, A. D. (1994) Cell-surface receptors for gibbon ape leukemia virus and amphotropic murine retrovirus are inducible sodium-dependent phosphate symporters. *Proc. Natl. Acad. Sci. USA* **91,** 7071–7075.
43. Harris, J. D. and Lemoine, N. (1996) Strategies for targeted gene therapy. *TIG* **12,** 400–405.
44. Russell, S. J., Hawkins, R. E., and Winter, G. (1993) Retroviral vectors displaying functional antibody fragments. *Nucleic Acids Res.* **21,** 1081–1085.
45. Fassati, A., Bardoni, A., Sironi, M., Wells, D. J., Bresolin, N., Scarlatto, G., et al. (1998) Insertion of two independent enhancers in the long terminal repeat of a

self-inactivating vector results in high-titer retroviral vectors with tissue-specific expression. *Hum. Gene Ther.* **9,** 2459–2468.
46. Ferrari, G., Salvatori, G., Rossi, C., Cossu, G., and Mavilio, F. (1995) A retroviral vector containing a muscle-specific enhancer drives gene expression only in differentiated muscle fibers. *Hum. Gene Ther.* **6,** 733–742.
47. Fassati, A., Takahara, Y., Walsh, F. S., and Dickson, G. (1994) Production of high titre helper-free recombinant retroviral vectors by lipofection. *Nucleic Acids Res.* **22,** 1117–1118.
48. Burns, J. C., Friedmann, T., Driever, W., Burrascano, M., and Yee J.-K. (1993) Vesicular stomatitis virus G glycoprotein pseudotyped retroviral vectors: concentration to very high titer and efficient gene transfer into mammalian and nonmammalian cells. *Proc. Natl. Acad. Sci. USA* **90,** 8033–8037.
49. Yee, J. K., Miyanohara, A., LaPorte, P., Bouic, K., Burns, J. C., and Friedmann, T. (1994) A general method for generation of high titer, pantropic retroviral vectors: highly efficient infection of primary hepatocytes. *Proc. Natl. Acad. Sci. USA* **91,** 9564–9568.
50. Takeuchi, Y., Cosset, F. L. C., Lachmann, P. J., Okada, H., Weiss, R. A., and Collins, M. K. L. (1994) Type C retrovirus inactivation by human complement is determined by both the viral genome and the producer cell. *J. Virol.* **68,** 8001–8007.
51. Rother, R. P., Squinto, S. P., Mason, J. M., and Rollins, S. A. (1995) Protection of retroviral vector particles in human blood through complement inhibition. *Hum. Gene Ther.* **6,** 429–435.
52. Lochmuller, H., Petrof, B., Pari, G., Larochelle, N., Dodelet, V., Wang, Q., et al. (1996) Transient immunosuppression by FK506 permits a sustained high-level dystrophin expression after adenovirus-mediated dystrophin minigene transfer to skeletal muscles of adult dystrophic (mdx) mice. *Gene Ther.* **3,** 706–716.
53. Miyake, K., Suzuki, N., Matsuoka, H., Tohyama, T., and Shimada, T. (1998) Stable integration of human HIV-based retroviral vectors into the chromosomes of nondividing cells. *Hum. Gene Ther.* **9,** 465–475.
54. Poeschla, E. M., Wong-Staal, F., and Looney, D. J. (1998) Efficient transduction of nondividing human cells by feline immunodeficiency virus lentiviral vectors. *Nature Med.* **4,** 354–357.
55. Graham, F. L., Smiley, J., Russel, W. C., and Nairn, R. (1977) Characteristics of a human cell line transformed by DNA from human adenovirus 5. *J. Gen. Virol.* **36,** 59–72.
56. Amalfitano, A., Begy, C. R., and Chamberlain, J. S. (1996) Improved adenovirus packaging cell lines to support the growth of replication-defective gene delivery vectors. *Proc. Natl. Acad. Sci. USA* **93,** 3352–3356.
57. McGrory, W. J., Bautista, D. S., and Graham, F. L. (1988) A simple technique for the rescue of early region I mutations into infectious human adenovirus type 5. *Virology* **163,** 614–617.
58. Horwitz, M. S. (1990) Adenoviridae and their replication, in *Virology,* 2nd ed. (Fields, B. N., Knipe, D. M., et al., eds.), Raven Press, New York. pp. 1679–1741.
59. Lee, M. G., Kremer, E. J., and Perricaudet, M. (1995) Adenoviral vectors, in *Molecular & Cell Biology of Human Gene Therapeutics.* (Dickson, G., ed.), Chapman & Hall, London, pp. 20–32.

60. Pauly, D. F., Johns, D. C., Matelis, L. A., Lawrence, J. H., Byrne, B. J., and Kessler, P. D. (1998) Complete correction of acid α-glucosidase deficiency in Pompe disease fibroblasts in vitro, and lysosomally targeted expression in neonatal rat cardiac and skeletal muscle. *Gene Ther.* **5,** 473–480.
61. Michael, S. I., Hong, J. S., Curiel, D. T., and Engler, J. A. (1995) Addition of a short peptide ligand to the adenovirus fiber protein. *Gene Ther.* **2,** 660–668.
62. Larochelle, N., Lochmuller, H., Zhao, J., Jani, A., Hallauer, P., Hastings, K. E. M., et al. (1997). Efficient muscle-specific transgene expression after adenovirus-mediated gene transfer in mice using a 1.35kb muscle creatine kinase promoter/enhancer. *Gene Ther.* **4,** 465–472.
63. Floyd, SS., Clemens, P. R., Ontell, M. R., Kochanek, S., Day, C. S., Young, J., et al. (1998) Ex-vivo gene transfer using adenoviral-mediated full-length dystrophin delivery to dystrophic muscle. *Gene Ther.* **5,** 19–30.
64. Acsadi, G., Jani, A., Massie, B., Simoneau, M., Holland, P., Blaschuk, K., and Karpati, G. (1994) Differential efficiency of adenovirus-mediated *in vivo* gene transfer into skeletal muscle cells of different maturity. *Hum. Mol. Genet.* **3,** 579–584.
65. Acsadi, G., Massie, B., and Jani, A. (1995) Adenovirus-mediated gene transfer into striated muscles. *J. Mol. Med.* **73,** 165–180.
66. Turner, G., Couture, L. A., Smith, A. E., Piper, T., Wells, D. J., and Dickson, G. (1994) Adenoviral vectors for gene transfer of full length human dystrophin cDNAs. *J. Cell. Biochem.* **18D(Suppl.),** W432.
67. Turner, G., Dunckley, M. G. and Dickson, G. (1997) Gene therapy of Duchenne muscular dystrophy, in *Dystrophin: Gene, Protein and Cell Biology* (Brown, S. C. and Lucy, J. A., eds.), Cambridge University Press, Cambridge, UK, pp. 274–309.
68. Yang, Y., Nunes, F. A., Berencsi, K., et al. (1994). Cellular immunity to viral antigens limits E1-deleted adenoviruses for gene therapy. *Proc. Natl. Acad. Sci. USA* **91,** 4407–4411.
69. Michou, A. I., Santoro, L., Christ, M., Julliard, V., Pavirani, A., and Mehtali, M. (1997) Adenovirus-mediated gene transfer: influence of transgene, mouse strain and type of immune response on persistence of transgene expression. *Gene Ther.* **4,** 473–482.
70. Simon, R. H., Engelhardt, J. F., Yang, Y., Zepeda, M., Weber-Pendleton, S., Grossman, M., and Wilson, J. M. (1993) Adenovirus-mediated transfer of the CFTR gene to lung of non-human primates: toxicity study. *Hum. Gene Ther.* **4,** 771–780.
71. Yang, Y., Trinchieri, G., and Wilson, J. M. (1995) Recombinant IL-12 prevents formation of blocking IgA antibodies to recombinant adenovirus and allows repeated gene therapy to mouse lung. *Nature Med.* **1,** 890–893.
72. Gooding, L. R., Elmore, L. W., Tollefson, A. E., Brady, H. A., and Wold, W. S. M. (1988) A 14 700 MW protein from the E3 region of adenovirus inhibits cytolysis by tumour necrosis factor. *Cell* **53,** 341–346.
73. Engelhardt, J. F., Litzky, L., and Wilson, J. M. (1994) Prolonged transgene expression in Cotton rat lung with recombinant adenovirus defective in E2A. *Hum. Gene Ther.* **5,** 1217–1229.

74. Bett, A. J., Prevec, L., and Graham, F. L. (1993) Packaging capacity and stability of adenovirus type 5 vectors. *J. Virol.* **67,** 5911–5921.
75. Ragot, T., Vincent, N., Chafey, P., Vigne, E., Gilgenkrantz, H., Couton, D., et al. (1993) Efficient adenovirus-mediated transfer of a human minidystrophin gene to skeletal muscle of mdx mice. *Nature* **361,** 647–650.
76. Vincent, N., Ragot, T., Gilgenkrantz, H., Couton, D., Chafey, P., Gregoire, A., Briand, P., Kaplan, J-C., Kahn, A., and Perricaudet, M. (1993) Long-term correction of mouse dystrophic degeneration by adenovirus-mediated transfer of a minidystrophin gene. *Nature Genet.* **5,** 130–134.
77. Stratford-Perricaudet, L. D., Makeh, I., Perricaudet, M., and Briand, P. (1992) Widespread long-term gene transfer to mouse skeletal muscles and heart. *J. Clin. Invest.* **90,** 626–630.
78. Deconinck, N., Ragot, T., Marechal, G., Perricaudet, M., and Gillis, J. M. (1996) Functional protection of dystrophic mouse (mdx) muscles after adenovirus-mediated transfer of a dystrophin minigene. *Proc. Natl. Acad. Sci. USA* **93,** 3570–3574.
79. Zabner, J., Couture, L. A., Gregory, R. J., Graham, S. M., Smith, A. E., and Welsh, M. J. (1993) Adenovirus-mediated gene transfer transiently corrects the chloride transport defect in nasal epithelia of patients with cystic fibrosis. *Cell* **75,** 207–216.
80. Clemens, P. R., Krause, T. L., Chan, S., Korb, K. E., Graham, F. L., and Caskey, C. T. (1995) Recombinant truncated dystrophin minigenes: construction, expression and adenoviral delivery. *Hum. Gene Ther.* **6,** 1477–1485.
81. Mitani, K., Graham, F. L., Caskey, C. T., and Kochanek, S. (1995) Rescue, propagation, and partial purification of a helper virus-dependent adenovirus vector. *Proc. Natl. Acad. Sci. USA* **92,** 3854–3858.
82. Parks, R. J., Chen, L., Auton, M., Sankar, U., Rudnicki, M., and Graham, F. L. (1996) Helper-dependent adenovirus vector system: removal of helper virus by cre-mediated excision of the viral packaging signal. *Proc. Natl. Acad. Sci. USA* **93,** 13,565–13,570.
83. Kumar-Singh, R. and Chamberlain, J. S. (1996) Encapsidated adenovirus minichromosomes allow delivery and expression of a 14kb dystrophin cDNA to muscle cells. *Hum. Mol. Genet.* **5,** 913–921.
84. Clemens, P. R., Kochanek, S., Sunada, Y., Chan, S., Chen, H. H., Campbell, K. P., and Caskey, C. T. (1996) *In vivo* muscle gene transfer of full-length dystrophin with an adenoviral vector that lacks all viral genes. *Gene Ther.* **3,** 965–972.
85. Monahan, P. E., Samulski, R. J., Tazelaar, J., Xiao, X., Nichols, T. C., Bellinger, D. A., Read, M. S., and Walsh, C. E. (1998) Direct intramuscular injection with recombinant AAV vectors results in sustained expression in a dog model of haemophilia. *Gene Ther.* **5,** 40–49.
86. Fisher, K. J., Jooss, K., Alston, J., Yang, Y., Haecker, S. E., High, K., et al. (1997) Recombinant adeno-associated virus for muscle-directed gene therapy. *Nature Med.* **3,** 306–312.

87. Acsadi, G., Dickson, G., Love, D. R., Jani, A., Walsh, F. S., Gurusinghe, A., Wolff, J. A., and Davies, K. E. (1991) Human dystrophin expression in mdx mice after intramuscular injection of DNA constructs. *Nature* **352,** 815–818.
88. Wicks, I. P., Howell, M. L., Hancock, T., Kohsaka, H., Olee, T., and Carson, D. (1995) Bacterial lipopolysaccharide copurifies with plasmid DNA: implications for animal models and human gene therapy. *Hum. Gene Ther.* **6,** 317–323.
89. Skarli, M., Kiri, A., Vrbova, G., Lee, C. A., and Goldspink, G. (1998) Myosin regulatory elements as vectors for gene transfer by intramuscular injection. *Gene Ther.* **5,** 514–520.
90. Mir, L. M., Bureau, M. F., Rangara, R., Schwartz, B., and Scherman, D. (1998) Longterm high level in vivo gene expression after electric-pulse-mediated gene transfer into skeletal muscle. *C. R. Acad. Sci. III* **321,** 893–899.
91. Decrouy, A., Renaud, J. M., Davis, H. L., Lunde, J. A., Dickson, G., and Jasmin, B. J. (1997) Mini-dystrophin gene transfer in mdx4^{cv} diaphragm muscle fibers increases sarcolemmal stability. *Gene Ther.* **4,** 401–408.
92. Decrouy, A., Renaud, J. M., Lunde, J. A., Dickson, G., and Jasmin, B. J. (1998) Mini- and full-length dystrophin gene transfer induces the recovery of nitric oxide synthase at the sarcolemma of mdx4^{cv} skeletal muscle fibers. *Gene Ther.* **5,** 59–64.
93. Wolff, J. A., et al. (1990) Direct gene transfer to mouse muscle *in vivo*. *Science* **247,** 1465–1468.
94. Schwartz, B., Benoist, C., Abdallah, B., Scherman, D., Behr, J-P., and Demeneix, B. A. (1995) Lipospermine-based gene transfer into newborn mouse brain is optimised by a low lipospermine/DNA charge ratio. *Hum. Gene Ther.* **6,** 1515–1524.
95. Vitiello, L., Chonn, A., Wasserman, J. D., Duff, C., and Worton, R. G. (1996) Condensation of plasmid DNA with polylysine improves liposome-mediated gene transfer into established primary muscle cells. *Gene Ther.* **3,** 396–404.
96. Dodds, E., Dunckley, M. G., Naujoks, K., Michaelis, U., and Dickson, G. (1998) Lipofection of cultured mouse muscle cells: a direct comparison of Lipofectamine and DOSPER. *Gene Ther.* **5,** 542–551.
97. Trivedi, R. A. and Dickson, G. (1995) Liposome-mediated gene transfer into normal and dystrophin-deficient mouse myoblasts. *J. Neurochem.* **64,** 2230–2238.
98. McCarter, G. C., Denetclaw, W. F., Reddy, P., and Steinhardt, R. A. (1997) Lipofection of a cDNA plasmid containing the dystrophin gene lowers intracellular free calcium and calcium leak channel activity in mdx myotubes. *Gene Ther.* **4,** 483–487.
99. Yanagihara, I., Inui, K., Dickson, G., Turner, G., Piper, T., Kaneda, Y., and Okada, S. (1996) Expression of full-length human dystrophin cDNA in mdx mouse muscle by HVJ-liposome injection. *Gene Ther.* **3,** 549–553.
100. Hart, S. L., Harbottle, R. P., Cooper, R., Miller, A., Williamson, R., and Coutelle, C. (1995) Gene delivery and expression mediated by an integrin-binding peptide. *Gene Ther.* **2,** 552–554.
101. Hart, S. L., Arancibia-Carcamo, C. V., Wolfert, M. A., Mailhos, C., O'Reilly, N. J., Ali, R. R., et al. (1998) Lipid-mediated enhancement of transfection by a nonviral integrin-targeting vector. *Hum. Gene Ther.* **9,** 575–585.

102. Blake, D. J., Tinsley, J. M., and Davies, K. E. (1993) The emerging family of dystrophin-related proteins. *Trends Cell Biol.* 4, 19–23.
103. Clerk, A., Morris, G. E., Dubowitz, V., et al. (1993) Dystrophin-related protein, utrophin, in normal and dystrophic human foetal skeletal muscle. *Histochem. J.* **25,** 554–561.
104. Campanelli, J. T., Roberds, S. L., Campbell, K. P., and Scheller, R. H. (1994) A role for dystrophin-associated glycoproteins and utrophin in agrin-induced AChR clustering. *Cell* **77,** 663–674.
105. Gee, S. H., Montanaro, F., Lindenbaum, M. H., and Carbonetto, S. (1994) Dystroglycan-α, a dystrophin-associated glycoprotein, is a functional agrin receptor. *Cell* **77,** 675–686.
106. Karpati, G., Carpenter, S., Morris, G. E., Davies, K. E., Guerin, C., and Holland, P. (1993) Localization and quantitation of the chromosome 6-encoded dystrophin-related protein in normal and pathological human muscle. *J. Neuropathol. Exp. Neurol.* **52,** 119–128.
107. Tinsley, J. M. and Davies, K. E. (1993) Utrophin: a potential replacement for dystrophin? *Neuromusc. Disord.* **3,** 537–539.
108. Pons, F., Robert, A., Marini, J. F., and Leger, J. J. (1994) Does utrophin expression in muscles of mdx mice during postnatal development functionally compensate for dystrophin deficiency? *J. Neurol. Sci.* **122,** 162–170.
109. Gilbert, R., Nalbanoglu, J., Tinsley, J. M., Massie, B., Davies, K. E., and Karpati, G. (1998) Efficient utrophin expression following adenovirus gene transfer in dystrophic muscle. *Biophys. Biochem. Res. Com.* **242,** 244–247.
110. Wilton, S. D., Dye, D. E., and Laing, N. G. (1997) Dystrophin gene transcripts skipping the mdx mutation. *Muscle Nerve* **20,** 728–734.
111. Dominski, Z. and Kole, R. (1993) Restoration of correct splicing in thalassemic pre-mRNA by antisense oligonucleotides. *Proc. Natl. Acad. Sci. USA* **90,** 8673–8677.
112. Dunckley, M. G., Eperon, I. C., Manoharan, M., Villiet, P., and Dickson, G. (1998) Modification of splicing in the dystrophin gene in cultured mdx muscle cells by antisense oligoribonucleotides. *Hum. Mol. Genet.* **7,** 1083–1090.
113. Derossi, D., Chassaing, G., and Prochiantz, A. (1998) Trojan peptides: the penetratin system for intracellular delivery. *Trends Cell Biol* **8,** 84–87.
114. Ye, S., Cole-Strauss, A. C., Frank, B., and Kmiec, E. B. (1998) Targeted gene correction: a new strategy for molecular medicine. *Mol. Med. Today* **4,** 431–437.
115. Brennan, K. J. and Hardeman, E. C. (1988) Quantitative analysis of the human alpha-skeletal actin gene in transgenic mice. *J. Biol. Chem.* **268,** 719–725.
116. Wang, Y., Xu, J., Pierson, T., O'Malley B. W., and Tsai, S. Y. (1997) Positive and negative regulation of gene expression in eukaryotic cells with an inducible transcriptional regulator. *Gene Ther.* **4,** 432–441.
117. Klamut, H. J., Gangopadhyay, S. B., Worton, R. G., and Ray, P. N. (1990) Molecular and functional analysis of the muscle-specific promoter region of the Duchenne muscular dystrophy gene. *Mol. Cell. Biol.* **10,** 193–205.
118. Davis, H. L. and Jasmin, B. J. (1993) Direct gene transfer into mouse diaphragm. *FEBS Lett.* **333,** 146–150.

119. Smith, T. G., Mehaffey, M. G., Kayda, D. B., et al. (1993) Adenovirus-mediated expression of therapeutic plasma levels of human factor IX in mice. *Nature Genet.* **5,** 397–402.
120. Huard, J., Lochmuller, H., Acsadi, G., Jani, A., Massie, B., and Karpati, G. (1995) The route of administration is a major determinant of the transduction efficiency of rat tissues by adenoviral recombinants. *Gene Ther.* **2,** 107–115.
121. Kessler, D. A., Siegel, J. P., Noguchi, P. D., Zoon, K. C., Feiden, K. L., and Woodcock, J. (1993) Regulation of somatic-cell therapy and gene therapy by the food and drug administration. *N. Engl. J. Med.* **329,** 1169–1173.

Index

C

D

F

J

L

O

P

FSC
www.fsc.org
MIX
Papier | Fördert gute Waldnutzung
FSC® C083411

Kolibri 360 GmbH
Ferdinand-Jühlke-Straße 7
99095 Erfurt, Deutschland
produktsicherheit@kolibri360.de